D0646679

long life

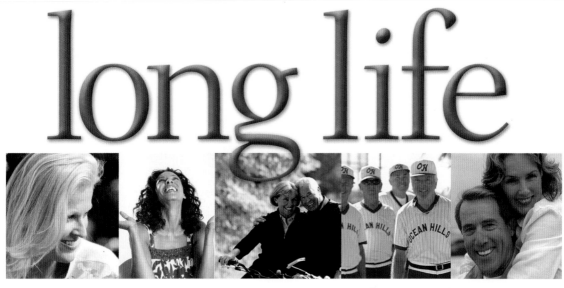

prescription

FAST AND EASY WAYS TO STAY ENERGIZED AND HEALTHY AT EVERY AGE

Based on More Than 500 Clinical Studies

Sarí Harrar AND *Debra Gordon*

Reader's
Digest

READER'S DIGEST ASSOCIATION, INC.
PLEASANTVILLE, NEW YORK / MONTREAL

Project Staff

Writers
Sarí Harrar, Debra Gordon

Editor
Neil Wertheimer

Contributing Editor
Marianne Wait

Exercise Editor
Selene Yeager

Cover Designer
Michele Laseau & Richard Kershner

Book Designer
Michele Laseau

Page Layout
Erick Swindell

Exercise Photographer
Jill Wachter

Research Coordinator
Kristina Swindell

Copy Editor/Proofreaders
Jane Sherman, Lisa Andruscavage

Indexer
Cohen Carruth Indexes

Administrative Assistant
Pamela DelSonno

Reader's Digest Home & Health Books

President, Home & Garden and Health & Wellness
Alyce Alston

Editor in Chief
Neil Wertheimer

Creative Director
Michele Laseau

Executive Managing Editor
Donna Ruvituso

Associate Director, North America Prepress
Douglas A. Croll

Manufacturing Manager
John L. Cassidy

Marketing Director
Dawn Nelson

The Reader's Digest Association, Inc.

President and Chief Executive Officer
Mary Berner

President, Consumer Marketing
Dawn Zier

Copyright ©2008 by The Reader's Digest Association, Inc.

Copyright ©2008 by The Reader's Digest Association (Canada) ULC

Copyright ©2008 by The Reader's Digest Association Far East Ltd.

Philippine Copyright ©2008 by The Reader's Digest Association Far East Ltd.

All rights reserved. Unauthorized reproduction, in any manner, is prohibited.

Reader's Digest and the Pegasus logo are registered trademarks of The Reader's Digest Association, Inc.

Library of Congress Data has been applied for.

ISBN: 978-0-7621-0768-1

Address any comments about *Long Life Prescription* to:

The Reader's Digest Association, Inc.
Editor in Chief, Health Books
Reader's Digest Road
Pleasantville, NY 10570-7000

To order copies of *Long Life Prescription,* call 1-800-846-2100.

Visit our website at **rd.com**

Printed in the China

1 3 5 7 9 10 8 6 4 2

US 4792/IC

Note to Readers

The information in this book should not be substituted for, or used to alter, medical therapy without your doctor's advice. For a specific health problem, consult your physician for guidance. The mention of any products, retail businesses, or Web sites in this book does not imply or constitute an endorsement by the authors or by the Reader's Digest Association, Inc.

Photography by Jill Wachter is ©Jill Wachter.

Additional Photography courtesy of Jupiter Images, RD Publications, and Getty Images.

The Key Truths
OF LONG HEALTH

Illness is *not* inevitable

Damage *can* be undone

Good health is a *choice* you make,
not a pill you take

Good health includes *happiness*

Good health *feels* great

To be healthy years from now,
be healthy *today*

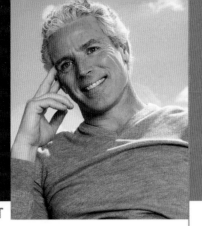
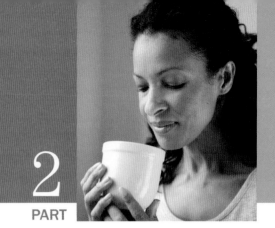

1 PART

2 PART

New Keys
to Health

Repairing
the Past

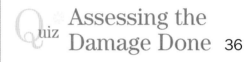
contents

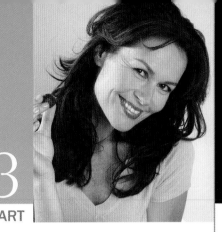

3
PART

Living
Healthy Today

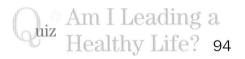
4
PART

Protecting
Future Health

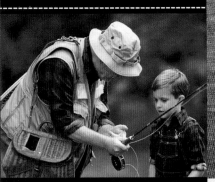

New Keys
to Health

Throw out all your old notions about aging. We are entering a

golden era of health in which we can live longer, healthier,

and more energized than ever before.

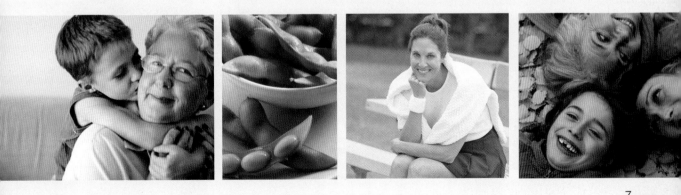

The Long Life Promise

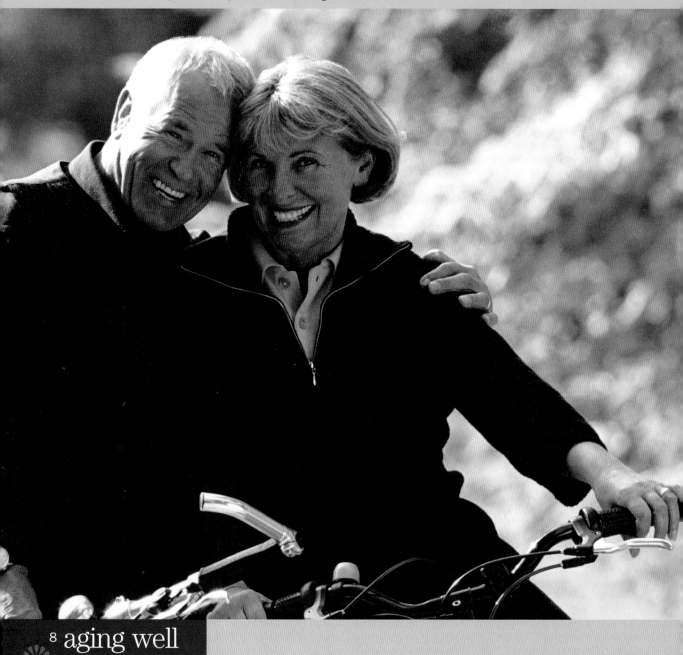

*You may not realize it, but fate has given you an extraordinary gift.
You have been born in a time and place in which people live longer than at any
time in human history. Compared with the vast majority of people who have
passed their time on this planet, you have been given on average 30 years
more life than they had. Do you realize the grandness of this?*

Until a century ago, the average person died in his or her forties. Before the 20th century, the cycle of life was much more compressed for most people. Your work life might have started at 8 or 10; by 15 you were a parent; by 30, you were a grandparent; and by 40, your body was broken, pain-filled, and in final decline.

Today, most people who turn 40 believe they have yet to get to the halfway point of their lives. Some are just becoming parents; others are finally launching their "real" careers. "To call 45 middle-age would have been ridiculous 100 years ago," says Dilip Jeste, MD, chief of the geriatric psychiatry division at the University of California, San Diego. Yet, he says, it may be just as ridiculous today.

"What *is* middle age?" he asks. After all, with an average lifespan of nearly 78, and with people 85 and older making up the fastest growing segment of the population in most countries, who's to say when we're really at the middle of our lives? Particularly when our wisdom, capabilities, and contributions are often just beginning to take flight in our forties and fifties?

Pete Townsend of the famed rock group the Who was only 20 years old in 1965 when he penned the words, "I hope I die before I get old," a phrase that became the rallying cry for an entire generation. More than 40 years later, Townsend and the Who are still releasing creative, high-intensity rock albums and touring the world. Their appearance might be older, but their energy and attitude aren't. The message: Being old no longer has much to do with the number of years you've lived.

So what is "old"? Old is your great-grandmother, who was bent, shaky, and mentally faded well before her time. Old are the people whose vitality long ago slipped away, leaving them in wheelchairs in nursing homes. Old is the lonely, tired senior who stays in the house and talks to the cats all day in between television shows.

As for the rest of us—we're just getting started.

The Goal: Long Health

Popular phrases like "anti-aging" and "long life" are deceptive. They imply that the goal of healthy living is to add more years to your life. And in fact, you *can* add even more years to your life by living a healthy, optimistic life. Some scientists hypothesize that the human body, when perfectly maintained, can comfortably last 120 years before naturally giving out.

But as mentioned, modern health care and lifestyles have already given you the opportunity to live to a ripe old age far beyond those of our ancestors. The goal today isn't merely extra years. It is *long health*.

Long health means that you are vibrant, creative, and energized at any age—be it 44, 58, 72, 85, or 94. It's understanding that although we all have to die one day, an infirm, sedentary life is not the inevitable final chapter of our lives. It means that you do not accept that the diseases of aging—heart disease, arthritis, insomnia, Alzheimer's, diabetes, and so on—are your destiny. Long health is living an active, healthy, happy, purposeful life—now and right up until your very final days.

Sounds ideal, doesn't it?

Better still, long health (as you will discover throughout this book) isn't achieved by swallowing pills, visiting doctors, or launching yet another formal exercise routine. Aging is neither a disease to be treated with medicine nor a process to be reversed through denial, sacrifice, or hard work. Instead, achieving long health is a process to be respected and enjoyed. As you'll read over and over, active, happy living each and every day is the path to long health.

In other words: The best path to being happy, energized, and healthy in the future is living happily, energetically, and healthily in the present.

So what is the first step to achieving long health? Recalibrating how you think about aging. Throw out notions that aging is a slow, sad decline toward death, and that your goal is merely to get to some artificial age threshold, like a high-stakes marathon race in which all that matters is reaching the finish line, no matter what torture it causes you.

The truth is that how long you live isn't the issue; it's how well you live. Nothing can break your heart more than seeing someone you love lying incontinent in a nursing home at age 72. Instead, wouldn't you rather see someone 72 still playing doubles tennis? Seventy-five and running for public office for the first time? Eighty-one and completing a 4-mile hike through a beautiful forest? These are not hypothetical examples; these are all activities that real people, real "old" people, are still doing and enjoying. Heck, there is even one centenarian who plays 18 holes of golf three times a week and consistently shoots 15 strokes under his age!

The thing is, these people didn't wait until their eighties to start golfing or hiking. Rather, at some point earlier on, they chose to live more actively and healthfully—perhaps in their youth, perhaps in retirement. That's the beauty of long-health living—the benefits and pleasures it delivers are both immediate and long term.

You are part of a generation that is redefining aging. It's already happening; when approximately 3,500 people with an average age of 80 were asked their ideas about aging, more than 60 percent said their opinions had changed in the past 20 years. Nearly all had thought about how they could age successfully instead of viewing aging as a negative thing. To them, freedom from disease, being able to function independently, and remaining actively engaged with life were critical components in successful aging.

In addition, more than 90 percent of this group listed "remaining in good health until close to death" as the most important component of successful aging. After that followed:

- Being able to take care of myself until close to the time of my death

- Remaining free of chronic disease

- Having friends and family who are there for me

- Being able to make choices about things that affect how I age, like my diet, exercise, and smoking

- Being able to cope with the challenges of my later years

- Being able to meet all of my needs and some of my wants

- Feeling satisfied with my life the majority of the time

- Being able to act according to my own inner standards and values

Notice anything missing? Less than a third chose "Living a very long time" as a component of successful aging. In fact, that statement was last on the list of 20 choices.

The New World of Aging

Obviously, we're heading into a new world of aging. There are no road maps or rules for this new world. But never fear: You won't be alone. Worldwide, the number of people 65 and older is increasing faster than any other demographic group, particularly in developed countries. By 2030, 12 out of every 100 people will be 65 or older, nearly double the percentage in 2000. In North America and Europe, that figure will be

1 out of 5 people. And throughout the developed world, those 85 and older are the fastest growing age group now.

In this new world, retiring to the golf course is being replaced with working part-time, flexible hours; active volunteering; and pursuing new interests and new friendships. Sedentary vacations like bus tours and cruising the islands are giving way to bike trips through wine country, volunteer missions to build houses in South America, and mini college semesters at Harvard to learn about the Middle East.

In this new world, you're less likely than your parents and grandparents to find yourself living with a disability or in poverty, and you are more likely to have completed college—all markers for successful aging.

This is a world in which you're accepting of the cosmetic changes time has wrought on your body, as long as your spirit remains robust. A world in which you finally figured out that there's more to good health than not being in bad health. And a world in which our old perceptions of aging—that cognitive decline and frailty are inevitable, for instance—have been turned on their head.

It's also a world in which the past *can* be changed, at least when it comes to harmful habits and activities. Even if you got frequent sunburns in your youth (remember baby oil?), drank a lot, or (gasp!) smoked pot, the damage can be managed and minimized, as you'll learn in the pages ahead. So yeah, maybe you wish you'd eaten less junk food, quit smoking earlier, done more to protect your bones and joints, and worried less, but it's never too late to change and to see the benefits of those changes. That's what *The Long Life Prescription* is all about.

Secrets of the Long-Lived

In the year 2000, the United Nations estimated that there were more than 180,000 people above the age of 100 throughout the world, a figure that will jump to 3.2 million by the year 2050. Still, estimates are that only 1 in about 10,000 people will reach this golden age. What's the secret?

If only we knew. Despite dozens of studies on centenarians, there doesn't seem to be a typical life pattern or history shared by these long-lived folks. Still, researchers say that they have found *some* similarities.

People who live to 100 and beyond tend to:

- Complain less about pain and discomfort than younger people with fewer disabilities, suggesting that centenarians are better at adapting to what life hands them
- Remain intellectually stimulated
- Maintain satisfying social relationships
- Keep their interests in creative activities
- Have few sleep problems
- Become anxious or depressed rarely
- Find great solace in their religious faith
- Be financially secure
- Believe that they can be happy
- Be extroverted

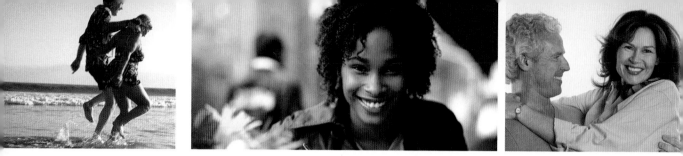

The Truth About Aging

If you rely on what you see on TV, in the movies, or in magazines, being old means frailty, infirmity, and dementia. But if you talk to the people actually doing research on aging, they'll tell you that popular culture has it all wrong. They're questioning every assumption about the effects of aging on our physical and mental health and finding some pretty surprising results.

Forget everything you ever thought you knew about aging and memory, says Sonia J. Lupien, PhD, who directs the Center for Studies on Human Stress at McGill University in Canada. She has a rather surprising argument for why we falsely believe older people have worse memories and declining learning abilities. To her, it's because the studies on which we base this opinion are deeply flawed.

You have to consider how the studies are conducted, she says. People have to come to a university setting, typically in the afternoon, where they're tested by a young graduate student. That's all well and good if you're one of the "young" participants. This group is typically composed of university students who know where they're going on campus, feel comfortable being tested by someone close to their own age, and prefer afternoon testing since they sleep late in the morning.

Now consider this from the perspective of one of the older participants. You have to drive or take mass transit to the university, figure out where to park, and navigate the campus until you find the room where the study is being conducted. You're confronted with someone young enough to be your grandchild who asks you a bunch of extremely personal questions, then puts you through the tests. And since you've been up since 6 a.m., afternoons are simply not your best time. You prefer to take a nap around 2 p.m. rather than a test (in fact, studies find memory is strongest in older people in the morning and in younger people in the afternoon).

So if you're an older person, Dr. Lupien says, the whole experience is unbelievably stressful. This is bad in two ways: First, the older you are, the more intensely your body reacts to stress; and second, stress and memory, as she and others have shown in dozens of studies, are like oil and water. The more acute stress you experience, the worse your memory.

Then there's the test itself. If you give older people words to memorize and tell them that you're evaluating their memory, they'll do poorly. If you give them the same words to memorize and tell them that you're evaluating the learning capacity of older adults, they'll do much better. Why? Because everyone—including that older participant—is conditioned to believe that memory gets worse with age. And you know the drill: If you think something *is*, then it will be.

Here's the important point: When researchers look more closely at the people taking the memory tests, they find that those who are in good physical health, educated, employed, and with a good income have memorization skills just as strong as that of people 30 years younger.

"Don't talk to me about any age-related impairment in memory until you take stress into account," Dr. Lupien says. In fact, she's doing just that. In a major study funded by the Canadian Institutes of Health Research, her 70-year-old research assistant asks the questions and conducts the memory tests in the morning in an off-campus location that the older people (but not the younger participants) have already visited for a pre-study cocktail party. "The young participants hate it," Dr. Lupien says with a grin.

Aging Truths, Aging Myths

What other myths about the physical and mental effects of aging are out there? Here are some big ones.

Creaky, achy joints are an inherent part of aging. Hardly. A more accurate statement would be that creaky, achy joints are an inevitable part of not exercising. Just ask researchers from Monash University Medical School in Australia. When they assessed 146 women ages 40 to 67 with no history of knee osteoarthritis or significant knee injury, and then compared their findings with the women's physical activity history, they found that women who exercised at least once every two weeks for at least 20 minutes had more cartilage in their knees, suggesting that they were less likely to develop arthritis.

Fragile bones and a bent posture are inevitable with age. One thing you'll learn from reading this book: *Nothing* is inevitable

with age except death. While osteoporosis is definitely a condition that's more prevalent in older people, it's also one that's very preventable. For instance, a study of 424 female centenarians found that only 56 percent had osteoporosis, and their average age at diagnosis was 87. That's not bad, particularly considering that these women grew up in a time long before we understood the benefits of diet and exercise on bone.

Your genes are the most important determinant in how well you'll age. Ha! If that were the case, then identical twins would age identically. But they don't. A major study from European and American researchers evaluated the lifestyle habits and medical history of 40 pairs of identical twins ages 3 to 74. As the twins aged, the researchers found, not only had their health taken different paths, but their genome changed from identical to one that showed several differences. Genetically speaking, the oldest pair of twins was the least alike.

How so? It all gets back to the "nature vs. nurture" argument. You might be born with the healthiest set of genes nature can provide; but how you live your life (the nurture part) determines how those genes behave over the next 90 years. It turns out that what you eat, how much physical activity you get, even your exposure to chemicals can change your genes through methylation—a process that plays an essential role in maintaining cellular function (changes in methylation patterns may contribute to the development of cancer).

You lose your creative potential as you age. Don't tell that to Gene Cohen, MD, PhD, who directs the Center on Aging, Health, and Humanities at George Washington University in Kensington, Maryland. Dr. Cohen, who is in his sixties, started a second career as a game-maker

aging Through the Decades

Here's a quick glimpse at some of the age-related changes that do occur as we move through our decades. It's a surprisingly short list: Most other common signs of "aging" have little to do with age, and everything to do with lifestyle.

20

- The first signs of age appear in your skin as the collagen fibers that keep your skin taut begin to weaken.

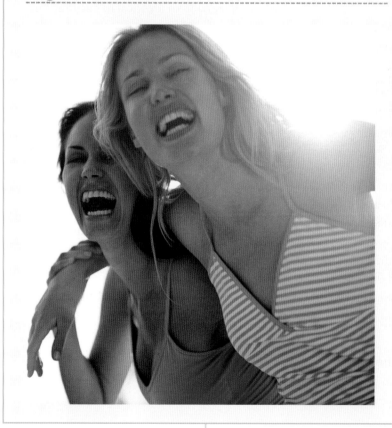

30s

- By the end of the decade, you may find your first gray hair. Men may find their hair color fading and their hair, well, disappearing.
- You've passed the halfway mark in terms of bone strength. During this decade, bone breaks down faster than it builds up.
- By the time you turn 39, you'll probably find it harder to maintain your weight with the same eating/exercising regimen you followed at the beginning of the decade. Your metabolism is slowing—time to pump up the physical activity.
- This is the time when women's fertility begins waning. It may take longer to get pregnant, and you may need to call in the experts for a little boost.

40s

- Gasp! Is that a wrinkle? Yes, this is the time of life when the sun you worshipped as a teen and in your twenties turns on you.

- By the middle of this decade, you're more likely to die of cancer than from accidents.

- By the end of the decade, you may find your days of rock 'n' roll have left sounds slightly muffled. Even if you were a classical-music aficionado, your eardrums have lost elasticity, affecting your hearing.

- Oh, and don't forget the reading glasses. The question is not "if" you'll develop presbyopia, a type of farsightedness, but "when." It occurs because the lens of your eye stiffens with age, making it more difficult to focus.

50s

- One day, you look down at your hands but see your grandmother's hands! Sadly, though, they *are* your hands, and all those brown spots and puffy veins are the result of years of sun exposure and the increasing inability of your skin to rid itself of gunk called lipofuscin—produced when free radicals build up in the skin.

- Early this decade, women will reach menopause. The average age of menopause in most countries is 52.

60s

- Even though you can't see it, you probably have small pockets throughout your intestines called diverticula. They won't bother you unless bits of digested food become caught in them, in which case they get inflamed and infected. To prevent this, make sure you get plenty of fiber.

- This is the decade in which men may find themselves having some urinary problems from an enlarged prostate.

- You should check in with your ophthalmologist; chances are that you have a cataract or two that needs removed.

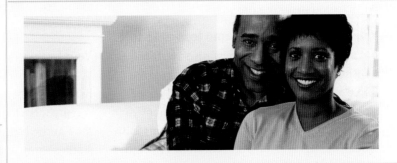

70s and 80s

- How you'll feel in your seventies and eighties really depends on how you spent the last six decades. If you never exercised, smoked, drank a lot, and considered late-night TV intellectual fare, you may find yourself frail with diabetes and heart disease, forgetting simple things, and fighting chronic pain from arthritis.

a few years back. He already has three intergenerational board games to his credit, two of which have been featured as works of art by the Smithsonian Institution.

Such creativity offers tremendous benefits for older people, he's found. For the past decade, he and his colleagues have been studying the impact of art and music participation on older adults. In one study of 168 healthy older adults, those who joined a choral group were in better health, used less medication, and had fewer falls after a year than a similar group of older adults that didn't join the chorale. The singing group also said they were less lonely, had a better outlook on life, and participated in more activities overall than the nonsinging group, which actually reduced the number of activities they participated in during the year.

You become less sexual and less able to have sex as you age. Hogwash, says Terrie B. Ginsberg, DO, of the New Jersey Institute for Successful Aging. In a major review of sexuality and aging, she notes that "contrary to many of our cultural and societal views of the aging individual, our aging population continues to enjoy their sexuality." The key is keeping yourself in shape. Impotence and reduced libido aren't related to age but to medical conditions that can, in most instances, be prevented, like high blood pressure, heart disease, diabetes, and depression. Something as simple as lifting weights a couple times a week can improve your sex life.

Here's the other thing: Sex doesn't only mean intercourse. When Dr. Ginsberg interviewed 166 people age 60 and older who lived in independent-living facilities, she found that about 60 percent had had regular physical and sexual experiences in the past year such as kissing, touching and holding hands, and hugging. However, all wanted more—and the main thing preventing them from having more was the lack of a partner. And yes, while sexual desire might ebb a bit as you age, that decline typically doesn't occur until age 75. Even then, it's usually related to whether you have a partner you're interested in, and how interested you were in sex most of your life.

Your brain stops developing after age 3. When this developmental myth was overturned in the 1990s, it created a seismic shift in the way researchers viewed aging. No longer could they look at the older brain as a static thing. Instead, studies show, your brain continues to send out new connections and to strengthen existing connections throughout your life—as long as you continue to challenge it. It really *is* the ultimate muscle in your body.

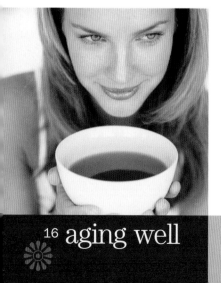

 Growing old doesn't cause you to have less energy, achy joints, or more frail bones. The culprit is simply not exercising.

Your brain shrinks with age. This myth began with studies in 2002 showing that the hippocampus, the part of the brain that controls memory, was significantly smaller in older people than in younger people. This never sounded right to Dr. Lupien, particularly after she conducted groundbreaking research in the late 1990s showing that chronic stress shrinks the hippocampus. Was it age or stress that was responsible for the shrinking brains of older people?

Probably stress. When she examined brain scans of 177 people ages 18 to 85, she found that 25 percent of the 18- to 24-year-olds had hippocampus volumes as small as those of adults ages 60 to 75. Her point: "Maybe the smaller hippocampus in the older person was already there when they were younger; possibly as a result of stress." In fact, other research she has conducted found that people born during the world wars have smaller hippocampuses than those born *between* the two wars, likely because those born during the wars were exposed to so much stress early in life.

Older people are cranky and unhappy. Not quite. When researchers from Heidelberg, Germany, interviewed 40 centenarians, they found that despite significant physical and mental problems, including the fact that 55 percent needed nursing care at least three times a day, 71 percent said they were happy, and more than half said they were as happy as they'd been at younger ages. Plus, when the researchers compared these 100+-year-olds to a group of middle-age people, they found that both groups were just as happy. Most important: Nearly 70 percent of the centenarians said they laughed often.

What does it all mean? It means there is no universal definition of aging. How you'll age is entirely up to you—and the time to begin writing that definition is today.

One Man's Secret

If anyone knows the secret to successful aging, it is the guru of successful aging, Robert Butler, MD, 80, President and Chief Executive of the International Longevity Center in New York City and founding director of the National Institute on Aging. "I work 80-hour weeks, walk five to six miles with a walking club on Saturdays and Sundays, work out on a treadmill in my library the rest of the week, don't smoke, and hardly ever drink," reveals Dr. Butler. A footnote: The Pulitzer Prize-winning author also just completed a new book.

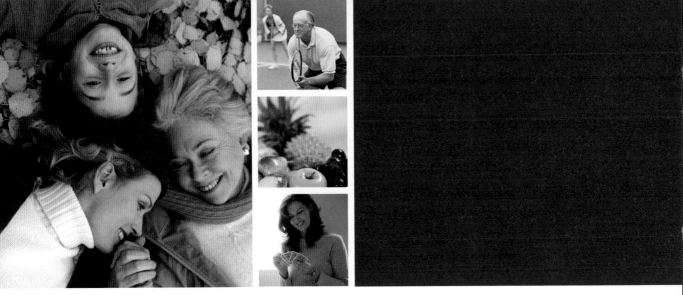

Seven Keys to Aging Well

A heaping plate of food—and a brimming social calendar. Freedom from diets—and plenty of time for fun and meaningful activities. A peek at the new science of aging reveals a new view of how to live long and prosper. And we're all for it.

With wisdom gleaned from some of the longest-living, healthiest cultures in the world, as well as new insights made possible by high-tech studies, researchers say that old views of aging are simply outmoded. Yes, our bodies change. But an inevitable slide in health as we age? Absolutely not! Each of us can live strong, healthy, vibrant, energetic lives for a long time to come. The key? Actually, there are seven of them. Read on—you may never see your bathroom scale, dinner plate, or friends in the same way again.

Be prepared for surprises. Only three of the seven keys involve nutrition and fitness. The other four are related to your attitude, optimism, and social interactions. As this book notes over and over, how you choose to live your life has far more impact on your health than any vitamin or pill. Philosopher René Descartes wrote the famous line, "I think; therefore, I am," but the new science of aging suggests that the important truth is really "How I think is how I am."

seven key

But First, the Runner Ups

The seven keys detailed in the pages ahead represent the best advice there is for living a healthy, happy, vibrant, long life. But in deciding on them, our experts also pointed to these five actions as being particularly beneficial for both long life and long health. So we proudly present these "silver-medal" pieces of advice first.

Drink lots of water. After age 60, your sense of thirst diminishes, so you may not even realize you're thirsty. The benefits of water are vast—topping off your tank with five to eight glasses a day can cut your risk of a deadly heart attack by as much as 54 percent and at the same time ease constipation, boost flagging energy, and even lower your risk of cancers of the breast, prostate, and large intestine, research suggests. By sipping more water throughout the day—and enjoying herbal tea and plenty of water-rich fruits and veggies—you'll give every cell in your body the fluids it needs.

Eat far more frequently. Having three meals and two or three snacks a day is a great way to fit in all the nutrition your body needs—and more. You'll keep your blood sugar lower and steadier to guard against diabetes and heart conditions associated with blood sugar problems. You'll avoid big portions and a starve-and-binge pattern that can lead to extra weight. And you'll have more chances to break bread with friends and family—an act that can be as nutritious for the mind and spirit as food is for your body. Let moderation replace deprivation, and you'll be happier and healthier.

Keep toxins out of your body. It's great to eat organic when you can. But it's even more important to avoid the common food additives and ingredients that are potent health wreckers: excess sodium, trans fats, saturated fat, sweeteners, and refined carbs. These five raise your blood pressure and "bad" LDL cholesterol, increase your risk of heart disease, put your blood sugar on a roller coaster, and even fire up body-wide chronic inflammation—a powerful risk factor for everything from heart disease and stroke to cancer and more.

Get the rest you truly need. Insomnia—annoying, exhausting, and mysterious—becomes a common experience as we age. Sleep patterns change radically after age 55, when your body clock resets itself and levels of melatonin and growth hormone drop. Medical conditions, prescription or over-the-counter drugs, eating patterns, exercise habits, time outdoors, and your bedtime routine all play important roles in your sleep as well. And because we often don't know how to adjust, an estimated 41 percent of women 80 and older experience insomnia, as do 23 percent of men 70 and older. Feeling sleepy all the time can be annoying and dangerous. It doesn't have to happen: Experts say it's still possible to be well rested if you work with, not against, your changing sleep cycles.

Learn to relax. In a stunning study that followed 202 women and men for more than 18 years, researchers found that those who practiced meditation had a 23 percent lower risk of dying from any cause during the study and a 30 percent lower risk of death from heart disease. Cutting stress can help your body heal faster, your mind function better, your digestion work better—and make every moment brighter and more pleasurable. You'll sleep better, too. The best news: You don't have to sit alone in a room saying *"Om … "* (though it does work!). Spending time with friends, walking in nature, and listening to favorite music with your spouse can all promote the deep relaxation we all need.

1 | Worry Less About Losing Weight

At some point a few decades ago, it became a widely held belief that you could be healthy—and attractive—only if you were lean. So, for much of our lives, we have gone about our business in a world obsessed with diet plans, mirrors, swimsuits, and belly fat.

As it turns out, the "overweight equals unhealthy" equation isn't quite that simple; even more shaky, particularly for mature adults, is the equation "losing weight equals better health."

In fact, new research shows that the drastic calorie-cutting strategies and scale watching that slimmed jiggly thighs in your twenties, thirties, or forties can set you up for bone fractures, weak muscles, and weight *gain* in your fifties, sixties, or seventies. Even worse, those popular weight-loss approaches fail to target the belly fat that causes serious weight-related health problems like diabetes and heart disease.

In fact, significant weight loss—either intentional or unintentional—can be life-threatening after age 60, experts are beginning to understand.

"Dieting or trying to return to an 'ideal' weight may not be the best recommendation for older women who aren't obese," says epidemiologist Matthew Reynolds, MS, of the University of Maryland School of Medicine, who has studied the health of older women who lose weight. "It's possible that maintaining body weight may actually keep you more robust and healthy later in life."

In one study of older women, those who maintained their weight for six years had a 13 percent chance of dying, but those who lost weight increased their risk to 22 percent. And women who had up-and-down weight swings during the study also had eye-opening results. "Fairly minor weight cycling—from 5 to 8 pounds for a 5-foot 5-inch woman—is associated with a significantly increased risk of death," says Jay S. Magaziner, PhD, director of the division of gerontology at the University of Maryland School of Medicine. "Even small changes should be taken seriously."

Experts aren't completely sure why weight loss cuts life short in older people. Obviously, some lose weight due to an underlying serious illness, but that's not the whole story. Dropping pounds on purpose, another study shows, is risky even for the *healthiest* older people. When University of California, San Diego, researchers tracked 1,801 women and men over age 71 from Rancho Bernardo, California, for 12 years, they found that women who lost weight were 38 percent more likely to die during the study, and men were 76 percent more likely to die.

Here's what we do know.

Losing weight means losing muscle. Older adults naturally have less muscle density than they did in their twenties, thirties, or forties. As a result, their metabolism slows and thus burns fewer calories throughout the day. Losing weight accelerates this process. If you lose 10 pounds on an old-fashioned low-cal diet, you'll drop 5 pounds of fat—and 5 pounds of muscle that you can't afford to lose, say experts at the Cooper Clinic in Dallas. The result: Losing that much

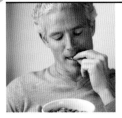

THE KEY Action

Eat for good nutrition and disease prevention. Do that, and your weight will take care of itself.

muscle will lower your metabolism even further, so you're burning 150 to 250 fewer calories a day.

Less muscle also means you'll be weaker, and your balance and flexibility won't be as fine-tuned—raising your odds for a fall. And once your diet ends, you're likely to regain lost weight as fat. If that fat's around your middle, it will pump out chemicals that fire up chronic, low-level inflammation throughout your body, raising your odds of developing insulin resistance, diabetes, heart disease, and even Alzheimer's disease and some forms of cancer.

Dieting threatens bones, too. When researchers at the University of Massachusetts in Boston followed 167 postmenopausal women for four years, they found that those who lost weight—either on purpose by dieting or because of illness—also lost a whopping 6 to 32 percent of their bone mineral density.

You'll never know you've lost bone density or muscle if you rely on the number on the bathroom scale. And your scale won't tell you if you're holding on to too much visceral fat—the kind packed inside your abdomen that raises the risk of diabetes and heart disease.

The best plan for almost everyone? Rather than eating to lose weight, focus on eating for good nutrition and disease prevention. Then get the exercise you need to build more smooth, dense, strong muscle. Plenty of dramatic studies prove that women and men as old as their late eighties and nineties who stick with a simple, safe, resistance-training program can build strength and agility, replace puffy fat with sleek muscle, and develop a renewed zest for life.

In one landmark study conducted at the Jean Mayer USDA Human Nutrition Research Center on Aging at Tufts University in Boston, 40 women ages 50 to 70 who traded their nonexercising routine for a twice-a-week weight-training program built muscle, lost fat,

Better Than the Bathroom Scale

If you need a number to help you judge whether your weight is healthy, skip the scale. Instead, try these two. (If your numbers are higher than they should be, be sure you're following a healthy eating plan and getting regular exercise.)

- **Your waist size.** Grab a tape measure. A waist that measures 34 1/2 inches or less for women or 40 inches or less for men is considered healthy. Anything higher could mean you're carrying around the type of visceral belly fat that raises your odds for diabetes and heart disease.

- **Your body fat percentage.** For this one, you'll have to visit a doctor, clinic, or fitness center that offers body fat analysis. For women over age 60, a healthy body fat percentage is 24 to 35. For men, it's 18 to 25 percent.

developed stronger bones, and became physically stronger than their daughters! These grandmothers were so excited about their new-found zing that they took up new hobbies—one moved 4 tons of topsoil, one wheelbarrow load at a time, to build a garden in her backyard. Another took up mountain biking. A third beat the study's lead researcher at bowling. Others tried inline skating and ballroom dancing.

They were slimmer, happier, stronger—and healthier. Yet the scale barely budged.

What if you find yourself losing weight without even trying? Do pay attention to the scale in that case—and tell your doctor. Unplanned weight loss could be a sign of dehydration, undereating, or severe loss of muscle or bone.

great advice

For a comprehensive guide to healthy eating, easy exercise, and smart appetite control, turn to the "Eat to Feel Good" and "Move to Feel Good" chapters.

Key 2 | Eat Fewer Calories— But More Food

That's no misprint. When nutrition researchers invited themselves over for dinner in kitchens across the globe—from Greece to Japan to the state of Pennsylvania—they discovered a tummy-satisfying secret to good health: Pile your plate high with vegetables and fruits, add respectable portions of beans and whole grains, and downplay high-calorie fare like cheeseburgers, cream sauces, and fatty meats.

The result: Fewer calories, more health-boosting antioxidants, and longer, happier, and more active and independent lives. "Ounce for ounce, people on Okinawa eat *more* food by weight than people who eat a Western-style diet," says Bradley Willcox, MD, of the Pacific Health Research Institute in Honolulu and lead researcher of the Okinawa Longevity Study. "They eat a lot of produce and grains and smaller portions of higher-calorie, higher-fat foods. It's the combination of high nutrition and lower calories that gives them a tremendous health advantage: Their risk for dementia, heart attacks, strokes, and cancer are among the lowest in the world."

Okinawans aren't starving. They eat about 1,800 calories a day. (In contrast, in many Western cultures, the average adult eats close to 2,500.) "Slight calorie restriction seems to prime the body for survival," Dr. Willcox says. "Just cutting back by 10 percent can have a dramatic effect. The theory is that this throws genetic 'master switches' so that more maintenance work gets done: Your cells invest more time and energy in repairing DNA; there's less oxidation (damage from rogue oxygen molecules called free radicals that leads to all sorts of diseases); and insulin, the hormone that tells cells to absorb blood sugar, becomes more effective."

We're not talking about starvation diets. Yes, eating extremely low-cal diets has extended the lives of earthworms in laboratories, but the jury's still out on whether this impractical, unpleasant, and even dangerous practice lengthens the lives of humans. Simply refocusing your food priorities by eating smaller portions of calorie-dense foods and copious amounts of plant-based foods is all you need to do.

More proof that choosing double portions of green beans (hold the butter) and saying "no thanks" to the cream sauce will have a big payoff: In a recent study of 980 older women and men, researchers at the Taub Institute for Research on Alzheimer's Disease and the Aging Brain at Columbia University found those who ate a high-calorie diet were 2.3 times more likely to develop Alzheimer's disease than those who consumed fewer calories and less fat. Meanwhile, University at Buffalo researchers have found that a single high-calorie meal boosts the body's production of unhealthy free radical molecules. These rogue oxygen molecules damage cells and cause low-level inflammation throughout the body. This type of

THE KEY Action

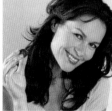

Eat as many vegetables, fruits, and whole grains as your appetite desires.

inflammation has been linked with a higher risk of diabetes, heart disease, high blood pressure, stroke, and even breast and prostate cancers. The scientists found that eating a fast-food breakfast sent a rush of free radicals into the bloodstream that remained at high levels for the next three to four hours—just in time for lunch.

"A high-fat, high-calorie meal temporarily floods the bloodstream with inflammatory components, overwhelming the body's natural inflammation-fighting mechanisms," says Ahmad Aljada, PhD, a researcher in the division of endocrinology, diabetes, and metabolism at the University at Buffalo School of Medicine and Biomedical Sciences. "People who experience repeated, short-lived bouts of inflammation resulting from many such unhealthy meals can end up with blood vessels in a chronic state of inflammation, a primary factor in the development of atherosclerosis."

What's happening? Digesting food requires oxygen. The more calories you consume, the more your body must digest—and the more free radicals are produced as a side effect. Foods loaded with saturated fat, trans fats, and refined carbohydrates seem to ratchet up the free radical production process. In contrast, Mother Nature's favorites—salads, steamed veggies, a dollop of brown rice or barley—don't. When Dr. Aljada's team tested the blood of volunteers who ate a meal packed with fruit and fiber, there was no increase in inflammatory free radicals.

The easiest way to eat more while getting fewer calories? Eat breakfast like a Greek, lunch like an Okinawan, and dinner like a Pennsylvanian. In Greece and on Okinawa, traditional diets call for a plate filled with three-quarters fruits and veggies and the rest whole grains and lean protein. And in recent studies at Pennsylvania State University, researchers found that people who ate diets richest in veggies, fruits, and whole

Getting Back to Natural

Think eating large amounts of meat is the natural human diet? Maybe if you live on the edge of the Arctic Ocean, where vegetables just don't grow, but not for the majority of the human race. Most of the large human populations evolved eating primarily fiber-rich, low-calorie vegetables, fruits, and beans. *That's* what natural is for us.

So return to your nutritional roots by doubling all of your daily vegetable and fruit portions and cutting the serving sizes of any fats, such as oil and butter, and high-fat and high-calorie foods, like desserts and fatty meats, in half.

You don't have to eat it raw. Try dropping handfuls of baby spinach into your soup at lunch, cook extra peas or carrots at dinner, and have a cup of fruit instead of a half cup at breakfast. Feeling full? Chunky veggies stretch your stomach, activating special "satisfaction sensors" that tell your brain you've had enough to eat. The bonus: Eating this way can save you hundreds of calories and dozens of grams of fat and flood your body with big doses of cell-protecting antioxidants.

grains typically took in 425 fewer calories per day, yet they were able to enjoy big portions (and didn't feel deprived) because they were choosing mostly low-calorie foods.

"That's a tremendous dietary advantage," Dr. Willcox says. "You're loading up on the foods that provide you with the most antioxidants, which protect against free radical damage."

great advice

For complete details on which foods to eat each day and in what amounts for optimal health today and tomorrow, turn to the "Eat to Feel Good" chapter.

Key 3 | Use Exercise as a Vaccine Against Aging

It's no secret that physical activity tones up muscles, protects bones, burns calories, and puts a happy bounce in your step. But recently, researchers uncovered a new, bonus benefit: Exercise acts as a powerful vaccine against the aging process itself.

When University of Florida exercise physiologists put healthy people ages 60 to 85 on weight-training programs for six months, then tested for signs of free radical damage, they were surprised by the results. By the end of the study, low-intensity exercisers had a drop in free radical damage, while high-intensity exercisers had a slight *increase*, and a control group of nonexercisers had a whopping 13 percent rise in free radical damage.

In a second University of Florida study, researchers found that fitting in an hour of activity a day for just three days raised levels of an important free radical–fighting compound called superoxide dismutase, produced by muscle cells throughout the body, including in the heart.

The scientists suspect that aerobic activities like walking and swimming help heart muscle better defend itself against the cascade of events that leads to a heart attack. The cycle begins when free radicals "oxidize" LDL cholesterol in the bloodstream. Over time, this damaged cholesterol accumulates on artery walls in the form of gunky, dangerous plaque. When your immune system detects the plaque, it sends in a cleanup crew, which attempts to whisk it away. If a pocket of plaque bursts, it can create blood clots that cause a heart attack. But if your heart muscle pumps out chemicals that disarm free radicals—like the superoxide dismutase pumped out by the heart muscle cells of exercisers—cholesterol never gets a chance to oxidize, and the process doesn't get started.

Of course, that's not the only reason to take a walk, try a few easy strength-training moves, or add extra bursts of movement to your day. Studies show movement can:

- Ease the ache of arthritis
- Lower your Alzheimer's risk
- Keep your bones strong
- Soothe anxiety
- Reduce your chances of developing diabetes
- Lower your odds for colon, breast, and prostate cancer
- Help you sleep better
- Boost your energy levels
- Help you achieve your healthiest weight
- Maintain muscle strength
- Improve balance and flexibility so you're less likely to fall

The flip side: Not exercising nearly doubles your risk of a heart attack, says Robert Nied, MD, a sports medicine specialist in California.

Even if you hated gym class and never exercised before, it's not too late to start. "People who go from no exercise to some exercise receive the biggest benefits," Dr. Nied notes. Adding some strength-training moves can have

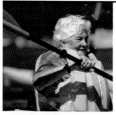

THE KEY Action

Add simple, natural, strengthening exercise to every day, even if just for a few minutes.

big benefits, too, he says. "Muscle strength declines by 15 percent per decade after age 50 and by 30 percent per decade after age 70," he notes. "However, resistance training can result in 25 to 100 percent strength gains or more."

"We don't place enough importance on the power of physical activity to keep older people healthy, active, and independent," says geriatrician Sonia Sehgal, MD, an assistant professor in the department of internal medicine at the University of California, Irvine. "There are so many wonderful benefits. And it's good to know that you don't have to sweat through a long, tough workout or run a marathon or hit the gym at 5 a.m. to get them. The kind of physical activity that really helps is whatever kind you enjoy and that you can do consistently—whether it's swimming, working in the garden, walking with friends, taking an easy exercise class, or trying something new like tai chi or yoga. You don't even have to do it for long periods of time. Getting 10 minutes in the morning, 10 minutes in the afternoon, and 10 minutes in the evening is all you need."

Forget the outmoded, macho adage "no pain, no gain." Sticking with a moderate, doable routine will give you the most anti-aging benefits. Like a flu vaccine that switches on your body's natural defenses, exercise actually works by unleashing a *helpful* amount of free radicals in your body. They're produced naturally by little energy-generating "machines" in your cells called mitochondria. Your body responds to this surge by pumping out more antioxidants and enzymes to mop up these villains. But if you exercise to the point of exhaustion, the burst of free radicals simply overwhelms your defenses. (That's one reason long-distance runners often get sick after a big race.)

Want to supercharge the benefits of your newfound fitness? Make it an everyday habit, like brushing your teeth or taking your multivitamin.

Exercise by the Numbers

No time, no inclination to get moving? With benefits like these, you can't afford not to. Getting 20 to 30 minutes of exercise most days of the week offers these amazing rewards.

3 lbs.	The amount of sleek, energizing, calorie-burning muscle you'll build
7%	The resulting boost in your metabolism
25%	The improvement in your body's ability to process blood sugar
1 to 3%	The increase in your bone density
55%	The improvement in your digestion
40%	The drop in your risk of dying in the next eight years
60%	The reduction in your risk of getting Alzheimer's

"When exercise is repeated regularly, the body promptly adjusts so that oxidative stress is eliminated or reduced," notes Sandra T. Davidge, PhD, of the University of Michigan. "A regular exercise habit seems to have an antioxidant effect."

Perhaps that's why the American College of Sports Medicine (ACSM) reports that exercise can dramatically ageproof your body: While nonexercisers see a 1 to 2 percent decline per year in all sorts of body functions after age 30, exercisers reduced that decline by 75 percent. "At 90 years old, a nonexerciser will have lost 70 percent of his or her functional ability, while an exerciser will have lost only 30 percent of functional ability—retaining 70 percent of his strength!" the ASCM notes.

great advice

For a fresh new look at exercise, as well as simple, at-home fitness routines for any age or exertion level, turn to the "Move to Feel Good" chapter.

Key 4 Find Something Interesting to Do

A retired real estate agent who tutors young children in reading. A housewife and mother of five grown children—and grandmom of eight—who travels the countryside with her oil paints and easel, capturing the wonders of nature in all seasons. A retired engineer, always fascinated by the dream of self-sufficient living, who heats his house with wood all winter—and splits every log himself.

Life is perpetually busy no matter what your age, where you live, or how well off you are. But the truth is, as careers reach their later stages, as children mature, and as home-improvement ambitions are fulfilled, time usually *does* become more available for adults moving through their fifties, sixties, and beyond.

With this time comes choices. The easy one is merely to relax: Watch more TV, eat out more often, talk on the phone as much as you want. The better choice, not only for your happiness but also for your health, is to discover something more meaningful to devote yourself to and pursue it wholeheartedly. Why? Following your bliss—whether it's joining a book group,

building hiking trails, or doing the things those folks above did—is more than just a pleasant pastime. A growing body of scientific research shows that doing something that interests you offers big mind-body benefits in your fifties, sixties, seventies, and beyond.

When Johns Hopkins University researchers compared the health of volunteer tutors within a large, urban school district with that of non-volunteers in the same city, ages 59 to 86, they found that 63 percent of volunteers had increased their activity level over the course of the year-long study, compared to just 43 percent of nonvolunteers. Volunteers boosted their weekly calorie burn by 25 percent because they were walking and climbing stairs more often as they went about their assignments; some who had been couch potatoes before joining the program even doubled their daily calorie burn, says study author Erwin Tan, PhD, an assistant professor of geriatrics at the university. They also reduced TV-watching time—perhaps because the burst of energy they got from volunteering inspired them to do more gardening and home maintenance (in contrast, many nonvolunteers were watching more TV by the end of the study). Volunteers' networks of friends expanded, while nonvolunteers' social circles shrank. And the volunteers were making a difference: The kids they tutored became better readers and had fewer behavior problems at school.

We're not saying you have to sign up to tutor kids every day or wash pots at a soup kitchen to find happiness and meaning. Plenty of research—and plenty more real people—prove that following everyday interests is a powerful antidote to aging. When psychiatrists at the University of California, San Diego, checked up on 500 adults ages 60 to 98 who were living independently, they got a pleasant surprise. By standard definitions of successful aging—which focus mostly on physical well-being—this group

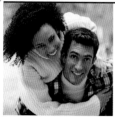

THE KEY Action

Make sure you do something every single day that improves you or the world.

had plenty of challenges. Most had coped with a tough health condition such as cancer, heart disease, diabetes, and mental health problems. Just 1 in 10 met the usual criteria for healthy, successful aging, the researchers noted.

The study volunteers, however, weren't buying into conventional wisdom. When they rated their own degree of successful aging on scale of 1 to 10 (with 10 being the top), the average score was a very happy 8.4. "People who think they are aging well are not necessarily the [healthiest] individuals," notes lead researcher Dilip Jeste, MD, chief of the university's geriatric psychiatry division. "In fact, optimism and effective coping styles were found to be *more* important to successful aging than traditional measures of health and wellness. Self-perception about aging can be more important than the traditional success markers."

That means getting involved, feeling the sense of flow that comes when you're absorbed in something—whether it's baking cupcakes, reading a novel, or playing a game with friends. In the study, for example, people who found time every day for hobbies, reading, and friends ranked their satisfaction with the aging process higher than those who were isolated and had fewer interests. And when Harvard University researchers tracked people over age 65 for 13 years, those who played games they enjoyed—whether poker, pinochle, or Monopoly—got as much stress relief and as strong a longevity benefit as people who exercised. (We hope you also exercise, though!)

The extra benefit of pursuing your interests: By cutting stress, it can lower your blood pressure and tame stress hormones that can wreak havoc with your blood sugar—thereby cutting your odds of having heart disease, high blood pressure, strokes, and diabetes. Not bad for an afternoon at the bridge table.

Finding the Right Opportunity

Sally Graber, 67, a retired bank manager, is intrigued by the idea of giving her time and talent to a worthy local organization.
But the options don't seem to fit: Some require too much time, others seem a little scary or even upsetting, while still others are downright dull. What to do?

"It's not always simple finding a good match," agrees John S. Gomperts, head of Experience Corps, a volunteer program that places tutors in schools in 19 US cities. "If you think it's going to be easy to find that thing that really turns you on and engages your passions, you'll be disappointed. It takes time. Don't be afraid to shop around—brainstorm about what you'd like to do first, then talk with organizations that might be able to use your talents. Audition prospective opportunities before making a commitment. Finding a good service spot is like searching for the perfect job: You may not get it right away, or it may take several tries. Visit in person or, better yet, try a one-time or short-term activity to see if the fit seems right."

"A lot of people have the desire to do work that serves the greater good, but they just don't have the opportunity during their regular working life," says John S. Gomperts, chief executive of Experience Corps, a volunteer program that places tutors in schools in 19 US cities. "People tell me all the time that volunteer work after retirement is the best thing they've ever done. It's a mini-career without the anxiety and economic concerns of regular working life, but it still has structure and colleagues and rewards."

great advice
For a complete understanding of the roles active living and personal engagement play in physical health, turn to the "Live to Feel Good" chapter.

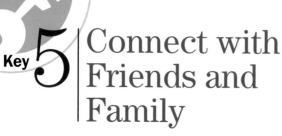

5 Connect with Friends and Family

Your spouse. Dear friends. Kids and grandkids. Longtime colleagues. Even Spot and Fluffy.

We hope plenty of loved ones—and pets!—spring to mind easily when you think about your personal support network. Close connections are a source of joy in the moment and offer a sturdy shield against the stress that can lead to health problems in the long term. Scientific journals are bursting with evidence that having friends around changes the biochemistry of your brain, pumping up feelings of joy and well-being that bolster immunity. The more close friends you have, the greater the odds that you'll be healthy and live longer, while being lonely puts you at risk for an earlier death, high blood pressure, depression, and accidents at home and on the road.

Experts are beginning to realize that we're hardwired for friendship. Back in the days when we lived in caves, being alone was perilous—no one was around to help fend off marauding wolves or forage for roots and berries if you were sick. Fast-forward to today: We're remarkably self-sufficient now, yet our ancient responses haven't changed one bit. When you're alone for too long (and the definition of "too long" is different for each of us), levels of the stress

hormone cortisol rise, ratcheting up your odds for heart disease, high blood pressure, depression, muddled thinking, and sleep problems. One University of California, Los Angeles, researcher has even documented that our brains register social isolation in the same way they register physical pain.

Yet keeping old friends close and building new connections is becoming a lost art. When Duke University researchers studied the social habits of 1,467 women and men in 1985 and again in 2004, they found that the number of people who had no close companions at all doubled—to 25 percent. Overall, the number of friends in whom study volunteers said they could really confide fell by one-third.

That's sad news for your heart, according to the scientists who run the world-famous Framingham Heart Study. When they checked on 3,267 men, they discovered that those who were the most socially isolated had the highest levels of interleukin-6—an inflammatory compound linked to cardiovascular disease. "Our analyses suggest that it may be good for the heart to be connected," says researcher Eric B. Loucks, PhD, an instructor in the department of society, human development, and health at the Harvard School of Public Health. "In general, it seems to be good for health to have close friends and family, to be connected to community groups or religious organizations, and to have a close partner."

A spouse or romantic partner may buffer stress best. In one study, brain scans revealed that women had milder reactions to a stressful event (in this case, a mild electric shock) while holding their husbands' hands than when they held strangers' hands—or no one's hand, a University of Virginia study found. Men who made love once or twice a week were 2.8 times less likely to have fatal heart attacks than men who made love less than once a month, report

THE KEY Action

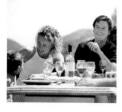

As best you can, fill your life with friendship, family, laughter, and love.

University of Bristol researchers who tracked the health of 914 Welsh men for five years.

Working on your relationship can make today sweeter and tomorrow healthier, too. Letting hostility and anger take center stage is a recipe for trouble. In a University of Utah study of 150 couples, those who deployed angry, mean-spirited verbal grenades had more heart-threatening atherosclerosis. The scientists uncovered the connection by videotaping the couples during a six-minute conversation about a sore marital subject. They also used a CAT scan to check their arteries for calcifications—an early sign of clogging. The surprising link: Husbands had a 30 percent higher risk of severe hardening of the arteries when either spouse was dominant or controlling; wives' risk rose 30 percent when either partner was hostile.

"People get heart disease for lots of reasons," says lead researcher Tim Smith, PhD, a professor of psychology at the university. "If someone said, 'What's the most important thing I can do to protect my heart health?' my first answers would be, 'Don't smoke,' 'Get exercise,' and 'Eat a sensible diet.' But somewhere on the list would be 'Pay attention to your relationships.' "

We're happy to report that furry, four-legged friends are part of the equation for a long, happy, sociable life, too. In one study of hard-driving stockbrokers, all of whom took ACE inhibitor drugs for high blood pressure, those who got a cat or dog reduced the size of stress-related spikes in their blood pressure readings by half. Six months after receiving their pets, study volunteers had their blood pressure measured while they tackled a high-anxiety challenge—such as talking their way out of a shoplifting accusation or soothing a client who'd lost $86,000 due to the stockbroker's poor advice. "Those who had pets went from 120 to 126 for systolic blood pressure [the first number in a blood pressure reading]. Those who had no

pets went from 120 to about 148," says lead researcher Karen Allen, PhD, a research scientist in the University of Buffalo's division of clinical pharmacology.

In a related study of 60 women and men caring for a brain-injured spouse, Dr. Allen found that caregivers who got a dog saw blood pressure rise only slightly during stressful times, while those without a dog saw systolic pressure jump a whopping 40 points when the going got tough.

The *Real* Health Givers

Think your doctor and dentist are the sole members of your personal health-care team? Take a second look. The real health protectors in your life may surprise you—and could include any of these folks, and more.

- **Your neighbor:** She's offered to start a morning walking club with you—why not say yes? Making a commitment to meet someone for exercise boosts the odds that you'll really do it. And walking with a friend provides soul-satisfying social time, too.

- **Your husband:** Every hug, smile, and "I love you" can cut your levels of brain- and body-threatening stress hormones.

- **Your dog:** Pets soothe stress, many studies show.

- **Your financial adviser:** Keeping your money organized and working for you lifts a big burden and eases your anxiety. Studies show that people who think they've got financial woes also have more health problems.

- **Your book group:** Discussing new ideas with good friends can cut your risk of Alzheimer's disease, research reveals.

great advice

For great ideas on how to increase social activity in your life, turn to the "Live to Feel Good" chapter.

Key 6 Focus on Loving Your Life

Back in the 1970s, 660 residents of Oxford, Ohio—all over age 50—agreed to take personality tests that revealed their true feelings about growing older. The optimists among them emphatically agreed with statements like "I have as much pep as I did last year," while the pessimists said morosely that gloomy sentiments such as "Things keep getting worse" rang true.

What happened next stunned researchers. Twenty-two years later, 50 percent of the optimists were still alive—but 73 percent of the pessimists had died. In fact, the "glass is half full" crowd lived 7 1/2 years longer on average than the "glass is half empty" group—a health advantage more dramatic than you'd get from quitting smoking, lowering high cholesterol, or getting high blood pressure under control.

Loving your life, research shows, is a lifesaver. Scientists have found that an optimistic attitude does more than put a smile on your face and make you good company. Studies show that it cuts your risk of getting sick when exposed to the common cold virus; reduces your odds of developing heart disease by 50 percent; and increases the likelihood that you'll recover from a heart attack, live longer after a cancer diagnosis, and even have fewer everyday health complaints such as upset tummies, intestinal distress, and breathing problems.

Staying happy and feeling in control in the face of life's challenges builds what experts call stress resiliency—a powerful health tool that you tap into whenever you take time to laugh, get in touch with your spiritual beliefs, or get together with loved ones. Without this near-magical force field, your mind and body can become steeped in stress hormones that lead to depression, fearfulness, and a higher risk of everything from colds and flu to Alzheimer's disease and heart disease; it can even make conditions like glaucoma, rosacea, and diabetes worse.

How can you get there? When Harvard Medical School researchers tracked the health, wealth, and happiness of 824 women and men from their teens through their eighties, they discovered that inheriting "good" genes or salting away a big nest egg were *not* the major predictors of bliss late in life. One of the real keys: a capacity for enjoying the moment. "The factors that made later life satisfying included the capacity to enjoy life for its own sake, and finding meaning and purpose," notes George Valliant, MD, a Harvard Medical School psychiatrist and author of *Aging Well: Surprising Guideposts to a Happier Life from the Landmark Harvard Study of Adult Development.*

Play is not an easy skill for a grownup to master, however. "We're wired from age 20 until age 65 to do things that other people will find valuable—that's how we get paid and how we get our own sense of worth," says Dr. Valliant. "All that has to change in later life. Men in my study were happiest when they could do things simply because they enjoyed them, not because other people would like what they did." Attaining this in-the-moment, who-cares-how-good-I-am bliss can be tricky. Dr. Valliant suggests taking lessons from little kids. "Fourth–graders know how to play. They don't have to be important. They don't

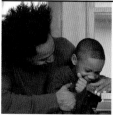

THE KEY Action

Constantly monitor yourself for negative, angry thinking and replace such thoughts with a reasonable sense of optimism.

get upset if their phone calls aren't returned. And they don't have to be paid for what they're doing," he says. He also holds up Winston Churchill as a good example of a guy who knew how to trade in drive and ambition in favor of fun at retirement. "Churchill was always looking for other people's esteem. He wrote beautifully and won a Nobel Prize for literature," Dr. Valliant says. "But as soon as he retired, he stopped writing and took up watercolors. It was simply something he enjoyed for himself."

We can't give you a paint-by-number plan for loving *your* life. It all depends on you and your unique beliefs, tastes, and interests. But we can offer some clues.

Laughter is important. It releases endorphins that create a feeling of joy and euphoria, erases stress and tension, and creates balance in your life no matter what's going on. And yes, there's a long-term benefit, too: Researchers at the University of Maryland School of Medicine found that laughter prompts the delicate inner lining of blood vessels to expand, increasing blood flow to the heart and other organs. (Stress causes blood vessels to contract.)

A sense of purpose and meaning matters. Studies show that faith, prayer, and the support of a friendly religious community can cut stress and improve your odds of recovering from illness. Having a rock-solid set of core beliefs seems to boost immunity, according to studies at the University of California, Los Angeles, and increase stress resilience as well.

Slowing down and letting go of the past can get you in the door to happiness. But if you cling to old dreams and goals that haven't been fulfilled, you can become bitter, says Stephen Treat, DMin, an instructor in psychiatry and human behavior at Jefferson Medical College in Philadelphia. "You can feel a lot of despair later

Half-Empty Thinking

Even if you're not a confirmed optimist, avoiding pessimism could help you avoid chronic stress and health problems, suggests an intriguing Ohio State University study. When researchers studied 224 middle-age and older adults, they found that those who agreed with statements like "If something can go wrong for me, it will" felt more stressed and anxious a year later than those who were neutral.

"It's not that optimism doesn't matter at all," says researcher Robert MacCallum, PhD, a professor of psychology at the university. "But pessimism has an impact above and beyond that of optimism."

Challenging negative attitudes could help. Don't beat yourself over the head if the little voice inside your brain persists in making comments like "This is just awful" or "Things never work out." You can't expect to become a Pollyanna overnight, and maybe you never should. Instead, teach yourself to counter with statements like "True, but now that I know what's happening, I can take steps to fix things" or "Despite this ache or pain, it's going to be a good day because I have [*insert three fun things that are on your schedule*] planned."

in life if you're still living off an original dream that never came true, such as being made vice president of your company. When you do that, you see your life as a failure. And you can't spend your time thinking about reality—about all the good things that have happened in your life. The goal is to keep changing, to look at yourself in new ways, and to change your dreams as you move forward in life."

great advice

For more on the extraordinary power of optimism and belief for helping you recover from and even prevent disease, turn to the "Live to Feel Good" chapter.

Stress Your Mind in Positive Ways

If you believe that mental fatigue, forgetfulness, fuzzy thinking, and even dementia and Alzheimer's disease are unavoidable in the years ahead, the new science of aging has an update just for you: By stressing your mind in productive ways, you can lower your risk of mental decline. And you don't need fancy computer programs or complicated "brain games" to do it—simple "brain calisthenics" (one neuroscientist calls then neurobics—aerobics for your brain cells) that involve new ways of doing everyday things are all it takes.

The idea behind neurobics comes from a remarkable discovery: During autopsies of 137 people with Alzheimer's disease, researchers realized that even though these women and men had all the brain plaques and tangles of full-blown Alzheimer's, their symptoms were much milder than they should have been. When the scientists looked further, they found a possible explanation: The patients' brains weighed more and had more neurons than usual, suggesting that they had "cognitive reserve"—a savings account of extra pathways that allowed them to function more normally for far longer.

Even more exciting: Neuroscientists have since found that people who use their brains more often—on the job and at play—seem to possess these brain-saving reserves. And they believe that stressing the brain in ways similar to the way we stress muscles during exercise can produce similar benefits—a stronger, fitter, more flexible brain. What helps: In one study of 1,772 older people with normal brain function, the odds of developing dementia dropped 12 percent for each leisure-time activity they were involved in. Those with the most activities were 38 percent less likely to develop thinking problems during the seven-year study. Exercise, spending time with friends, and intellectual pursuits all helped, but activities that required the most concentrated brain power, such as reading, doing crossword puzzles, and playing games that call for strategizing, were the most protective.

While "bad stress" leads to depression and cognitive problems (and even physical ailments), this "good stress" seems to help the brain by stimulating nerve cells, increasing blood flow, and boosting production of neutrophins—chemicals that protect brain cells. While you're at it, give your body a dose of good stress, too: Exercise increases levels of a chemical called brain-derived neurotrophic factor (BDNF), which acts like brain fertilizer. This chemical increases the number of connections between neurons, helps spur the growth of new blood vessels in the brain, may aid in the growth of new neurons, and protects existing nerve cells in the brain from free radical damage.

Adding neurobics to your mix of brain-healthy pursuits could make an even bigger difference, believes Lawrence Katz, PhD, a brain researcher at Duke University Medical Center and a member of the Dana Alliance for Brain Initiatives. "Your brain is activated by your senses, and you encounter new stimuli all the time," Dr. Katz notes. "Activities that involve

THE KEY Action

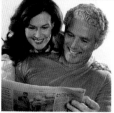

Challenge your brain every day through puzzles, reading, thinking, problem solving, and conversing.

one or more of your senses in a new way, such as getting dressed with your eyes closed, or that combine two or more senses in unexpected ways, such as listening to a piece of music while smelling an aroma, can strengthen synapses between nerve cells and make brain cells produce more brain growth molecules."

Just going through regular daily routines won't help your brain stay strong and flexible, simply because you're so used to them that your brain's virtually on autopilot when you brush your teeth, make the morning coffee, and do all the other daily things that never vary. By breaking the routine, you stimulate unused parts of the brain.

While you can buy fancy computer programs and sign up for pricey brain-training classes, experts like Dr. Katz say you can get similar results without spending a dime. Love crossword puzzles or Sudoku games? Try more challenging ones. Are you a lifelong lover of books? Practice fixing things around the house. Cross-train. Get out of your comfort zone. Expect to feel challenged and even a little bit out of your depth—the idea is to push the mental envelope.

Does it really help? Consider this evidence. In the 20-year-long Bronx Aging Study of nearly 500 women and men, those who engaged in mentally stimulating activities, such as games or even dancing, four times a week were up to 75 percent more likely to stay mentally sharp than those who stayed on the sidelines. And a 5-year study of 3,000 people who went through just 10 hours of training in memory, reasoning, or processing speed still had slightly sharper thinking skills five years later. Participants said that making phone calls, taking medications, and other activities requiring memory and judgment were somewhat easier—a gain experts hailed as proof that if you use your little gray cells, you won't lose them.

When Left Is Right

Become left-handed for the day—or, if you're normally a lefty, write and eat with your right hand. Brain scientists say that switching hands activates a big network of brain cell connections, circuits, and even regions that normally don't get used when you write out the grocery list, stir the scrambled eggs, or spoon up mushroom soup.

There are many other instant ways to stimulate new brain connections in fresh, beneficial ways. For example:

- Figure out in your head how to say the name of everyone in your family backward (Thomas becomes Samoht, for example).

- Similarly, read a whole sentence from the newspaper or a book backward.

- Play music? Start at the very end of a piece of sheet music and play the song backward.

- Multiply numbers in your head. Start with two-digit numbers multiplied by a single digit (for example, 82 times 7) and work up to multiplying by two digits.

- Do counting challenges. For example, count by 13s up to 390.

Does all of this sound silly? It's not! Challenging and even frustrating changes in thinking patterns can help strengthen brain wiring and build new networks in ways that will preserve sharp thinking for longer.

great advice

For more on keeping your memory and other brain skills sharp, see the "Preventing Memory Loss" chapter.

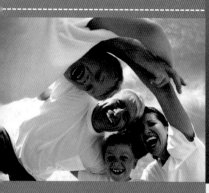

Repairing
the Past

The human body has an astounding capacity for healing and regenerating. That includes the ability to undo many of the wrongs of your youth. Here's how.

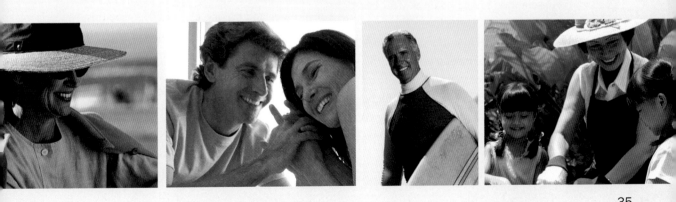

Assessing the Damage Done

Do you believe—actually, do you know—that you can live a longer, healthier, more-energized life, no matter what your current situation? The power to make that come true is already within you, and the guidance you need to succeed is within these pages.

But it's time for some honesty. Decades of abuse to your health is not always easily fixed. For you to take charge of your health, it means coming to terms with your past.

Over the next 56 pages, this book does something that few health books do: Looks backward. First, you'll discover the fascinating science of how your body repairs and rejuvenates itself. Then you'll explore the habits and lifestyle choices that might have damaged your health along the course of your life. Finally, you'll find out which can most influence your future health and what exactly you need to do to minimize that risk.

Be prepared for a few surprises. Some are good: For example, many vices from your younger, wilder days have less of a lingering effect than you might think. But there are challenging learnings as well—that some lifestyle choices, such as a disregard for the summer sun in your youth, can have lingering health effects decades after the damage occurred.

To start on this journey into your health's past, there are some tough questions for you to answer. On the facing page is a checklist that probes the unhealthy habits and choices you made during three periods of your life: youth, young adulthood, and the past few decades. Check off all the statements that are mostly or entirely true.

This isn't a quiz—there are no right or wrong answers; there are no assigned points to your responses; and no one else needs to see this. Instead, use the list as a personal catalyst. If you've checked off a lot of items, your need to remediate past health sins is more urgent. If you've checked off just a few, congratulations! That means that you have little holding you back from achieving the longer, healthier life you desire.

Hard Questions about My Past

My Youth

- ☐ I frequently got sunburned.
- ☐ I had one or more serious injuries.
- ☐ My home life was not happy or supportive.
- ☐ I snacked a lot on junk food.
- ☐ I regularly ate fast food or frozen dinners.
- ☐ I was frequently sick with colds or flu.
- ☐ I lived with smokers.
- ☐ I lived in a polluted neighborhood.
- ☐ I had a major debilitating disease.
- ☐ I watched television every night.
- ☐ I was frequently angry or hostile.

My Teens and Twenties

- ☐ I smoked cigarettes.
- ☐ I smoked marijuana.
- ☐ I regularly got drunk.
- ☐ I had sex with many partners.
- ☐ I snacked a lot on junk food.
- ☐ I regularly ate fast food or frozen dinners.
- ☐ I gained lots of weight.
- ☐ I regularly stayed up much of the night.
- ☐ I rarely exercised.
- ☐ I lived an isolated existence.
- ☐ I was frequently depressed.

The Past 20-30 Years

- ☐ I smoked cigarettes.
- ☐ I smoked cigars.
- ☐ I regularly got drunk.
- ☐ I had sex with many partners.
- ☐ I had poor romantic relationships.
- ☐ I got divorced.
- ☐ I had a very stressful job.
- ☐ I had workaholic tendencies.
- ☐ I spent myself deeply into debt.
- ☐ I rarely took vacations.
- ☐ I was frequently frustrated, cynical, or angry.
- ☐ I rarely exercised.
- ☐ I lived an isolated existence.
- ☐ I gained lots of weight.
- ☐ I watched lots of television most days.
- ☐ I was a frequent user of painkillers or sedatives.
- ☐ I ate ice cream, cake, or doughnuts most days.
- ☐ I lost touch with most of my old friends.
- ☐ I rarely saw a doctor.

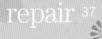

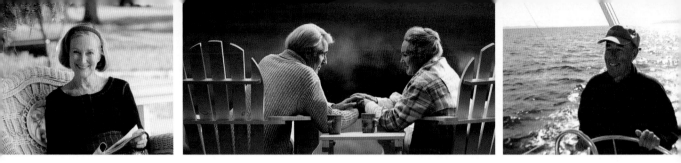

One, Two, Three...Four

Your birth certificate says that you're 53 ... or 67 ... or 81. But thanks to your body's amazing ability to continuously regenerate, many of your "parts" are far younger.

You see, a natural function of your body is to create new cells to replace those that have worn out. Your body generates new blood cells, new skin cells, new hair, and new cells for your digestive organs. In fact, most every part of your body is being replaced to some extent, each and every day.

Did you know that the muscles in your legs and the tissue within your gastrointestinal system are only about 15 years old? The red blood cells that deliver oxygen to every cell in your body are only four months old, on average. And the cells on the surface of your skin have a lifespan of just two weeks.

This is pretty motivating, isn't it? If our bodies are constantly rebuilding ourselves, then we all have the chance to greatly improve our bodies and, by extension, our health—starting this very moment.

How well will your body's regeneration system do the job? That's where you come in. While cell turnover naturally slows with age, giving your internal "mechanic" the right parts for the job (healthy food) and staying away from age-robbers that slow regeneration (such as too much fat, sugar and calories; smoking; too much alcohol; and excess stress) will make all the difference.

Teach Your Body to Repair

So how can you help? As it turns out, your body has different regeneration modes. We'll call the less helpful one the "slow mechanic" and the optimal one the "young mechanic". You can choose which body-repair mechanic will do the work, experts now believe. The key? Exercise.

Without physical activity, experts now suspect, your body surmises that it is winter—literally. Remember that your genetic coding isn't based on life as it is lived today, but as it was lived many thousands of years ago. And if you were sitting around day after day back then, it usually meant it was the cold-weather season, with you and your family huddled together inside for warmth, long past the season for running around gathering berries and hunting wild game. And that meant that your body needed to shift into hibernation mode; in fact, your top priority would be to burn as few calories as possible. So the slow mechanic took over, doing minimal work and allowing your bones to thin, your muscles to weaken, and more.

But if you get up and move around every day, your genetic coding says, "Aha! I need stronger bones and muscles, more brain cells to figure out how to hunt that wild boar, and a stronger cardiovascular system to keep it all supplied with oxygen and nutrients while I forage for nuts and berries in the woods." Then, the young mechanic gets to work, bolstering key body systems and creating strong new cells.

"You choose how healthy your body will stay," notes geriatrician Robert Stall, MD, of Buffalo. "You can depend on medications or allow unhealthy changes to happen, or you can do all you can to keep your body healthier and stronger as your first step. And it works—after I turned 50, my blood pressure started to creep up. My doctor gave me a prescription, but first I worked on losing weight and exercising more—and I lowered it. I made my cardiovascular system younger and stronger."

Another important way to make sure that the young mechanic is the one doing the work is to stay happy and socially connected. People who do this live longer and healthier, even after major life-threatening health problems such as a heart attack or a breast cancer diagnosis. In contrast, anxiety and isolation seem to switch on the old mechanic, raising your odds for developing more complications and perhaps even dying earlier.

"When I was a child, there were two older men in my neighborhood with the same medical problem: bone cancer. But how they handled it was radically different," says psychologist Michael J. Salamon, PhD, director of the Adult Developmental Center in Hewlett, New York. "One guy would come out and shoot hoops with the kids. The other man stayed in his house. The guy who was out living life, being with people and enjoying himself, lived about six years longer. Being involved with living keeps us happy, and young."

A New Body Every Day

Inside a research lab at Stockholm's Karolinska Institute, researcher Jonas Frisen, PhD, has borrowed a technique normally used to date ancient archeological treasures and focused it on the human body. Dr. Frisen checks levels of radioactive carbon-14 in cells, using this high-tech system to determine the age of various cells and tissues. He announced recently that while some tissues in the human body date from before birth, others arrived on the scene less than a month ago.

Cells that face lots of wear and tear, such as skin cells, red blood cells, and those that line the stomach and intestinal tract turn over quickly. The liver, which detoxifies every food, beverage, and drug you ingest, replaces all its cells in less than 18 months.

The oldest tissues in your body? The muscle cells of your heart; the inner lens of the eye, which forms before birth; and the nerve cells of your brain's cerebral cortex. Dr. Frisen estimates that the average age of the cells in your body is 7 to 10 years old—making you a youngster at any age.

Just as astonishing, other researchers have been turning up new evidence that some surprising parts of the body can regenerate. Scientists at Harvard Medical School recently discovered that in mice, the insulin-producing cells of the pancreas could regenerate—exciting news that could one day help people with type 1 and even type 2 diabetes regrow a natural insulin supply instead of relying on medication. Meanwhile, experts at New York Medical College have found that human hearts have a limited, though impressive, ability to grow new cells—a skill scientists hope one day to exploit to help survivors of heart attacks and congestive heart failure develop stronger, better-functioning tickers.

The biggest news of all came a decade ago, when neuroscientists turned the conventional wisdom about brain cells upside down. Once, experts agreed that the human brain didn't grow new nerve cells—we received a lifetime supply at birth (or grew the rest soon after, as the brain developed in early childhood). With age, these cells grew weak and began to die... and that was that. But now, we know that at least in some areas, your brain can develop stronger connections and even brand-new cells (provided, of course, that you call in the young mechanic!)

Bottom line: Your body has a vast capacity for repair—and you don't have to be a scientist in a lab to experience the benefits.

Maximizing Regeneration

There are four strategies that have proven to be the best for nurturing your body's repair system—and ensure that the young mechanic is doing the work. These are strategies that keep coming up in this book—in this case, for maximum body rejuvenation, in other cases, for maximum disease prevention, healing, energy, mood, and beyond. Hopefully, with each new mention, you become increasingly convinced of their powers to give you long life and long health.

Strategy 1: Exercise

The new Fountain of Youth: A daily walk plus three strength-training sessions each week. As mentioned, exciting research is proving that physical activity flips the youth switch, signaling your body to grow younger as it repairs, maintains, and regenerates itself. Among the key body systems that benefit:

- **Muscles.** In one research study, 70-year-olds who performed regular strength-training exercise were as strong as 28-year-olds who didn't work out. Skip exercise and you'll lose muscle strength with every passing year.

- **Brain.** Once, experts believed that age-related drops in memory and cognitive skills were the inevitable result of dying brain cells. Now, scientists know that the brain can strengthen old cells and generate new ones. Exercise releases a fertilizer-like substance called BDNF.

- **Heart.** A heart-threatening lifestyle—replete with high-fat foods, too many calories, little exercise, and smoking—can leave you with stiff, clogged arteries 40 years older than your biological age. Aging also weakens the heart's ability to contract and pump blood. Exercise makes heart muscle contract more forcefully, makes arteries more supple, and slows atherosclerosis.

- **Bones.** Your skeleton grows lighter with time. But research shows that strength-training pumps up the body's natural bone-building system so that bone density increases. Without it, you can lose 2 percent of density per year, raising your risk for fractures.

Strategy 2: Shed Stress, Make Connections

People's brains are hardwired to live in groups. After all, that's where safety was in prehistoric times. And so when we're isolated, our stress levels rise; to our subconscious minds, prolonged periods of isolation aren't safe or natural, and so our brains respond by producing stress chemicals to goad us into action.

Some proof of the powerful influence that stress reduction and social connections can have on your body's repair system:

- Men who survive a heart attack are four times less likely to die from a second heart attack if they come home to family members than if they come home to an empty house or apartment.

• Women with more friends and relatives in their lives are more likely to survive heart disease and cancer than those with few.

• People with heart disease who had been anxious, but then lowered their stress levels, significantly cut their risk for a heart attack, according to one Harvard Medical School study.

Strategy 3:
Supply the Correct "Parts"

A Volvo won't run with replacement engine parts pulled from a beaten-up, low-quality car. And your body won't be able to repair itself with the wrong parts, either. Every time you swallow junk food, refined sugars, refined grain products like white bread, trans fats, and highly processed foods, you're doing just that. Nature's top-of-the-line parts list for the human body are all the nutrients you'll find in good fats, whole grains, fruits and veggies, lean protein, and dairy products (go low-fat to help control calories and saturated-fat levels).

The proof it works:

• Every daily serving of veggies you add to your diet cuts your heart disease risk by 4 percent (or more) and your stroke risk by 3 to 5 percent.

• Just five servings of fruits and veggies a day lower diabetes risk by 39 percent.

• Subjects age 70 and older who ate the most produce, in one Australian study, had the fewest wrinkles.

• People who ate whole-grain cereal every day, during a Harvard School of Public Health study, were 17 percent less likely to die over the next several years from any cause, and 20 percent less likely to die from cardiovascular disease than those who skipped this important repair food.

How Old Are You, Really?

Here are the average ages of the cells in your body, based on new studies.

Stomach lining	5 days
Tastebuds	10 days
Skin surface	2 weeks
Eyelashes	2 months
Red blood cells	4 months
Liver	300–500 days
Bones	10 years
Rib muscle	15.1 years
Stomach	15.9 years (excluding the lining)
Cerebellum	2.9 years younger than you are
Inner eye lens	Older than you are

Strategy 4: Nix the Stuff That Interferes with Repair

Smoking. Exposure to secondhand smoke. Drinking to excess. This bad stuff thwarts your body's regeneration efforts. The upside: Study after study proves that your body's repair system goes back to work the moment you give them up:

• Within minutes of stopping smoking, your lungs and cardiovascular system begin repairing themselves. Blood pressure falls closer to a healthier level within just 8 hours. Within 24 hours, your heart attack risk begins to fall. Within a month, your lungs will work better. (You'll read much more on the benefits of quitting smoking in the pages ahead.)

• Your brain can repair itself even after damage inflicted by heaving drinking. In a study from the University of California, San Francisco, researchers found that alcoholics who stayed sober for nearly seven years performed as well as nonalcoholics on brain-function tests.

• Heart attack rates among nonsmokers plummeted when a smoking ban was instituted in restaurants and bars in one mid-size Montana town—something researchers attribute to a drop in exposure to secondhand smoke.

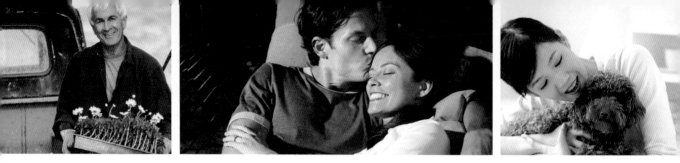

A Doctors' Poll

Take control. Don't put off healthy changes. But above all, stop worrying and start enjoying life.

When the health editors of Reader's Digest asked nine doctors who specialize in anti-aging to rank the impact of dozens of lifestyle habits—past and present—on future health, their answers were both intriguing and amazing.

As expected, the informal expert panel took a serious stance on notorious health-wreckers such as tobacco smoking, drinking to excess, and being too sedentary. But these doctors and psychologists were equally concerned about *hidden* health threats—stuff like worry, unhappy relationships, and debt.

Plenty of research suggests that these extra-strength stresses can lower immunity and raise risk for everything from diabetes to heart disease to migraine headaches and more. The result? The panel in some instances ranked these seemingly unrelated-to-health issues ahead of better-known health risks such as not exercising, breathing secondhand smoke, and ignoring troublesome medical symptoms as the most dangerous to your future.

Their fixes surprised us, too, going beyond the conventional wisdom of "eat more vegetables" and "get more exercise" to emphasize the pleasurable. Good company, relaxation, vacations, and fun, they told us, are as important for a healthy future as that whole-grain bread you had at breakfast this morning or the walk you plan to take with your best friend this afternoon.

The Deadliest Health Sins

Among current bad health habits, eight out of nine doctors rate these three as having the potential to cause significant harm:

- Smoking
- Chronic anger, stress, or worry
- Feeling out of control at home or in your relationships

"Certainly smoking is the biggest killer," notes geriatrician Robert Stall, MD, of Buffalo, one of the panelists. "My feeling is the tobacco companies are the biggest drug cartel in the world, killing more people than all illicit drugs combined."

Tobacco smoke makes risk for lung cancer and heart attack skyrocket, but that's only the beginning. "Smoking is the most destructive habit when it comes to lung health," Dr. Stall notes. "It triggers conditions like emphysema and chronic obstructive pulmonary disease [COPD], where you're literally suffocating. It's as if you're holding your nostrils shut so that you can barely get any air through, and breathing that way every moment of every day. It's torturous."

What was the next tier of unhealthy habits? More than half the doctors identified the following as having the greatest chances of causing you significant health harm in the future:

- Not having a regular exercise routine
- Breathing secondhand smoke regularly
- Drinking to excess (that is, until it's unsafe to drive) on a weekly basis
- Needing sleeping pills in order to fall asleep most nights
- Gulping large quantities of sugary soda every day

Being stuck in an unhappy relationship—with your spouse or with your own body—got top rankings, too. Experts said that ignoring warning signs and symptoms of potential health problems could be as damaging as living with a spouse or partner with whom you fight or maintain an icy silence.

Food faux pas set off alarms, too. All of the experts agreed that noshing regularly on high-calorie, high-fat, high-salt, fast-food meals could cause moderate to significant health effects. And eight out of nine saw similar risks for those who skimped on veggies or rarely drank plain old water—as well as those who filled up on meat, pastries, candy, or ice cream. Dieters, beware: Gaining and losing the same 10 to 20 pounds over and over again was deemed dangerous by most. So was skipping breakfast.

What happens after meals mattered, too. Do you brush and floss? Eight out of nine said that neglecting dental health could be the cause of moderate to significant harm—an opinion corroborated by research linking gum disease with more chronic inflammation and a higher risk for diabetes, heart disease, and even stroke.

Hurting Your Health

The panel of surveyed doctors rated the following ongoing habits, eating patterns, and attitudes as most harmful to present and future health.

Habits

1. Smoking cigarettes
2. Spending yourself deeply into debt
3. Needing sleeping pills to get a good night's sleep
4. Drinking too much to drive at least once a week
5. Taking painkillers every day

Eating Patterns

1. Drinking a lot of soda
2. Eating four or more meals a week at fast-food restaurants
3. Eating ice cream, cake, doughnuts, or candy bars every day
4. Rarely eating vegetables
5. (tie). Skipping breakfast most mornings

Losing and gaining back the same 10 to 20 pounds, over and over again

Lifestyle Choices

1. Being angry, worried or stressed more than happy
2. Feeling a loss of control over home, career, or family
3. Living in an unhappy relationship for some time
4. Ignoring most health problems and symptoms
5. Not exercising beyond everyday living

What's Done May Not Be Done

One thing we all worry about is which habits and activities from our past could most affect our current and future health. While none of the seven choices the doctors considered raised much concern, this is the order they chose:

1. Getting sunburns frequently
2. Getting drunk a lot
3. Smoking marijuana regularly
4. Living in a heavily polluted area
5. Having major injuries
6. Having a major illness
7. Having many sexual partners

Why did the experts come down harder on current bad habits than on health sins from your past? Was a current soda habit really worse than getting drunk in your twenties? Turns out that the answer is usually yes. "We all have a health reservoir called functional reserve—it's the extra capacity that helps protect us against illness, helps us recover when we get sick, and maintains body functions," Dr. Stall notes. "As we get older, this reserve naturally lowers. And if you add insults such as smoking, drinking too much, overeating, or avoiding exercise, the threshold is lowered even further. You can maintain a bigger safety cushion between health and disease, even in your eighties and nineties, if you eat well, exercise, and relax."

The experts also weighed in on 21st-century vices. Eight out of nine thought too much debt, too much coffee, and too much intense, competitive driving could have moderate to significant health effects. Six warned that skipping vacations isn't a good thing, and seven were concerned that being a workaholic could have health-damaging consequences. (Plenty of researchers agree, too.

Missing out on rest and relaxation is a major risk factor for heart attacks.)

Rating Your Past

What would be the worst health mistake you made in your youth? It probably was NOT drinking too much, using marijuana, or even having had lots of sexual encounters with different partners. Yes, most of the experts rated these as having moderate to significant power to harm your present or future health, but an innocent and often-unavoidable risk earned the top spot: Frequent sunburns in childhood or adolescence. (Research confirms that early sunburns—an unfortunate consequence of days spent in the open air and sunshine, without the benefit of sunblock—are an important risk factor for skin cancer later in life.)

Meanwhile, more than half of the panel thought that several other unavoidable childhood health experiences—a major illness, accident, or exposure to pollution—could also play important roles in shaping your future health. Research confirms that all three can shape the course of well-being decades later, yet studies show that most survivors of childhood illnesses and accidents don't receive the follow-up care they need (and long-term effects of environmental toxins are still often not well-known).

The panel said that it would be difficult to undo damage caused by childhood health exposures. But that's not the end of the story. Keeping up with recommended screenings for everything from skin cancer to lung health to sexual well-being remains the smartest way to catch potential trouble early.

Health and Emotions

It's impressive that "worrying less and having more fun" earned the number five spot when the experts listed their favorite ways you can add more healthy years to your life. On the flip side, it was also surprising that eight of the nine ranked feeling out of control and feeling worried, stressed, or angry most of the time as sources of significant harm.

But the results didn't surprise psychologist and researcher Michael J. Salamon, PhD, director of the Adult Developmental Center in Hewlett, New York. Dr. Salamon, one of the doctors who took the Reader's Digest survey, says his own research illuminates the power of feelings and attitudes to extend life. "In a study, we surveyed older people about their life satisfaction, then went back 10 years later to see how they were," he says. "What we found was that those with the highest life-satisfaction scores were much more likely to still be alive a decade later than those who had had the lowest scores. Something was going on with the way they approached life."

A growing stack of research confirms the connection. Stress, unhappiness, loneliness, and hostility have been linked with higher levels of stress hormones, higher blood sugar levels, and even more clogged arteries. "The people who were still alive had an accepting attitude. One person told me, 'You bless the bad as well as the good'", Dr. Salamon notes.

If you think the satisfied people were simply richer or more popular or maybe started the study in better health, Dr. Salamon has news for you. "We found no correlation between health or wealth or popularity and satisfaction," he says. "It's purely attitude. If you don't have a happy personality naturally, you can cultivate satisfaction by acknowledging your innate grumpiness and making an effort to appreciate the good things in your life."

The Top Six Fixes

When asked which activities would be most likely to add healthy years to a person's life, the doctors had numerous responses, but these six came out on top:

1. Exercising more
2. Quitting smoking
3. Eating more fruits and vegetables
4. Eating less junk food and fatty food
5. Worrying less and having more fun
6. Sleeping more

The Fix: Take Charge Today

More good news: The experts thought most current lifestyle mistakes are moderately easy or downright simple to fix. Among the easiest in their estimation were: Taking more vacations, cutting back on TV watching, eating more veggies, drinking more water, having breakfast, cutting back on sodas and sweets, and having less coffee. Slightly more challenging were: Getting more exercise, seeing your doctor more often, calling a halt to yo-yo dieting, and reducing meat consumption (to make room for healthy main dishes with beans and grains).

Toughest to change: smoking, a dependence on sleeping pills, and an ingrained fast-food habit. Their best advice: Just do it.

"It's never too early to start taking good care of yourself, but it's never too late, either," one survey-taker wrote. "There will always be some benefit." Added another: "This is not unique advice, but ... today is the first day of the rest of your life. [You] are in charge of caring for yourself and enjoying each day."

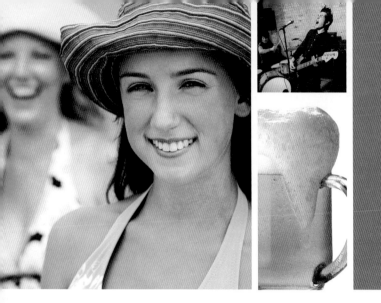

Erasing the Damage

When it comes to health, some sins of our past are not so easily forgiven.

As it turns out, several youthful indiscretions have a potentially long-lasting effect on our bodies. That was our discovery after reviewing a mountain of medical research and interviewing doctors about such excesses as binge drinking, marijuana smoking, and having multiple sex partners.

But there is a very positive side to the story. By halting bad habits and embracing healthier ones, you can *in every case* minimize the risks those past deeds pose, to the point where statistically, they become truly minimal. In fact, five straight days of eating ice cream or cookies in the past week likely has far more bearing on a person's health than any escapades of 30 years earlier, experts made clear.

So it's time to put concerns about your past to rest. In the following pages, we closely examine 35 habits and lifestyle choices of your distant and recent past, and explain how they might effect your health of today and tomorrow. More important, we reveal the best ways to mitigate any damage the habit or lifestyle caused, to make sure that what's done is finally done. Because when it comes to health, you want your best to begin today, and to only increase with age!

erasing the da

I'm a former smoker, but I quit a year or more ago.

DAMAGE DONE

If you've kicked the habit, you are to be congratulated and admired. Breaking an addiction to the nicotine in tobacco isn't easy. With each smoke-free year that passes, you lower your odds for heart disease, serious breathing problems, and cancers of the lungs, mouth, throat, esophagus, bladder, and possibly the pancreas, too.

But you may not be in the clear yet. Your heart and lungs remain at higher risk of disease than that of a nonsmoker for up to 20 years after you quit.

Can I Undo It? Absolutely.

You'll see immediate health improvements shortly after quitting, but the full benefits of quitting take years to reap. Your heart disease risk drops by 50 percent within a year after you kick the habit; but it's not until 15 years later that your risk for heart disease and stroke fall to the level of someone who's never smoked. As for lung cancer: After 10 smoke-free years, your risk is about one-third to one-half that of continuing smokers; it falls to nearly that of someone who's never smoked within 20 years.

Good news: If you take additional steps to improve your health beyond staying smoke-free, you can accelerate the recovery and end up even more immune to the diseases most linked to smoking.

+ BENEFITS

Your skin will look younger and less wrinkled than someone who continues to smoke. You're saving money (cigarettes can be expensive!) and life's little pleasures—the taste of good food, the smell of spring flowers, the sensation of taking in a big lungful of fresh, rain-washed air—are yours to enjoy again. And then there's the big one: lowered risk of most life-threatening diseases.

Repair Plan

Be vigilant. Habits and addictions do not die easily. Even if you've been smoke-free for years, it might take just one weak moment to restart your habit. Always be mindful of the benefits of not smoking and the self-respect you've earned in kicking the habit, and do not let yourself be tempted.

Stay away from secondhand smoke. Passive smoking nearly doubles your odds for a heart attack—and may be even more risky for former smokers whose lungs and cardiovascular systems are still recovering from past insults. Avoiding smoke at home, at work, and when you're out socializing is the biggest preventive step a former smoker can take, say Harvard Medical School experts.

Eat lots of fruits, veggies, and whole grains. These natural foods are packed with cell-shielding antioxidants that further protect against heart disease, stroke, and several forms of cancer. Bonus: You get extra vitamins and cholesterol-lowering fiber.

Get checked. Stay up-to-date with blood pressure and cholesterol checks. Make regular appointments with your doctor in advance so you don't forget.

Monitor lung health. Stay alert for signs of lung problems, such as persistent coughing, shortness of breath, and chest pain. Tell your doctor right away if you have these.

■ FOR MORE ON OVERCOMING BREATHING PROBLEMS, SEE PAGE 366.

My skin is freckled and worn from a youth spent in the sun.

DAMAGE DONE

Nearly 80 percent of lifetime sun damage occurs before age 18. The more sun exposure you had, the more likely you are to face wrinkles, splotches, freckles, and skin discolorations when you look in the mirror after age 50. Even more dangerous is your heightened risk for skin cancer in later decades.

Your odds of developing skin cancer are higher if you have pale skin, blonde or red hair, and/or blue eyes: all signs that your skin has low levels of protective melanin. If you endured three or more blistering sunburns before age 15, you're at higher risk for melanoma, the most deadly form of skin cancer. Five early sunburns doubles it. Having a job that kept you outdoors for at least three summers during your teens or twenties—such as lifeguarding, being a camp counselor, or working on a farm, in a park, or at a construction site—increases your chances as well.

Oddly, so does a history of being careful. If you were one of the first to jump on the suntan-lotion bandwagon in the 1950s and 1960s, you may have felt free to stay on the beach longer because the lotion kept you from burning quickly. What you didn't know was that, until recently, most tanning lotions and sunscreens only protected against UVB rays and did nothing to guard skin from damaging UVA rays. UVA rays are weaker but penetrate deeper into the skin and may play a role in triggering melanoma; experts know for sure that they contribute to skin aging, wrinkling, the development of brown spots, and blotching.

Can I Undo It? Regrettably, no.

Sun damage cannot be reversed. But you can take steps to prevent further damage, to reduce your odds for developing skin cancer, and for spotting potential cancer in its earliest, most treatable stages.

+ BENEFITS

Taking steps now will help you prevent further damage to your skin and help ensure early detection of skin cancers. You'll also experience reduced skin inflammation, meaning less strain on your immune system.

Repair Plan

Hide from the sun. Avoid the sun during peak UV radiation hours, usually 10:00 A.M. to 4:00 P.M.

Buy a "broad spectrum" sunscreen with a sun protection factor (SPF) of 15 or greater. Look for one that protects against UVA and UVB rays. Ingredients that block UVA include benzophenone, oxybenzone, sulisobenzone, titanium dioxide, zinc oxide, and butyl methoxydibenzoylmethane (also called avobenzone and known by the trade name Parsol 1789). If you love to swim, buy a sunblock marked "waterproof"—it will provide protection for at least 80 minutes even when you are swimming or sweating. Sunblocks marked "water resistant" protect for just half that long.

Slather it on 30 minutes before sun exposure. Use an ounce—about a shot-glassful—and cover all body parts exposed to the sun. Reapply every two hours and always after swimming or sweating.

Invest in a broad-brimmed, crushable hat. Carry it with you in your purse, tote bag, or pocket when you're not wearing it.

Use lip balm with sunblock in it. Lips are very sensitive to the sun, but we often forget to tend to them when we go outside. When you apply your sunscreen, put on some sun-blocking lip balm as well.

Buy wraparound sunglasses. Make sure that your sunglasses protect against UVA and UVB rays (check the label) and wear them year-round. Glasses that wrap around the sides of your temples help protect you even more.

Have an annual skin check performed by a dermatologist. Studies show that a skin doctor is more likely than your family doctor or gynecologist to spot trouble.

Ask your family doc and your gynecologist to be on the lookout. The more doctors who check your skin, the higher your chances of finding cancerous spots in their earliest, most treatable stages.

Check your own skin regularly. After a shower or bath, take a hand mirror into a well-lit room and examine your entire body—including between your toes. Becoming familiar with your own birthmarks, moles, and blemishes will allow you to spot changes and potentially dangerous newcomers at your next check.

Watch for danger signs. Classic melanomas may show up as blackish/brownish splotches or moles with irregular edges. But this lethal cancer can also be red, pink, or waxy, or it can be a sore that just won't heal. Other warning signs include itching, bleeding, sensitivity to touch, or obvious growth.

Be extra-careful in the sun if you take medications. Any of the following medications can make your skin more sensitive to sun damage: tetracycline, sulfa drugs and some other antibiotics, naproxen sodium, tricyclic antidepressants, thiazide diuretics (used for high blood pressure and some heart conditions), and sulfonylureas (a form of oral antidiabetic medication). Check with your doctor for any medications you take that could increase your vulnerability.

■ FOR MORE ON MANAGING SKIN PROBLEMS, SEE PAGE 295.

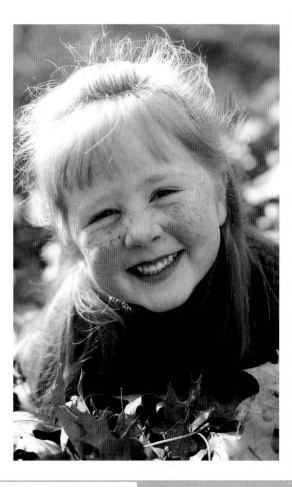

I used to smoke marijuana in my youth.

DAMAGE DONE

More than you realize. Marijuana smoke contains 50 to 70 percent more carcinogenic hydrocarbons than tobacco smoke, plus high levels of an enzyme that converts certain smoke components into their most potent, cancer-causing forms. Combined with the fact that marijuana smokers inhale more deeply and hold smoke in their lungs longer than cigarette smoke means that regular pot-smokers may have an even higher risk for lung cancer than former cigarette-smokers.

But that's not all. Researchers at Canada's McGill University have found that long-term cannabis-smokers lose molecules called CB1 receptors in blood vessels inside the brain. This can lead to reduced blood flow and to memory and concentration problems, long after you've stopped smoking. It may also double or even triple your risk for cancers of the head and neck, according to a study that compared the health histories of 173 cancer patients and 176 people who were cancer-free.

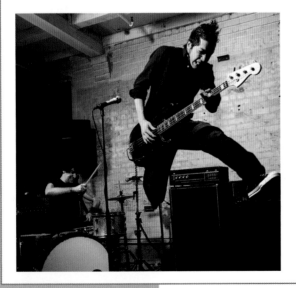

Can I Undo It? Unknown.

There are no studies that show the long-term health effects of a short-lived marijuana habit. But healthy living, including avoiding all forms of smoke, likely will reduce what lingering damage your youthful indiscretion caused.

+ BENEFITS

You can work toward having a much lower chance of stroke and cancer.

Repair Plan

Don't smoke cigarettes. Just because tobacco is legal and marijuana isn't doesn't make it healthier. As noted, nothing is worse for your health than a smoking habit of any kind.

Eat well. A diet packed with fruits, vegetables, and whole grains can help cut your risk for stroke—and may help lower your risk for lung and other cancers.

Avoid secondhand smoke. Passive smoking is risky for the lungs of former cigarette-smokers. The same goes for former marijuana-smokers, too.

Get checked. Make regular appointments with your doctor so you stay up-to-date with blood pressure and cholesterol checks.

Stay alert for signs of lung problems. Tell your doctor right away if you have persistent coughing, shortness of breath, or chest pain.

■ FOR MORE ON PREVENTING CANCER, SEE PAGE 328.

I used to get drunk a lot.

DAMAGE DONE

Again, more than you might realize. Even if your drinking days are far behind you, alcohol's effects on your health could linger for decades. In one study of 3,803 women and men, former drinkers reported more depression, heart problems, chronic bronchitis, and diabetes after age 40 than did current social drinkers. They also felt less energetic and said their health problems interfered more often with social activities.

Heavy drinking in your twenties can raise your heart disease risk by 36 percent later in life—perhaps due to an enlarged heart muscle, high blood pressure, or to a lifestyle (then and now) that doesn't include much exercise or enough healthy food. If you ever binge-drank, such as downing an incredible 25 drinks in a day—even just once—researchers say your later odds for heart disease could be seven times higher than normal.

Bingeing can also increase a man's later risk for prostate cancer by 64 percent—especially in men who have type 2 diabetes. In women, a history of heavy drinking may increase breast cancer risk, especially if the drinking happened in midlife. The reason? Alcohol seems to alter hormone levels that may fuel the growth of some types of breast cancers. Irritation caused by drinking may also increase your odds for cancers of the head and neck for about 10 years after you stop.

Can I Undo It? Yes.

There's plenty you can do to help your body repair alcohol's damage, and to offset added risks. Experts are just beginning to look at how much of drinking's physical and mental effects can be reversed. Proof that the body can heal:

In one study of nearly 1,600 people, former drinkers' risk for cancer of the esophagus dropped to normal after a decade.

+ BENEFITS

Choose to replace your overindulgent past with a healthy present and future, and the benefits are widespread. You'll protect yourself from heart disease and several forms of cancer. You'll feel more energized and upbeat. And you'll give your self-esteem a huge boost as well, knowing that you've greatly improved the person you are.

Repair Plan

Quit smoking. Former drinkers are often smokers—one study found that they were 31 percent more likely to smoke cigarettes as current drinkers were. Follow the advice on pages 58 and 59 to help you kick the habit.

Get the cancer screenings you need. Follow your doctor's advice for regular mammograms and clinical breast exams for women, prostate-cancer screenings for men.

Stay on top of heart health. Work with your doctor to keep blood pressure, cholesterol, and triglycerides at healthy levels. Also get regular blood sugar tests to screen for diabetes.

Eat plenty of fruits and vegetables. Eating well and exercising regularly help offset your added risk for heart attack, stroke, diabetes, and even some cancers.

Beware of signs of depression. Understand that depression could be related in part to your wild past. Talk with your family doctor about seeing a therapist.

I had a major illness when I was young.

DAMAGE DONE

It is human nature to believe in full recoveries and happy-ever-after endings, particularly when it comes to children. But the reality is that major diseases cause lasting damage to children's bodies, even when recovery seems complete.

The reasons are varied. For example, survivors of childhood cancers may face more risks from the treatments they underwent than from recurrences of cancer itself. Harsh chemotherapy drugs and radiation damage healthy cells throughout the body. The result: You're three times more likely to have a chronic health problem as someone who's never had cancer, and eight times more likely to have a severe condition, says a study of 10,000 Canadian and American survivors of pediatric cancers.

If you had rheumatic fever as a child, you have a 40 to 80 percent chance for developing pancarditis—inflammation of the heart that can damage the valves that help control the flow of blood through your heart. You also have a higher risk for arthritis, especially in your fingers. If you've had lifelong asthma, long-term use of inhaled corticosteroids could increase your risk for brittle bones and fractures later in life. Survivors of childhood polio (cases of polio peaked in the early 1950s) often experience progressive muscle weakness with age.

Can I Undo It? Unfortunately, no.

You can't erase the lingering damage of a major childhood disease. But you can live healthy and, by doing so, reduce risks of new disease. You can nip any emerging problems if you work with your doctor to stay current with health screenings, something only 20 percent of people who survived a major childhood illness do.

+ BENEFITS

Healthy living has many benefits, but for those who had major challenges as a youth, the mental rewards of a healthy, active adulthood are particularly sweet. Plus, by being mindful of the long-term effects of your past challenges, you'll catch related health problems earlier, when they're most treatable.

Repair Plan

Tell your doctor about your medical history. Ask what screenings you need now. Knowing your childhood disease challenges helps a doctor know what to watch for and how to help you achieve better health.

Lead a healthy life. Good food, ample exercise, a healthy attitude, and life-affirming habits like getting plenty of sleep, water, and relaxation are the ticket to long life and good health for everyone, but particularly those whose bodies have been challenged. Make the mental commitment to health, and you will find that your past might become increasingly irrelevant to your future.

Add an oncologist to your personal medical staff. If you had a childhood cancer, make an appointment with an oncologist to get the latest information about long-term effects of your earlier illness and treatments—and what you need to do to protect yourself from future health problems.

Get protective care if you had rheumatic fever. You may need to take a special course of antibiotics before having any type of treatment or procedure—even dental cleaning—that could allow bacteria to get into your bloodstream.

Be smart about bone health. Get enough calcium, vitamin D, and weight-bearing exercise to protect your bones.

I had some major injuries when I was young.

DAMAGE DONE

Most childhood injuries—from a skinned knee when you fell off your bike to a bumped head when you fell out of the neighborhood tree house—heal swiftly, causing no further problems. But more serious injuries—the result of car accidents or major sports injuries—can have consequences that show up or grow worse later in your life.

Childhood fractures can change the way bones finish growing. About 15 percent of injuries to a child's or teen's growth plate—the vulnerable area of growing tissue at the ends of long bones—can slow future growth of arm or leg bones. While a slight difference in the length of your arms won't cause problems, even a tiny discrepancy in leg length could. Foot pain, knee pain, hip pain, and lower back pain have all been linked with small leg-length differences that can be difficult to detect on your own.

Knees are especially vulnerable. Growth-plate injuries at the knee can lead to crooked legs and knee pain. And if you ever tore your anterior cruciate ligament—the key ligament that keeps knee joints stable—you may be at higher risk for arthritis later in life.

If you were a serious high school or college athlete who experienced more than two concussions, you may now be at higher risk for headaches, depression, and memory problems as well as sleep problems, mood swings, ringing in the ears, and poor concentration.

Can I Undo It? No.

But you can take important steps to compensate for some problems and to prevent future damage.

+ BENEFITS

You'll have less joint pain and, perhaps most important, less chance of a recurring injury.

Repair Plan

Have your legs measured by a professional. Ask your family doctor, an orthopedic surgeon, back specialist, or podiatrist to measure your legs if you've had ongoing foot, knee, hip, or lower back pain. A difference in leg lengths could be the cause—and might be corrected with something as simple as an orthopedic lift in your shoe.

Tell your doctor if you had multiple concussions earlier in your life. This can help her make decisions about treating memory, sleep, and mood problems.

Protect your head. If you had several concussions earlier in your life, skip sports and activities that could cause more damage if you fall, such as roller skating or ice skating. Be sure to wear a helmet if you bike or ski.

Exercise regularly, but not too intensely. Stronger muscles can take some of the strain off of once-injured joints, and properly exercised joints get lots of nourishment and care from your bloodstream and immune system. Exercise also helps prevent the rise of arthritis and other aches and pains of aging. Avoid high-impact exercise, however, which can actually hurt or aggravate existing joint conditions.

■ FOR MORE ON MANAGING JOINT PAIN, SEE PAGE 284.

DAMAGE DONE

If your wild days are well behind you, so are most of the immediate risks for sexually transmitted diseases. There is one important exception: The more sexual partners a woman has had, the higher her odds for developing cervical cancer at any age. Cervical cancer is caused by some strains of the human papilloma virus (HPV). A persistent, silent infection could linger for years before the cancer is discovered: Slightly more than 20 percent of women with cervical cancer are diagnosed when they are over 65 years old.

Your odds for developing cervical cancer after an HPV infection double if you're also a smoker, if you ever used oral contraceptives for 5 years or longer (your risk may rise four times above normal if you were ever on The Pill for longer than 10 years), if you've given birth to several children, if your mother or sisters have had cervical cancer, or if you've had any illness that lowers your immunity.

If you've resumed an active sex life with new partners, or have had more than one partner in the past few years, here's something else to consider: Your knowledge of sexually transmitted diseases (STD) may be dangerously out of date. Some doctors are beginning to report an upswing in STD infections in their older patients, as more single or even newly married older people enjoy new intimacies. The rules for safe sex have changed radically in the past 15 years—you may need to catch up.

Can I Undo It? No.

You can't "undo" an HPV infection, but you can get tested and treated (with surgery or other procedures). If you're sexually active again, you can learn new preventive rules to protect yourself.

+ BENEFITS

You can have a greater sense of control and safety in your intimate relationships. Plus, being proactive will greatly lower your risk for STDs and help catch signs of cervical cancer earlier.

Repair Plan

Get double-tested if you are a woman. Both a PAP smear and an HPV check are imperative to detect cervical health issues. PAP smears test for early warning signs of cervical cancer, but can miss precancerous cells 25 to 50 percent of the time. In contrast, an HPV test looks for the actual cause of cervical cancer: the 13 potential strains of this nasty, carcinogenic virus. If you test positive, you can have infected cells removed early, before damage is done.

Get tested every three years. Even if you are not currently sexually active or you have negative PAP and HPV results, get tested. It takes at least three years for a new HPV infection to begin causing cells to change in precancerous ways. Cutting-edge cervical cancer–screening guidelines suggest that rechecks every three years, with another PAP and another HPV, are sufficient to catch problems. (But continue to see your gynecologist every year for a pelvic exam and clinical breast exam!)

Ask your gynecologist about the HPV vaccine. Studies are underway to see if this vaccine helps prevent the development of cervical cancer in women up to age 55. It was first recommended for teens and young women only. Check with your doctor about its effectiveness for you.

Ask if you can stop testing. If you are over 70 years old and have had three or more normal PAP tests in a row in the past 10 years plus at least one negative HPV test—and you have had no new sexual partners in at least 3 years—it may be safe to stop cervical cancer screenings. Additionally, If you've had a total hysterectomy, you may be able to skip cervical cancer checks. If you still have your cervix or if the surgery was done to treat cervical cancer or precancer, continue to have checks regularly. Ask your doctor.

Have a fruit salad and a yellow, orange, or red vegetable every day. Studies suggest that getting plenty of the powerful antioxidant beta-carotene— from food, not supplements—may cut your risk for developing cervical cancer.

Play by the new rules. Sexually active again? Don't be fooled by the proverbial wisdom of your age: Your odds for contracting an STD are not much different than those of a teen or 20-year-old who's just becoming sexually active. You'll need condoms (even if risk of pregnancy is nil). It's also a good idea to ask your partner a few tough questions: Are you HIV-negative? Do you have herpes or other STDs? Have you had other sexual partners recently? While such questions once seemed out of line, today's sexual landscape is much more open and honest. Use your maturity to ask them in a sensitive, appropriate way. And if you don't like the answers—or trust them—it's still okay to say no.

Watch for signs of STDs. Call your doctor if you develop rashes, blisters, sores, itching, pain, fever, discomfort during sex, or an unusual discharge.

Be honest with your doctor. Your doc may not realize that you're active … or be reluctant to ask. Tell her if you've had new sexual partners or are in a new relationship so that she knows to be concerned about sexual health issues.

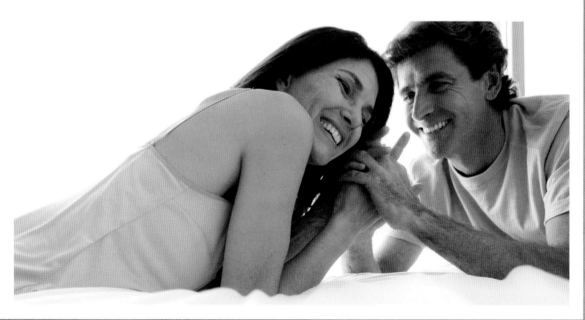

I grew up in a heavily polluted area.

DAMAGE DONE

Children's lungs are more vulnerable to damage from air pollution and excess ozone than adults' lungs, since they are still developing and growing. The result is a high propensity for lung-related disease for those with constant exposure to smoke and pollution. This was vividly revealed in a study that compared healthy children in a heavily polluted area of Mexico City against similar kids raised in rural Mexico. X-rays of the children's lungs revealed that more than half of the city kids already had lung damage that may be predictive of future problems.

Another study shows that exposure to pollution for many years can raise your lung cancer risk by as much as 24 percent and can be as destructive as breathing secondhand tobacco smoke. In a different study that tracked 500,000 people from 100 cities for 16 years, researchers found that dirty air also increased the risk of dying from heart disease by 6 percent or more. The more polluted the air, the higher the death rates.

Can I Undo It? No.

Damage done to young lungs doesn't get repaired by your body. But there's plenty you can do to keep your lungs healthy and to protect against future damage.

+ BENEFITS

Achieving better lung health means improved, deeper breathing. Delivering better-quality air to your lungs results in greater stamina and overall energy, too.

Repair Plan

Avoid smoke and dirty air. The only way to consistently avoid polluted air is to live far from heavy traffic, smokestack factories, and highly crowded neighborhoods. Not everyone has that choice, however. If you must live in an urban area, there are still many things you can do. Pay attention to the pollution forecast for the day, especially on hot summer days when there may be higher levels of ozone in the air. Explore better air filtering for your home. Take frequent trips out of the city. Stay indoors during peak traffic times.

Don't smoke. Tobacco smoke irritates fragile, already-vulnerable lung tissue.

Pay attention to lung health. Call your doctor right away if you have chest pain or aches when you inhale or exhale or if you are coughing up blood. These, along with unexplained weight loss, can be symptoms of lung cancer, as can shortness of breath, a hoarse voice, difficulty swallowing, pain under your ribs, and/or swelling of your face or neck.

Watch for COPD. See your doctor if you're coughing frequently, wheezing, have frequent lung infections, or have a lot of mucus. These symptoms can be a sign of a complex breathing problem that doctors call chronic obstructive pulmonary disorder, or COPD.

Exercise. It strengthens muscles that help you breathe.

Eat lots of fruits and vegetables. The antioxidants can help protect lungs from future damage.

Learn to control your breathing. If you have COPD, your doctor or a respiratory therapist can teach you how to relax when you're feeling short of breath.

■ FOR MORE ON BETTER BREATHING, SEE PAGE 366.

I enjoy a good cigar every now and then.

DAMAGE DONE

Even if you don't inhale, smoking the occasional cigar raises your odds for heart disease and a wide variety of cancers. While no one's figured out the precise risk, consider this: Because cigars are bigger than cigarettes, take longer to smoke, use tobacco that's aged and fermented, and are rolled in slower-burning wrappers, a single large cigar emits up to 20 times more ammonia, 5 to 10 times more cadmium (a carcinogenic metal), and up to 80 to 90 times more highly carcinogenic nitrosamines.

"All smokers, whether or not they inhale, directly expose the lips, mouth, throat, larynx, and tongue to smoke," says a definitive U.S. National Cancer Institute report on cigar smoking. "In addition, smoke constituents in the saliva are swallowed into the esophagus."

If you smoke one or more cigars every day, you've raised your odds for heart disease, serious lung problems, and a wide variety of cancers on virtually every part of your body that is exposed to tobacco smoke, from your lips, tongue, mouth, and throat to your esophagus, larynx, and lungs. The more you smoke, the higher the risk: while one or two cigars a day doubles your risk for cancers of the mouth; puffing three or four raises your risk more than 8 times above normal; smoking five or more cigars a day boosts it to 16 times higher than that of nonsmokers.

Can I Undo It? For the most part.

If you've been an occasional smoker, quitting will probably wipe out most cigar-related risks within a few years. If you've been a heavy cigar smoker for years, however, your heart disease and lung cancer risk may not fall to that of a nonsmoker's for decades.

+ BENEFITS

Stop smoking cigars and you will not only lower your risk for mouth and lung cancers but also you'll have more money in your pocket. Your colleagues will appreciate that you no longer have cigar breath, and your clothes, car, and house will smell significantly better.

Repair Plan

Commit to never buying cigars again. When you run out of your current stock, switch to a healthier pastime, such as a sipping a good glass of wine. Unlike cigarette smoking, smoking cigars is usually an occasional vice, not a dependency, making quitting a little easier.

Don't buy into the cigar culture. While it might seem that the occasional cigar with the fellows is bold, classic, even elegant, it isn't. There are many better ways to show solidarity with your friends and associates and without doing such harsh damage to your body.

Downsize. Can't give up the occasional cigar? Smoke the smallest size possible.

Monitor for the effects of past smoking. Get regular blood pressure and cholesterol checks to catch heart disease risks as early as possible. Tell your doctor about your smoking history and watch for warning signs of possible lung cancer, such as constant chest pain, shortness of breath, or coughing up blood.

Be sure your dentist checks for oral cancers. Stay alert for oral cancer warning signs such as a sore on your lips, gums, or inside your mouth that won't heal; a thick spot in your cheek; numbness; difficulty swallowing; or a feeling that something's caught in your throat.

DAMAGE DONE

As far as health goes, no popular habit on this planet is as harmful as smoking. Cigarettes directly cause 30 percent of heart disease deaths, 30 percent of cancer deaths, and a whopping 80 to 90 percent of all lung cancers. They also increase people's risk of developing mouth, throat, esophageal, bladder, and possibly pancreatic cancer. No wonder smoking is officially the number one cause of preventable deaths in the developed world.

As few as 8 cigarettes per month—just 100 in a year—raises your smoking-related lung-cancer risk, especially if you've kept it up for years. In fact, any smoking raises your risk. In a study of British doctors, smoking just 1 to 14 cigarettes a day raised risk 8 times higher than normal, smoking 15 to 25 cigarettes raised risk 13 times, and smoking more than 25 per day pushed risk up 25 times.

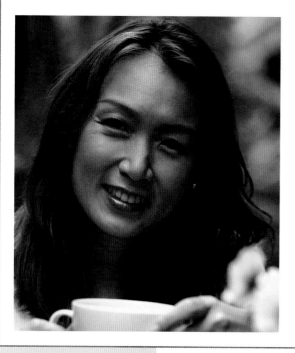

The 4,000 chemicals in tobacco smoke are lethal for your cardiovascular system—raising your odds astronomically for heart attacks, strokes, and high blood pressure. Chemicals in tobacco smoke increase cardiovascular risk by strangling the body's oxygen supply, making artery walls stiff, slashing levels of "good" HDL cholesterol, and making blood platelets stickier and more likely to form heart-threatening clots.

Then there's lung damage. Smoking can trigger or exacerbate short-term breathing problems including bronchitis and asthma attacks. Smoking is also closely linked to chronic obstructive pulmonary disorder, or COPD—a cluster of incapacitating airway problems. This disorder, which is essentially the combination of chronic bronchitis and emphysema, is one of the fastest-growing and most debilitating lung issues among older people. In fact, it is the fourth leading cause of death in the United States—and 80 to 90 percent of cases are linked to smoking.

Can I Undo It? Yes.

No matter how long or how much you've smoked, you can reverse much of the damage—if you stop smoking once and for all. When researchers at Memorial Sloan Kettering Cancer Center in New York City checked the health histories and lung scans of 18,172 current and former smokers, they discovered just how powerful quitting can be. According to their data, a 51-year-old woman who'd smoked a pack a day for 29 years, and then quit, cut her risk for developing lung cancer within 10 years to less than 1 percent.

Your lungs and cardiovascular system begin repairing themselves within minutes of your last cigarette. Within eight hours of your last cigarette, your blood pressure begins falling to a healthier range and high levels of toxic carbon monoxide gas in your bloodstream drop. In a day, your heart attack risk begins to fall. Within two days your sense of taste and smell sharpen. Within a month, your lungs will work better and you should be coughing less, feel more energetic, and have less congestion and shortness of breath.

+ BENEFITS

Quitting smoking has countless health benefits. Significantly reduced threat of cancer or heart disease, an improved sense of taste and smell, better endurance, and fewer colds and infections are just a few. In addition to feeling better physically, you will also reap confidence-boosting rewards like fresher breath, younger-looking skin, and no more tobacco smell on your clothes.

Repair Plan

Treat it like an addiction, not a habit.
Nonsmokers—and oddly, many smokers themselves—often fail to understand how thoroughly addicting smoking can be. Ending a long-running smoking habit cannot be done casually. It is hard to do—for some, brutally hard. Before stopping, smokers need to prepare themselves mentally and physically for a challenging road ahead. They need to have a strategy, a support team, and a Plan B if some of the methods they intend to rely on fail to deliver.

Ask your doctor about a smoking-cessation drug.
Two drugs—an antidepressant called buprion and a withdrawal-easing drug called varenicline—have been shown in studies to increase a quitter's chances for success.

Get support. Counseling, an online support group, or a local nonsmoking group can all help. So can telephone hotlines you call if you suddenly get the urge to light up again. And of course, enlist your friends, family, and co-workers, as appropriate, to get you through to the smoke-free life.

Take care of yourself. Get plenty of sleep, exercise every day, drink plenty of water, and stay busy. Healthy living delivers rewards that help replace whatever benefits smokers feel they get from the habit.

Time it right. Plan to start your life as a nonsmoker during a calm period—not over the holidays or when you're under a lot of stress.

Eat lots of fruits and veggies. Studies show that smokers and former smokers who eat plenty of produce, in a variety of brilliant colors, have lower rates of lung cancer. The reason? Probably the protective antioxidants in fresh fruits and veggies.

Try "nicotine fading." If nicotine cravings have kept you from quitting in the past, this longer-term, slower quitting technique could help. Use a nicotine patch or gum to help you become accustomed to life without cigarettes as you gradually step down your nicotine exposure. Keep using the patch or gum for as long as you need to, making sure to follow the package directions.

Remember, a lapse isn't a failure. Most successful quitters have lapsed many times. Use the lapse to discover your personal obstacles to quitting, and create a plan for dealing with your needs. If you use cigarettes to relax, try a walk, a stretch, a phone call, or a piece of fruit instead. If a cigarette was part of your after-meal routine, replace it with a cup of tea.

■ FOR MORE ON BETTER BREATHING, SEE PAGE 366.

I take painkillers and sedatives as a matter of course.

DAMAGE DONE

While these drugs can be beneficial when taken for legitimate health problems, long-term habitual use can cause more problems than it solves. Taking nonsteroidal anti-inflammatory drugs (NSAIDs) such as ibuprofen or aspirin for arthritis or muscle pain can, over time, raise your risk for ulcers, gastrointestinal bleeding, high blood pressure, and heart attack. Each year, the side effects of long-term NSAID use cause nearly 103,000 hospitalizations and 16,500 deaths in the United States alone.

Taking headache pills on a regular basis can lead to rebound headaches as the drug's effects wear off and blood vessels surrounding your brain begin to swell again.

Meanwhile, prescription pain relievers and sedatives can become a habit before you realize what's happened. The number of older people who overuse opioid-based pain pills has nearly doubled in the last decade, experts say. And the use of calming drugs called benzodiazepines is also on the rise. Often prescribed for insomnia or after an emotionally upsetting experience, these tranquilizers and sleeping pills can leave you feeling confused and prone to stumbling and falling if you take them in higher-than-prescribed doses or for too long. Since they make you feel good, you may want to take more or keep on taking them. Why that's dangerous: As you age, your body metabolizes drugs more slowly, so you actually get the desired effects with a lower dose.

The biggest danger from prescription pain pills and tranquilizers is hidden addiction. Do you:

- Use over-the-counter pain relievers most days for painful joints, a bad back, or persistent headaches?
- Continue to use powerful prescription pain killers long after the surgery or injury that led to the initial prescription?
- Feel compelled to take a sedative frequently to ease anxiety or beat insomnia?

If you answered yes to any of the three, then it's probably time for a new strategy. If you think that you may be addicted to prescription pain pills or sedatives, tell someone—and talk with your doctor. Signs include the inability to stop taking them, hoarding and hiding pills, worried family members, or using more than one doctor or pharmacy in order to get more pills.

Can I Undo It? Yes.

New pain-relief strategies can ease muscle, joint, and head pain with fewer pills—and fewer side effects. And kicking the sedative and prescription pain pill habit is possible with commitment and support. Once the pill-taking has ceased, your body will quickly rebound from their effects.

+ BENEFITS

You'll spend less money on medications. You may cut your risk for heart and high blood pressure problems as well as gastrointestinal ulcers and bleeding. You'll be more alert—and you'll have the satisfaction of knowing that you've beaten a drug dependency.

Repair Plan

Watch for warning signs of GI trouble. If you take over-the-counter pain relievers regularly and have any pain or bleeding, call your doctor right away.

For chronic pain—such as arthritis or back pain—switch to acetaminophen. It doesn't cause stomach irritation and, in studies, didn't raise blood pressure the way NSAIDs do.

Save ibuprofen for flare-ups of severe, short-term pain. It's generally safe to take for up to 10 days, but not more!

If you must take ibuprofen on a regular basis, protect your stomach. Guard against bleeding and ulcers by taking a drug called a proton-pump inhibitor, which blocks the production of irritating stomach acid.

For frequent headaches, see your doctor about a migraine-stopping drug. Many headache-prone people have migraines, which can be stopped quickly with the right medication.

Check out alternate pain-relief strategies. For arthritis pain, strategies could include weight loss, gentle exercise, acupressure, and adding more omega-3 fatty acids to your diet. For back pain, exercise and stress relief are tops. For headaches, avoid triggers such as certain foods, drinks, and situations (stress, sleeplessness, getting too hungry).

Take the right dose of all prescription drugs. If you're not sure, call your doctor or pharmacist.

Don't take habit-forming drugs for more than four months. Challenge your doctor any time they want to put you on painkillers, depressants, or sedatives for a prolonged period. Express your concern about their long-term effect, and be honest if you believe that you might be susceptible to addiction—particularly if they work well!

Watch for the hidden signs. There are clues that you're taking too much of a tranquilizer, or have taken it for too long. These include memory loss or forgetfulness, excessive sleepiness, feeling emotionally numb or unresponsive, and frequent falls or stumbling.

Get help if you can't stop taking a pain reliever or tranquilizer. There's no shame in asking for assistance from family members, friends, or your doctor.

■ FOR MORE ON AVOIDING CHRONIC PAIN, SEE PAGE 333.

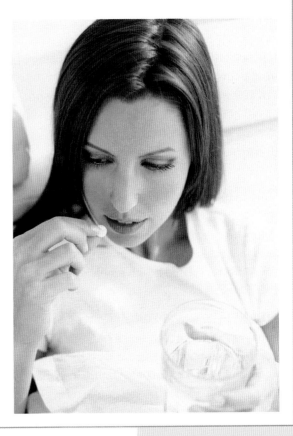

I watch a lot of television.

DAMAGE DONE

The more TV you watch, the higher your odds for being overweight and developing type 2 diabetes. In one study of over 9,000 women and men, normal-weight people watched about 2.3 hours of TV a day, while overweight people watched 2.6 hours and the obese watched 3 hours or more. The connection? More screen time means less activity and increased eating.

In the same study, people who watched more than 2 hours of TV a day ate 150 more calories per day, downing more pizza, more sugary soft drinks, and more high-fat, high-calorie, low-fiber processed snack foods than those who watched less TV. Small wonder, then, that a Harvard School of Public Health study of 37,000 men found that those who watched lots of TV—40 hours or more a week—were three times more likely to develop diabetes as those who watched less than 10 hours a week. Watching 21 to 40 hours doubled the risk.

If you watch TV instead of keeping up with an old hobby, visiting friends, or stretching your mind, you may also hasten memory loss, research shows.

Can I Undo It? Completely.

By turning TV time into active time, and by committing to a healthy TV/activity balance, you can burn more calories, become more fit, and reduce your odds for related health problems quickly.

+ BENEFITS

You'll have a fitter body and more time for sleep plus more energy, better mood, sharper mind, and more social connection, which may even help you gain more self-confidence.

Repair Plan

Follow the 2/30 rule. Experts suggest watching no more than two hours of TV a day—and doing at least 30 minutes of exercise every day.

Set a no-repeat rule. That is, never watch something you've watched before. If you find yourself watching that same ol' cop show or prison movie late at night, instantly turn it off!

Set a "no channel surfing" rule. Turn on the TV only when there is something you truly want to watch. If you are turning on the TV without any particular show in mind, take that as a sign that you need to be more active.

No snacking in front of the TV. It's far too easy to eat hundreds of calories' worth of chips and barely realize it. In fact, many weight-loss programs smartly advise you to never allow food to go beyond your kitchen table. That also means no snacking in bed, and no candy bars while paying the bills.

Exercise while you watch. Walk in place, do sit-ups, or try the Easy Does It! strengthening and stretching program, beginning on page 200, while your show is on. Or, drag your treadmill into the TV room and move while you watch your favorite show.

Clean during commercials. Empty wastebaskets, vacuum a room, put in a load of wash ... it can add up to 20 minutes' worth of calorie-burning chore time every hour. When you're finished, your home will shine—and you will have saved hundreds of calories by moving instead of snacking. Added bonus: You won't have to watch all the food commercials designed to make you want to overeat.

Resolve to leave home more often. See more friends, do more interesting things, and stimulate your mind every day.

■ FOR MORE ON GETTING FIT THE EASY WAY, SEE PAGE 172.

I snack all the time, whether or not I'm hungry.

DAMAGE DONE

Losing touch with your body's natural hunger and satisfaction signals can lead to chronic overeating—and unhealthy extra pounds that can lead to diabetes, heart disease, and other serious conditions. When Swedish researchers compared the eating habits and weight of 4,359 people, they found a consistent pattern: Overweight people ate more snacks than normal-weight people. And if you snack on junk foods, you're also flooding your body with trans fats and saturated fats, excess sodium, and sugars and refined carbohydrates.

Can I Undo It? Yes.

With determination, anyone can fix bad eating habits, and anyone can get to a healthier, more natural weight. By acknowledging the psychological issues behind your snacking habits, you'll find that there are other choices besides eating that provide what you need. And by paying attention to your hunger signals and switching to healthy snacks, you can boost nutrition, control cravings, lose weight, and avoid energy slumps.

+ BENEFITS

Your weight will fall to a healthier level. You'll replace unhealthy trans fats, saturated fat, sugar, refined carbohydrates, and extra sodium with nutritious, high-fiber fare.

Repair Plan

Reacquaint yourself with hunger. If you've lost touch with feelings of hunger and of satisfaction, try postponing eating until your stomach is truly hungry and your body is craving fuel. You might be surprised at how long the wait is!

Before you eat, rate your hunger on a 1-to-10 scale. On the hunger scale, 1 is "starving, feeling light-headed"; 5 is "comfortable"; and 10 as "so full I feel sick." Your goal: Eat only when you reach a 3.

Stop eating well before you're stuffed. Finish when you reach a 6 on the hunger scale—just a little bit full. You'll eat less—and be truly hungry again in time for your next meal or snack.

Satisfy emotional hunger the right way. So much of snacking is related to stress, boredom, even sadness or depression. If you need a psychological boost, don't turn to chocolate. Treat yourself to relaxation or fun: Take a walk, call a friend, or make plans to socialize. Express anger, frustration, sadness, and other emotions to a confidant, a journal, or the person who's triggering your feelings.

Put a stop to mindless eating. If snacking is simply a long-held bad habit that helps you get through the day's routine, it's time to ban chips, ice cream, pretzels, and all other snack food from every room except the kitchen or lunchroom. If you can't take a break, and chewing and drinking are comforting to you, turn to sugarless gum and tea or ice-cold water to satisfy your needs.

Replace junk food with real food. Throw away chips, crackers, cookies, and candy. Instead, stock fruits, veggies, whole-grain crackers, nuts, and low-fat or fat-free dairy products. Make your snacks beneficial to your health.

Plan snacks like real meals. Try healthy, high-fiber fruits and fresh vegetables such as baby carrots or cherry tomatoes, and for a more substantial snack, perhaps some whole-grain crackers with a dab of peanut butter. Put your snack on a plate, pour a glass of water or a cup of tea, and sit at the table to enjoy it.

■ FOR MORE ON HEALTHY EATING HABITS, SEE PAGE 108.

DAMAGE DONE

Alcohol can be a tonic—or toxic. If you've enjoyed a glass of wine with dinner throughout the years or the occasional cocktail at a party or beer after work with friends, you're a moderate drinker. For you, alcohol delivers benefits: In more than 100 studies, moderate drinkers enjoyed a 25 to 40 percent reduction in heart attacks, ischemic (clot-caused) strokes, peripheral vascular disease, sudden cardiac death, and death from all cardiovascular causes. Why? Alcohol in moderate amounts raises levels of "good" HDL cholesterol and discourages the formation of small blood clots that can lead to heart attacks and strokes. It may even help protect against type 2 diabetes and painful gallstones.

But if you drink to excess on a regular basis, alcohol can be a poison. Women who regularly consume two or more drinks a day and men who regularly down three or more are at higher risk for liver damage; pancreatitis (inflammation of the pancreas); various cancers including those of the liver, mouth, throat, larynx, and esophagus; high blood pressure; and depression. Women, who are more sensitive to alcohol's inebriating effects and its long-term health effects, may develop heart disease, brittle bones, and even memory loss. Just two drinks a day can, over time, raise your odds for breast cancer. In a study from the Fred Hutchinson Cancer Research Center in Seattle, women who followed a two-drink-a-day routine for 20 years and were still drinking had a three times higher risk for hormonally sensitive breast cancers than nondrinkers.

Several studies have found a higher risk of prostate cancer among men who consume a lot of alcohol or who have been longtime drinkers.

Too much alcohol can pack your liver with fat—and can lead to a reversible liver problem called alcoholic hepatitis or to irreversible scarring called cirrhosis.

The list continues: If you've been drinking to excess for years, you may need screening and treatment for thinning bones or an enlarged heart. Alcohol can also age your brain, making memory and thinking problems worse.

Can I Undo It? For the most part.

Soon after you cut back or quit, your digestion will improve; your stomach won't have to cope with the irritation caused by the alcohol and the excess stomach acids it triggers. You'll sleep more soundly. Your blood sugar will be lower and steadier. Your blood pressure may fall toward a healthier range. Even your brain will bounce back if you cut back or stop drinking. In a study from the University of California, San Francisco, researchers found that alcoholics who stayed sober for nearly seven years performed as well as nonalcoholics on brain function tests. Even if you have liver damage, cutting back on alcohol and eating a healthier diet could help your liver regenerate itself to some degree.

+ BENEFITS

Without a doubt, you'll have a healthier liver and cardiovascular system. Since you are limiting your alcohol intake, you will have a far-reduced risk of automobile accidents. You'll also feel more energetic and probably have better relationships with your family and friends if drinking has caused problems in the past.

Repair Plan

Stick with healthy limits. That's two or less alcoholic drinks per day for men, one for women. Health dangers begin to rise for people who drink more than that.

Reserve alcohol for meals. You're more likely to slowly sip a beer or a nice glass of wine if you're enjoying it along with a good meal. At parties or before you eat, stick with iced tea, water, or sparkling water with a splash of lemon or lime.

Drink for flavor, not to get drunk. For a teenager, feeling drunk might seem novel and cool. As a mature adult, there is no sound reason ever to get drunk. If you discover that you are drinking for the effects of the alcohol—be they to escape a bad day, give you courage in new situations, or merely to be "one of the gang"—stop immediately. Work hard to find a healthier coping mechanism.

If you can't stop, acknowledge the addiction. If you can't stick with a healthy drink limit, if you drink secretly, or if you need more alcohol to get the same "drunken" effect, it's time to get help. You may have an alcohol-use disorder. Talk with your doctor and contact a support group such as Alcoholics Anonymous for the support you'll need to make a healthy change.

Take health screenings for bone density and cancers seriously. Drinkers should talk with their doctors about whether they need more frequent screenings for cancers of the mouth, throat, esophagus, liver, breast, and colon.

Liver damage? Get a liver-health plan. Your doctor should discuss a high-calorie diet to help your liver regenerate. You may also need medications for related health problems including high blood pressure, bleeding blood vessels, fluid retention, and itching.

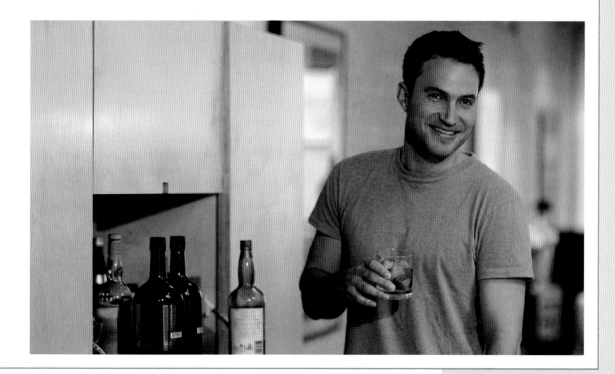

I have spent myself deeply into debt.

DAMAGE DONE

Money worries can have serious health consequences. In a Rutgers University telephone survey of 3,121 women and men, half admitted to having stress about money, 23 percent said their anxiety was severe, and 12 percent called it overwhelming. The damage? Survey-takers said financial stress contributed to high blood pressure, depression, insomnia, headaches, digestion troubles, aches and pains, ulcers, excessive smoking and drinking, and gaining or losing weight.

In an Ohio State University study of 1,036 people, those with a higher proportion of their income tied up in credit card debt also had more health problems than those living with a lower debt-to-income ratio. "Any one of us who has debt knows that it can cause stress in our lives, and it makes sense that this stress may be bad for our health," notes lead researcher Paul J. Lavrakas, PhD.

Can I Undo It? Yes.

But let's be honest: It's not easy. Getting yourself out of debt is analogous to losing large amounts of weight: It takes time, the process can be hard on your ego and your lifestyle, you must be constantly vigilant, and it is easy to revert back to old habits. But for those who succeed—and many people do—the results are stunning.

+ BENEFITS

You are going to feel more in control of your life with less stress and fewer worries. You'll be able to sleep better, stop overeating, and have fewer headaches. Finding ways to curb your spending and focus on the simple joys in life will help improve your relationships.

Repair Plan

Learn about money management. You can't master your money if you don't understand the rules and methods of personal finance. Find a book, magazine, or Web site that speaks to your level of understanding and learn all you can about credit cards, mortgages, electronic banking, budgeting, and investing.

Put your credit cards on ice. Literally. Put them in a cup, add water, and place it in the back of the freezer so you can't use them. It's just one clever way to get you to immediately stop increasing your debt.

Create a budget. How much money is coming in each month? How much are you spending on essentials, and how much are you spending on frivolous purchases and entertainment? An hour of honest assessment of your spending habits can go a long way toward showing you a better path.

Pay at least the minimum amount due each month on all your bills. And pay more than the minimum payment on your highest-interest credit card. After you've paid off your highest-interest card, move to the next.

Automate good money habits. Today you can have paychecks deposited directly into your accounts, small amounts automatically diverted to savings accounts, and bills paid automatically from your accounts. The more you can use technology to improve your money management, the better.

Change money priorities. Banish shopping as a form of entertainment. Instead, go for a walk, take up a hobby, meet with friends, or try a craft project. Identify the things you want to spend on in the future—vacations, a retirement home, a new car—and start savings programs for each.

I'm a workaholic.

DAMAGE DONE

Nonstop thinking about your job. Never-ending work e-mails and phone calls, at all times of the day and night. Repeatedly prioritizing work over family, friends, and personal pleasures. Workaholics are people who are out of balance with life. And that imbalance is unhealthy—workaholics are at risk for stress-related high blood pressure, heart disease, overweight, and type 2 diabetes.

A workaholic's biggest health threats: Stress and self-neglect. In one British study of small business owners, those who worked the longest hours were the most likely to cancel doctors' appointments or to wait and "store up" illnesses so that they wouldn't have to take as much time off to see the doctor. And thanks to fatigue and overscheduling, one in five never exercised. If you feel chained to your desk, you're probably not eating well, either.

You're also missing out on the joys of life—and the experiences and relationships that can sustain your health and happiness in the years ahead. In one study of 1,000 women, researchers found that those who were married to worka-holic men were more likely to divorce and had fewer happy feelings about their relationship.

Can I Undo It? Yes.

It takes just one thing: convincing yourself to do it. Half the battle is in your mind. As with any habit or addiction, once you truly commit to pull back and regain the balance you once had, changing is a simple, step-by-step process, with measurable benchmarks and outcomes.

+ BENEFITS

You'll enjoy the novel concept of having time for yourself, your family, and your friends. You'll get better, more-restful sleep and have less stress. You will likely lose weight and have a healthier heart. It's all about balance.

Repair Plan

Set a quitting time—and stick to it. That means telling all the people you work with that between certain hours, you are not going to be available, and enforcing that by not answering the phone or responding to e-mails.

Make healthy eating and exercise a priority. Put them on your calendar and keep these "health appointments" with yourself as religiously as if they were meetings with an important client.

Fill your free time in ways you enjoy. If you cut back on work only to sit in front of the television, you will go back to working. Instead, commit to social activities, family time, cooking, or a home project. Fill your time in a way that's more fun than work, and you will help end your work addiction.

De-stress before, during, and after work. A few minutes of stretching, deep breathing, or yoga helps release tension and keep priorities straight. Tend to your mental health a little better, and you'll quickly see the world in a new way.

Turn off the electronics. The combination of wire-less communications technology and worldwide corporations mean that you can instantly plug into work at any time, at any place. Fight this urge! When you are not working, turn off your cell phone, your laptop, your blackberry device, and any other electronics that link you to your work world.

■ FOR MORE ON A HEALTHY, HAPPY LIFESTYLE, SEE PAGE 236.

I drink a lot of coffee or caffeinated beverages.

DAMAGE DONE

Minimal. For most of us, years of coffee drinking will have no ill-effects—in fact, surprising research suggests that coffee-drinkers have a 30 to 60 percent lower risk for type 2 diabetes. But if you're extra-sensitive to caffeine, drink several cups per day of supercharged espresso or cappuccino, or have cut nutritional corners elsewhere in your diet, a highly caffeinated lifestyle could pose some health problems. Downing more than four cups of regular coffee (or as few as two espressos or other high-caffeine javas) can cause anxiety, insomnia, and nervousness. Experts say that once your body is used to caffeine, it probably doesn't affect blood pressure. But some research suggests that in the short term, the amount of caffeine in two to three cups of coffee can raise systolic blood pressure (the top number) by 3 to 14 points and diastolic blood pressure (the bottom number) by 4 to 13 points.

Can I Undo It? Yes.

Since caffeine's effects are relatively short-lived, cutting back will lessen them in a day or two.

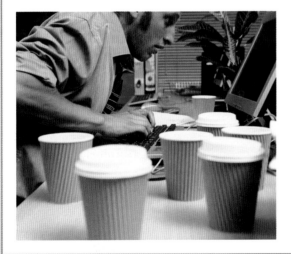

+ BENEFITS

You'll feel calmer, sleep better, and know you're protecting your bones from fracture risks.

Repair Plan

Skip caffeinated coffees, teas, and soft drinks after noon. If you drink caffeinated drinks for their energizing effects, drink them in the morning and leave it at that. Caffeine lingers in your system for three to seven hours. A cup after lunch could create sleep problems at bedtime.

Avoid caffeinated drinks for a few days before your next blood pressure check. If your numbers drop after cutting caffeine, consider switching permanently to decaffeinated versions of your favorite drinks.

Get plenty of calcium. If you love coffee but hate dairy products, baby your bones by taking enough calcium supplements to get 1,200 milligrams of calcium a day. Also schedule a bone-density test. Studies show that coffee-loving women who also got less than 740 milligrams of calcium a day (the amount in two glasses of skim milk and a half-slice of American cheese) lost bone density faster than women who drank less coffee—or got more calcium. If that's you, make up for lost time by increasing your calcium intake and getting a bone-density scan to see if you need help bolstering your bones.

Switch to decaf slowly. If caffeine is jangling your nerves, but you love the taste, buy a bag of decaffeinated coffee and one of your favorite caffeinated blends. Mix a little decaf into your morning brew. Over the course of a month, add more and more decaf and less and less caffeinated. Your taste buds will adjust, and you'll feel less anxious without all that caffeine.

I eat ice cream, cake, or doughnuts every day.

DAMAGE DONE

A lot. In the early 1800s, we ate about 15 pounds of sugar per year. But by the turn of the 21st century, sugar consumption for people with modern diets reached nearly 160 pounds per year—with serious consequences for health and weight. A steady diet of sugar, fat, and refined carbohydrates means that you're eating far more empty calories than you should, yet getting less of the high-fiber, high-nutrition foods like fruit, vegetables, and whole grains that your body needs. It also puts your blood sugar on a roller coaster, swinging between dizzying highs and energy-draining lows—and leaving you with intense cravings for even more sugar.

The combination of high calories, low fiber, and a dearth of vitamins, minerals, and protective antioxidants work together to raise your odds for heart disease, stroke, a prediabetic condition called insulin resistance, Alzheimer's disease, some cancers, and even sexual problems. In one Dutch study of 16,000 women, those who ate the most sweets and refined carbohydrates had an 80 percent higher risk for heart disease than those who ate the least.

Can I Undo It? Yes.

Saying "no thank you" to cakes, cookies, doughnuts, and candy can reduce sugar cravings and improve energy levels in a matter of days.

+ BENEFITS

Better moods—no more irritability caused by blood sugar fluctuations. You'll manage to attain a healthier weight and lower risk for heart disease, diabetes, and other blood sugar–related problems.

Repair Plan

Make healthy substitutions. Rather than swearing off sweet treats, start by choosing some healthy alternatives. Fruit is a terrific choice, particularly watermelon, peaches, and berries. All are sweet and satisfying. Instead of ice cream, have no-fat frozen yogurt or fruit ices. Instead of cake, have a cookie and fruit.

Splurge weekly, rather than daily. Allow yourself a moderately sinful dessert once a week. That way, you don't have to feel deprived.

Ask yourself why you're treating yourself so often. So much of snacking is out of habit, boredom, or stress. The best rule of all is to find healthier ways to fulfill emotional needs than through food. Take a walk, call a friend, do a stretch, read a joke. Limit your food intake to satisfying hunger.

Start a new after-meal routine. Go for a walk instead of having dessert. Or, if you still want a family dessert ritual, schedule it for 60 minutes after the main meal, when the kitchen has been cleaned up and everyone has done something active. Then choose something healthy, like watermelon or cantaloupe slices.

Make your kitchen a sugar-free safety zone. Don't keep treats, or even sweet baking ingredients, such as chocolate chips, in the house. Instead, go out for an occasional dessert.

Don't rely heavily on artificial sweeteners. It's far better to retrain your taste buds to appreciate the natural sweetness of fruit than to maintain your unnatural craving for refined sugar.

■ FOR MORE ON HEALTHY CARBOHYDRATES, SEE PAGE 108.

I usually skip breakfast.

DAMAGE DONE

More than you realize. Missing breakfast can have serious consequences for your weight, your energy levels, and even your blood sugar.

Breakfast-skippers tend to weigh more than people who eat breakfast, studies show. Skipping the first meal of the day leaves your metabolism in "sleep mode"—a thrifty state intended by Nature to get your body through the 12 hours or more between dinner and the break of day. Munching a piece of morning toast or crunching a bowl of bran flakes signals to your metabolism that it's time to kick things up a notch by burning more calories. Skipping the fuel keeps your metabolism on low, which can lead to weight gain and feeling sluggish.

You've also created a starve-now-indulge-later eating pattern. Breakfast-skippers tend to overeat later in the day.

Breakfast-avoiders may also be at higher risk for diabetes—perhaps because they tend to eat fewer whole grains, produce, and dairy products.

Can I Undo It? Yes.

Starting a breakfast routine is easy. And the moment you do, you take a major step toward fixing the problems it has caused, including excess weight and unhealthy blood sugar swings.

+ BENEFITS

Eating breakfast will result in more stable blood sugar. This means fewer food cravings and hunger pangs later in the day. Because you are re-fueling your body early on in the day, you'll have more energy in the morning, and you may find that you start to control your weight easier, too.

Repair Plan

Work with your body. Not hungry first thing in the day? Wait an hour or two and then have a piece of toast with peanut butter, a bowl of cereal, or some fruit, a hard-boiled egg, and a glass of milk.

Eat foods you like. Breakfast foods are a marketer's creation, nothing more. There's no rule that says you have to start the day with them. Have a sandwich, a bowl of soup, or last night's leftovers, if that is your pleasure.

No time? Make a portable breakfast sandwich. One great combination is peanut butter and banana on whole-wheat. Any kind of protein between two pieces of bread would work. Bring along a piece of fruit and you're set. If you like milk, add a cup of skim milk, poured into a take-along coffee mug with a lid.

Grab an energy bar and cup of yogurt. Together they are the perfect amount of nutrients and calories to start your day. And both are instantly ready for eating.

Have a smoothie. For the ultimate on-the-go breakfast, whirl low-fat yogurt, frozen berries, half a banana, a little orange juice, and some honey in a blender. (For more volume, add ice cubes before blending). It tastes like ice cream, but is packed with fiber, calcium, protein, and antioxidants.

Set things up in advance. Get breakfast ready the night before, so that you can eat it at the kitchen table in 10 minutes or less. Pour cereal into bowls, set out silverware and cups, set up the coffeepot, and wash, chop, and refrigerate fruit.

I lose and then gain back the same 10 to 20 pounds, over and over.

DAMAGE DONE

More than you think. Experts say this common dieting phenomenon (also known as yo-yo dieting or weight cycling), can alter your body composition in frustrating and even dangerous ways. Repeated weight gain and loss lowers the amount of muscle mass you have. This raises your body-fat percentage, lowers your body's ongoing calorie burn, and reduces your body's ability to regulate blood sugar. All this is a set-up for more weight gain and related health problems.

Muscle mass declines naturally with age; moving into your later years with a deficit due to weight cycling can leave you even weaker and more prone to balance problems. And if the extra body fat you've gained has settled around your midsection, you'll be at higher risk for heart disease and diabetes. Meanwhile, other researchers have found that yo-yo dieters have lower levels of "good" HDL cholesterol.

If you've followed fad weight-loss plans—from the grapefruit diet to the low-carb craze to the low-fat craze—you may also have skimped on important nutrients like calcium or protein or the cornucopia of vitamins and antioxidants in fruit, veggies, and whole grains.

Can I Undo It? Yes.

Switching to a consistently healthy diet will end the yo-yo weight effect, and adding strength-training to your routine will rebuild muscle mass and get your metabolism back to where it belongs. All this can be achieved within a few months.

+ BENEFITS

The obvious benefit is a sleeker, stronger, more-energetic body—thanks to strength training. Exercising will also improve your balance and prevent falls. Better nutrition will aid in lowering your risk for heart disease, diabetes, and dying prematurely.

Repair Plan

Give up fad diets! It's time to convince yourself once and for all that formal diets don't work. Science shows over and over that short-term regimens or gimmicks to lose pounds fast aren't healthy or sustainable. Eat healthy foods in healthy portions, and you'll naturally get to a stable, appropriate weight for your body. Talk with your doctor about what's right for your age and body type.

Give up your feast-or-famine eating style. Instead, plan to have three normal-size meals a day, and three small snacks, too. Never allow yourself to get very hungry.

Focus on portion control. Most fad diets are built on demonizing certain foods or overstating the importance of others. But at the end of the day, only one thing matters for weight—whether you are eating too many calories. So rather than focusing on *what's* on your plate, learn first to focus on *how much* is on your plate. Portion control is the best method of all for losing weight. Learn to eat a little less at your meals, and the pounds will slowly but permanently disappear.

Rebuild lost muscle mass. Muscle is crucial to long-life living, and if yo-yo dieting has weakened you, you have an obligation to yourself to regain strength. To start, try our fitness plans in our "Move to Feel Good" chapter. Do something to challenge your muscles each and every day.

I drink a lot of soda or other sweetened drinks.

DAMAGE DONE

Surprise! Our panel of doctors rated this as the worst daily food habit of all. But they're right: Sipping lots of sugary sodas as well as fruit drinks, sweetened iced teas, and other soft drinks is a setup for weight gain, diabetes, brittle bones, and more.

When Harvard School of Public Health researchers looked at the diets and health of tens of thousands of women, they found that those who drank at least one sweetened soft drink a day had twice the risk for type 2 diabetes as women who downed soft drinks less than once a month. The culprit? Extra calories … and all that sugar. Downing a few hundred excess liquid calories a day seems to be responsible for a hefty weight gain: Women who drank soft drinks put on more than 10 pounds in just four years. On contrast, women who quenched their thirst with water, milk, and unsweetened (or diet) drinks gained far less weight, the study found. In a study from Finland, people who drank the most sugary beverages had a 68 percent higher risk for type 2 diabetes.

Think of soft drinks as liquid candy—a sneaky source of calories that does little to fill you up, but is certain to fill you out. In a Purdue University study, researchers found that when volunteers drank roughly three cans of soda a day—totaling 450 in calories—it didn't have any impact on how much they ate at meals. In contrast, when they munched jelly beans, they automatically ate less throughout the day.

Soft drinks can also weaken your bones—most likely because the more sweet sips you take, the less likely you are to also be drinking bone-protecting, calcium-rich milk. In one Tufts University study, women who had more than three cola drinks a day had 4 percent lower bone mineral density at the hip. Experts suspect that phosphoric acid in colas interferes with natural bone-building in the body, even if you're getting plenty of calcium.

Can I Undo It? Yes.

You can fix the damage, and you can kick the soft drink habit. But it's harder than you might think. We have programmed our taste buds to crave sweetness, and so weaning ourselves off sugar can be difficult. Like any habit, it takes persistence to truly break it forever.

+ BENEFITS

Cutting back on soda will result in lower, steadier blood sugar levels, which means a lower risk for diabetes, heart disease, and stroke. Eliminating the 150 calories for each soda from your diet will help you lose weight or maintain your weight. And since soda can etch the surface of teeth, you'll have stronger tooth enamel for better dental health.

Repair Plan

Quench thirst with water. Treat soda and sweetened fruit drinks strictly as snacks. For thirst, drink water.

Carry water with you. Start the day with a large bottle of cold water, and constantly replenish it as the day goes by. You'll find that it is a very effective way to cut back on sugary drinks.

Think through your daily beverage intake. After water, daily drinks that are good for your health include coffee, tea, milk, natural unsweetened fruit juices, and even wine. Spread those out through the day, and you diminish the need for sodas.

Discover the art of iced tea. Brew your own fruity, herbal iced tea the easy way—drop four tea bags in a quart of filtered water, refrigerate overnight. Give it extra zing with a spritz of lemon juice and enjoy as much as you wish as a replacement for water.

Bypass diet versions of sodas and sweetened juices. Diet sodas are one way to wean yourself off of a soda habit, but they should be a temporary solution, not a permanent one. There's new evidence that having more than one a day raises your risk for metabolic syndrome, a prediabetic condition that also threatens your heart.

Sweeten your milk. Indulge in a cup of cocoa every day: Add a tablespoon of pure cocoa and a teaspoon of sugar to a cup of skim milk, heat and enjoy. One teaspoon of sugar is a fraction of the sugar in most sodas.

Make a rule: Just water at restaurants. Save calories—and money—by skipping sodas at restaurants. This is particularly true at fast-food restaurants: get a bottle of water, not soda, with your combo meal.

Particularly avoid caffeinated cola. Colas containing caffeine were associated with lower bone mineral density than decaf versions in one study. One alternative: Home-brewed iced tea, made with black tea for a little caffeinated pick-me-up.

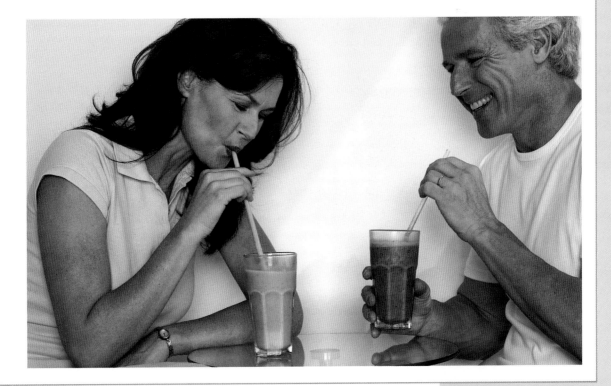

I rarely drink water.

DAMAGE DONE

If you barely drink any water, you may be living on the verge of dehydration—or flooding your body with hundreds of extra calories a day if you instead are drinking mostly juices and soft drinks.

Even mild dehydration can make you feel tired. It can also lead to constipation. Over time, dehydration can raise your risk for a heart attack simply because your blood may be slightly thicker and more likely to clot. If you're taking a diuretic to control your blood pressure, or you take laxatives, you may need to drink extra water to maintain a healthy fluid balance in your body. Dehydration can happen faster with age, because your body already contains about 10 percent less water than it did when you were younger—so there's less of a safety margin.

Can I Undo It? Yes, immediately.

Developing a water-drinking habit is easy, and it will quickly improve your health and energy levels.

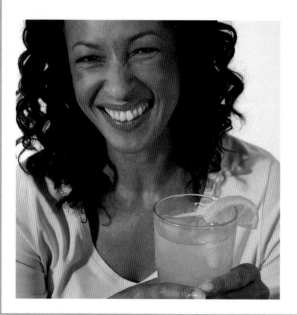

+ BENEFITS

Hydrating your body gives you more energy, plus, you'll have a lower incidence of confusion and dizziness, with less risk of falling. Simple water will aid in digestion and lead to a lower risk of heart disease.

Repair Plan

Aim for five to six glasses of pure water, herbal tea, and juice per day. Sparkling water or club soda with a splash of juice or a spritz of lemon counts, too. Experts no longer believe that everyone needs eight glasses per day.

Eat juicy fruit. Enjoy watermelon, oranges, peaches, berries ... the juicier, the better.

Check your urine every time you relieve yourself. If it's pale and has almost no odor, you're probably getting plenty of fluids. If it's dark, strong-smelling, or you simply don't urinate very much or very often, you probably need to drink more water.

Always have a glass of water first thing in the morning, and with each meal and snack. Don't wait until you feel thirsty to have a drink—sense of thirst grows fainter after age 60, but your need for fluids remains the same or increases.

Drink when you're active. Have a glass of water before you exercise, every 20 minutes while you exercise, and again when you're finished.

Treat yourself to a fruit Popsicle on a hot day. You need an extra glass of water on a hot day, and the fluid in a fruit pop will fill the bill.

Stay alert to signs of mild dehydration. These include sudden thirst, fatigue, a headache, dry mouth, muscle weakness, dizziness, and light-headedness. At the first symptom, start drinking water.

I rarely eat vegetables.

DAMAGE DONE

Significant. If you routinely shun salads, pass up the peas, and banish broccoli from your plate, you've denied your body fiber, folic acid, and antioxidants that help guard against heart disease, diabetes, cancer, memory loss, and stroke. Chances are good that you've filled your plate with extra potatoes, bread, or rice and, as a result, may have put on extra pounds and elevated your risk for a prediabetic condition called insulin resistance, too.

Can I Undo It? Absolutely.

Finding veggies you like—or new ways to prepare and serve the ones you've been avoiding—can lower your blood pressure, decrease levels of "bad" LDL cholesterol, smooth out your blood sugar, improve your digestion, and perhaps even lower your risk for lung cancer. Several well-designed studies show benefits in as little as four weeks. Every serving of veggies you add to your day cuts your heart disease risk by 4 percent (or more) and your stroke risk by 3 to 5 percent.

+ BENEFITS

The benefits of adding vegetables to your diet are immeasurable, but some of the biggest ones include: better digestion. stronger bones, and a lower risk for heart attack, high blood pressure, stroke, and some cancers. But that's not all: You may end up with fewer wrinkles!

Repair Plan

Start with "nibble" vegetables. The easiest way to reintroduce yourself to vegetables is to munch on pleasant, crunchy raw choices like cucumbers, carrots, celery, and tomatoes. Getting into that habit will make it easier to move on to cooked vegetables.

Have a salad at every lunch and dinner. It's hard not to like crunchy lettuces with a tasty dressing. Start each meal with a salad, and you'll not only greatly increase your vegetable intake but also lower your appetite for the rest of the meal.

Put more vegetables into your stews, soups, and casseroles. There is no reason that your world-famous chili can't be bolstered with diced carrots, celery, peppers, onions, and even green beans.

Add a little fat. Ready to start preparing veggie side dishes? A dab of olive oil, a teaspoon of margarine, or a sprinkle of Parmesan brightens the flavor of cooked broccoli, spinach, green beans, squash, and other veggies. Fat boosts absorption of nutrients, too.

Sip your veggies. Low-sodium tomato juice or vegetable juice counts as a vegetable serving.

Double the lettuce and tomato on your sandwich. And use a dark green lettuce, such as romaine, or switch to baby spinach for an extra-nutritious punch.

Buy pre-sliced. No time to chop? Pre-cut carrots, broccoli, cauliflower, green beans, and more are waiting for you in the produce section of your supermarket. So is shredded cabbage. Take advantage—let someone else be your sous chef! Just microwave, steam, or sauté.

■ FOR MORE ON GETTING MORE PRODUCE INTO YOUR DIET, SEE PAGE 110.

I get many of my meals at fast-food restaurants.

DAMAGE DONE

Significant. A steady diet of double cheeseburgers and fries washed down with an oversize soda or milkshake often leads to a bigger waistline and other related health problems. When University of Minnesota researchers tracked 3,031 women and men for 15 years, they found that those who ate fast food twice a week compared to less than once a week gained 10 extra pounds and were twice as likely to have a prediabetic condition called insulin resistance.

What no one could see: Thanks to the type of fats used until recently in French fries and deep-fried offerings at fast food restaurants, frequent diners may also have raised their heart attack risk by 25 to 100 percent. Trans fats raise "bad" LDL cholesterol, lower "good" HDLs, raise blood fats called triglycerides that contribute to hardening of the arteries, and fire up inflammation—an immune-system response that's involved in the build-up of fatty plaque in artery walls. There's also evidence that a steady fast-food diet packs more fat around your abdomen, raising your odds for heart disease and diabetes still higher. Eating fried chicken pieces and French fries on a regular basis could double your heart risk.

Can I Undo It? Yes, with commitment. It will take permanent lifestyle changes that won't be easy at first. Fast food is super-convenient, surprisingly inexpensive, and thanks to all its fat, salt, and sugar, undeniably tasty. Healthy eating takes more time and thought, and in some cases, more money. But the health benefits of making the switch will be immediate and substantial.

+ BENEFITS

In addition to losing extra weight, slimming your waistline, and protecting yourself from heart disease and diabetes, you'll save several dollars a day if you make your own meal instead of buying fast food.

Repair Plan

Wean yourself off slowly. Most people cannot end a habit cold turkey, and that holds true for fast-food consumption. Cut back a little per week, and each time you go, buy a little less than you used to and start ordering the healthier choices like fruit slices or yogurt parfaits.

Start off by cutting out the soda. As discussed earlier, soda consumption really hurts your health. And fast-food restaurants love to serve up monster-size cups of soda. Switch to milk, coffee, or bottled water to save hundreds of unneeded calories.

Switch from burgers to chicken. In particular, switch to grilled chicken. These sandwiches are usually one of the healthiest choices on a fast-food menu. Get dressing on the side and use just a tiny bit.

Switch from fries to salad. Those fries are cooked in pure fat, and are covered in salt. Fast-food salads may not have the crunch of a French fry, but they are more satisfying than you might realize, and they are considerably more healthy.

End the impulse visits. The worst health sin is to spot a drive-thru window, and impulsively turn in for a quickie hamburger, even if you aren't all that hungry or it's not mealtime. Put a firm halt to these kinds of mad meals and noshes.

Switch to grocery stores. On the road and need a fast meal? Go to a grocery store and get some fruit, a cup of yogurt, a prepared salad, and maybe a six-pack of sushi. Every major grocery chain has responded to the need for fast meals with lots of healthy choices. You likely can eat a greater volume of food and consume fewer calories.

Try local sandwich shops. Wherever you go, privately owned sandwich shops are there. Walk in, order a turkey on whole-wheat and a salad on the side, chat it up with the owner, and leave with a much healthier meal—and the good feeling of supporting an entrepreneur.

Make your own. You can eat with confidence in your own kitchen. How about leftover roast beef on a crusty roll, a handful of plump cherry tomatoes, crunchy carrots, and a fresh orange? Wash it down with unsweetened iced tea.

Get your health tested. Eating frequent fast-food restaurant meals is indicative of a generally unhealthy lifestyle. If you want to switch to the healthy side, get to a doctor soon for a full battery of health screenings. Finding out the damage that has been done can be strong motivation for ending your fast-food restaurant visits. Likely your doctor will test your cholesterol, triglyceride, and blood sugar levels, as well as other vitals.

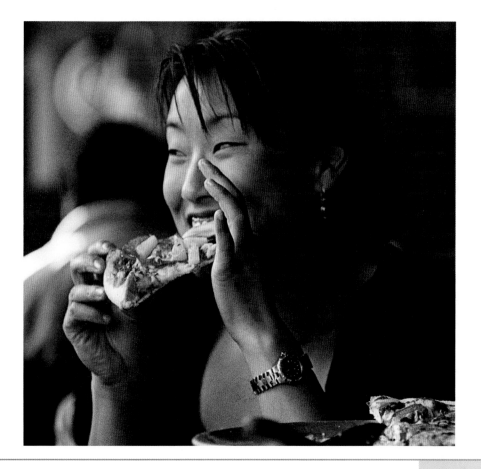

I have a nice piece of meat for dinner most days.

DAMAGE DONE

A tender steak or juicy pork chop is one of life's simple pleasures. But a growing stack of research links daily red meat consumption with a higher risk for cancers of the breast, colon, pancreas, and prostate—as well as greater odds for painful, inflammatory arthritis. Eating lots of meat may also raise heart disease risk, especially for people with diabetes.

In one study of 150,000 women and men, those who ate 2 to 3 ounces of red meat a day were 30 percent more likely to develop colon cancer than those who had less. Overall, when compared to vegetarians, meat-eaters have a 40 percent higher risk for a range of cancers. Why? It could be that meat simply lacks the fiber, antioxidants, and other nutrients found in fruits, vegetables, beans, and whole grains, putting meat-eaters at a nutritional disadvantage. But there appears to be more: The fat in meat boosts human hormone production, which could fuel some breast and prostate cancers. And experts also think that when meat is cooked at high temperatures—grilling, for example—compounds called heterocyclic amines (HCA) and polycyclic aromatic hydrocarbons (PAH) form that seem to raise cancer risk.

Then there is the portion issue. A "nice piece" of meat too often means a slab that is three to six times the size of what is considered a healthy serving. Meat inherently contains lots of fat, so lots of meat often means a high-calorie diet that could be adding pounds to your frame.

Can I Undo It? For the most part.

While you cannot reverse cell damage that may be caused by HCAs and PAHs, there's plenty you can do to lower your future risks. For example, eating fish and poultry (plus plenty of produce and whole grains) rather than red meat, potatoes, and refined grains could lower your heart disease risk by nearly 25 percent.

+ BENEFITS

You'll broaden your taste in food; save money if you buy beans instead of meats for some meals; and most important, cut your risk for cardiovascular disease and some cancers.

Repair Plan

Set a goal of eating three or fewer meat-centered dinners a week. Go with chicken, seafood, or vegetarian entrées the rest of the nights.

Skip processed meats like breakfast sausage and lunchmeats. Filled with salt, chemicals, preservatives, and fat, there's evidence that these may raise diabetes risk.

Automatically order fish when dining out. It's an easy way to get an extra serving of this super-healthy protein.

Use meat as an ingredient, not as an entrée. That means using meat in salads, stews, soups, or stir-fries, rather than serving up as a single hunk.

Grill smarter. To reduce creation of unhealthy PAH and HCA chemicals, use low-fat meats, trim fat, and use low-fat marinades to avoid flare-ups from fat drippings.

Stay current with colon cancer screenings. You need checks regularly after age 50. Talk with your doctor about which type of check is right for you.

■ FOR MORE ON EATING MORE LEAN PROTEIN, SEE PAGE 146.

I tend to ignore health problems and symptoms.

DAMAGE DONE

It's one thing to be neglectful of one's health when things are going fine. But to ignore symptoms and "let nature take its course" when health problems emerge is highly risky. Your immune system can battle back against minor infections well enough, but beyond that, nature taking "its course" often means you get worse, not better. Everyday symptoms like headaches, lethargy, dizziness, or chronic coughs can often be indicating the emergence of more serious diseases—including life-threatening heart attacks, strokes, and cancers.

Yet, people ignore symptoms all the time. In a recent survey of 1,100 men, 30 percent said they wait as long as possible before taking troubling symptoms of any kind to the doctor's office. The problem with waiting? You lose the opportunity to get small health problems treated before they become big health problems. Catching many cancers early boosts your chances for survival significantly. Reversing high blood pressure, high cholesterol, or high blood sugar as soon as possible lowers your odds for fatal heart attacks, strokes, and a wide range of scary, diabetes-related complications such as kidney failure, blindness, and amputation due to infections in feet and legs. Even ignoring a seemingly small problem like bleeding gums could raise your risk for serious gum infections, which contribute to diabetes and heart disease.

Can I Undo It? Possibly.

If you have your health, then you are lucky—no clear damage has come about as a result of your self-neglect. Still, get yourself to a doctor today! A full checkup and a new approach to health, in which you are highly mindful of your body's health signals, are in order.

+ BENEFITS

Early diagnosis of chronic problems is worth far more than you can imagine. So is losing the uncertainty related to your undiagnosed symptoms and health problems. These benefits far outweigh the financial and emotional costs of consulting a doctor.

Repair Plan

Change your attitude. So many men—and plenty of women too!—have an I-don't-need-a-doctor attitude, as if suffering in silence is a virtue and going to see a doctor a defeat. It's time to change that. Just as success in business almost always relies on a team, so does success in health. Your doctor is essential to your achieving long life and long health. Treat him or her as a welcome participant in your successful future.

See your doctor at least as often as your car sees the auto shop. That means at least once per year. Ask for an annual physical with a blood workup. Women should also see their gynecologists.

Don't forget your eyes and your teeth. Once a year is the minimum for seeing your eye doctor and your dentist, too.

Resolve to take aches and pains seriously. Pain specialists agree that early pain relief is best. Left alone, chronic pain can create hard-to-break feedback loops in your brain.

Set a two-week limit. Do you have an odd-looking mole? An abnormal bulge? Unusual bloating? Take any strange symptom to your doctor's office if it persists for more than two weeks.

I'm often in locations that have smoke in the air.

DAMAGE DONE

Considerable. Eight hours of exposure to other people's smoke—at work, at home, or out with friends—is as damaging to your cardiovascular system and lungs as smoking a pack of cigarettes a day. After just 30 minutes, secondhand smoke makes platelets in the bloodstream stickier and more prone to clotting. Every year, secondhand smoke causes an estimated 60,000 deaths from heart disease and 3,000 from lung cancer. If you grew up in a household with smokers, your own lung cancer risk is 3 to 11 times higher than normal. It also raises your risk for respiratory infections and even nasal sinus cancer—and could elevate your odds for cancers of the cervix, breast, and bladder.

The fallout for your cardiovascular system is even worse. When Harvard University researchers tracked the health of 32,046 non-smoking women for 10 years, they found that those who regularly breathed in other people's smoke at home or at work were 91 percent more likely to have heart attacks than those who weren't exposed. Clearly, secondhand smoke kills.

Can I Undo It? Absolutely.

The proof: When the town of Helena, Montana, banned smoking in public places in 2002, heart attack rates among residents fell 58 percent in just six months. Just as with a smoker's, your body will begin purging the poisons and returning to a healthier state within hours after you stop breathing in smoke.

+ BENEFITS

Removing yourself from smoke-filled environments results in reduced risk for heart attack. Earlier detection of COPD will help ensure that you can receive treatments to stop lung damage. The same is true for lung cancer: Catching it early will increase your odds for successful treatment. Bonus: You'll feel better, your clothing and hair won't smell like smoke, and your eyes won't burn from smoke exposure.

Repair Plan

Insist that the smokers in your life step outside. There are only two ways to deal with smoke in the air: Get rid of the cause of smoke or remove yourself from the location. Today, most cultures call for smokers to accommodate nonsmokers, and not the other way around. So don't feel awkward asking the smokers among you to take it outside.

Patronize smoke-free restaurants and bars. The onus isn't just on smokers to accommodate you, though; you should also choose social places where smokers don't congregate. An increasing number of restaurants are either entirely smoke-free or segregate smokers.

Get tests if you have been extensively exposed to secondhand smoke. If there were smokers in your household when you were young, or if at any time in your life you were heavily exposed to daily smoke, talk with your doctor about screenings for lung cancer and for a breathing problem called chronic obstructive pulmonary disease (COPD). Your doctor might use computed tomography (CT) equipment to get a detailed picture of the interior of your lungs, or check your lung function to see how much air you're breathing in and out—and how much oxygen you're absorbing.

■ FOR MORE ON IMPROVED BREATHING, SEE PAGE 366.

I get sunburned a few times each summer.

DAMAGE DONE

Unquestionably some, potentially a lot. If you love sunbathing or make an effort to maintain a golden-bronze tan, you've unwittingly contributed to the aging of your skin. Sunbathing destroys the elastic fibers that keep skin looking firm and smooth. That leads to earlier wrinkles, blotches, freckles, and discolorations. More important, sunburns contribute significantly to cancers of the skin.

If you've augmented sun-kissed color with trips to the tanning salon, beware: Using tanning beds doesn't, as advertisements suggest, build up a "safe" base tan—it *raises* your risk for skin cancer and wrinkles. In a study from Brown University Medical School, researchers found that tanning-bed aficionados were as much as 2 1/2 times as likely to develop one of the three common forms of skin cancer as people who don't use tanning beds. Some beds put out higher levels of ultraviolet (UV) rays than the UV levels emitted by the midday summer sun.

Can I Undo It? No.

Sun exposure, especially if your quest for the perfect tan has left you sunburned, damages skin in ways that cannot be repaired. But there's plenty you can do to prevent further damage—and to spot skin cancers in their earliest, most treatable stages.

+ BENEFITS

Protecting your skin results in softer, suppler skin with fewer wrinkles and less discoloration. The main advantage, however, is your lowered risk for skin cancer.

Repair Plan

Schedule an annual skin check by a dermatologist. Your doctor will inspect you for moles, growths, and any other unusual skin changes. If any are spotted, your doctor likely will test a small sample to determine the nature of the growth. Ask your family doctor and gynecologist to be on the lookout for suspicious moles, too.

Always wear sunscreen when outdoors. Keep high SPF (sun protection factor) sunscreens by your back door, in your car, in your purse, or anywhere else handy. Get in the habit of spending the 30 seconds it takes on the way out the door to rub some on your face, scalp, and exposed arms and legs.

Stay safe in the sun. Stay in the shade or wear a broad-brimmed hat, sunglasses, long sleeves, and pants during peak sunburn hours, 10:00 A.M. to 4:00 P.M.

At the beach, wear a sun-protection water shirt. Surfers do. They are the equivalent of a high SPF sunblock lotion, and they don't wash off in water!

Get your glow from a self-tanning product instead of the sun. Tanning creams and gels can give your skin a bronzed look without the cancer risk.

Know a danger sign when you see it. A melanoma may be blackish/brownish with irregular edges—but it could also be red, pink, or waxy, or it could be a sore that just won't heal. Other warning signs include itching, bleeding, sensitivity to touch, or obvious growth. Basically, anything that doesn't look right to you on your skin deserves to be checked by a doctor.

Sip green tea. There is some evidence that polyphenols in green tea may protect your cells against cancer-causing sun damage.

■ FOR MORE ON HEALTHY SKIN, SEE PAGE 295.

DAMAGE DONE

Surprisingly high. A study of 105 middle-age British government employees found that women and men with more marital worries had higher levels of the stress hormone cortisol as well as higher levels of stress and high blood pressure—factors that raise risk for heart attack and stroke.

When University of Utah researchers studied videotaped conversations between 150 husbands and wives—and also scanned their blood vessels—they found that spouses whose exchanges were angry and mean-spirited were also 30 percent more likely to have arteries clogged with heart-threatening plaque. Other studies show that an unhappy relationship can raise your odds for weight gain, depression, lowered immunity, stomach ulcers, and heart disease risk.

In contrast, a happy marriage may protect your health because spouses imitate each other's healthy habits. When Brigham Young University researchers checked up on 4,746 married couples ages 51 to 61 years old, they found that couples mirror each other's health status: A man in his early fifties in excellent health had a very low chance of having a wife in fair or poor health. But a fiftysomething man in poor health had a 24 percent chance of being married to a woman with so-so health and a 12 percent chance of being married to a woman in poor health. Why? Couples live in the same environments when it comes to food, exercise, and stress reduction. They also share emotional stresses.

Can I Undo It? Probably.

If your union has been unhappy or hostile for a long time, pay extra attention to your mental health and your heart health. Creating a happy marriage can lead to a longer, healthier life: A University of Pittsburgh study of 7,524 women ages 65 and older found that simply being married cut their risk of dying over a six-year period by 17 percent. Why? Married people are more likely than single people to take simple health-promoting steps on a daily basis such as eating breakfast, wearing seat belts, getting physical activity, having regular blood pressure checks, and not smoking. And be patient: In another study, most unhappy couples who simply stayed together were very happy within five years.

+ BENEFITS

Happy marriages deliver on most every conceivable health benefit: lower risk of major diseases, longer life, less stress. Then there are the emotional benefits: happiness, fun, joy, intimacy. A close, loving relationship is among the best things in life for your long-term health.

Repair Plan

Stop expecting perfection from your mate. Experts say most couples—even those in happy marriages—have 6 to 10 areas of disagreement that may never be resolved. Your marriage may not be broken at all—just normal!

Keep your love account in the black. According to various experts, it takes 5 to 20 positive statements to outweigh the damage wrought by a single negative remark—or even by a steely squint or impatient harrumph! Do more of the former, less of the latter.

Don't try to change your partner. When things aren't going right, change the way *you* act. Marriage experts say that trying to force your partner to change rarely works, and worse, it creates lots of resentment. If you take good-hearted steps to improve, it'll be noticed—and often, will cause your spouse to respond in kind.

Touch. Human touch triggers the release of feel-good endorphins—for giver and receiver alike.

Study the art of small acts of love. You know how to push Mr. or Mrs. Right's hot buttons, and if you think about it, you know how to push his or her joy buttons, too. That doesn't just mean sex, but it's not a bad place to start. Greet him with a glad-to-see-you hug and kiss when you get home. Surprise her by delivering coffee, bedside, some rainy Thursday morning.

Spend time together every day. You clear your schedule for hair appointments, favorite TV shows, and your book group—how about your spouse? Spend 20 to 30 minutes a day chatting together about your daily lives, your dreams, your plans. And make time for intimacy—even if it means scheduling it in day planner.

Skip the blame game. Setting your partner up as the bad guy ignores the 80 to 90 percent of him or her that's really wonderful. Criticism, contempt, confrontation, and hostility don't help anything. Instead, express concerns by calmly and honestly talking about how you feel.

Listen carefully to your spouse. Don't try to defend yourself or argue ... just respect what he or she has to say. This alone can go a long way toward ending the fights and finding a healthier common ground.

Raise concerns when you both have time and energy to discuss them. Late at night, when you're rushing out the door, or when you are hungry isn't the right time.

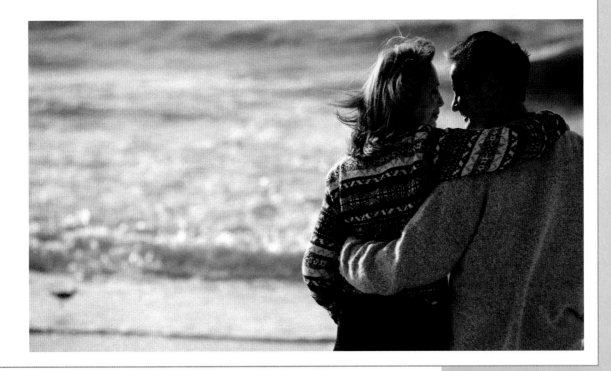

I've lost touch with most of my old friends.

DAMAGE DONE

If you read the opening chapters of this book, you know already where the science stands here—positive social connections are crucial to your health. Unless you're the rare loner who truly thrives on going solo, spending too much time by yourself or having too few friends to confide in and socialize with can, over time, raise your odds for heart disease, high blood pressure, depression, muddled thinking, and sleep problems.

Why? Loneliness raises levels of stress hormones in the bloodstream and as a result, may play a role in firing up chronic inflammation—a risk for heart disease, diabetes, and even some forms of cancer.

The biggest danger posed by having too few friends: It becomes a habit that could rob you of happiness in the future, when you may need it most. In one University of South Florida study of 354 people in their seventies, those whose health declined felt far happier and more satisfied with their lives if they still had a social life. And in a Canadian study that tracked older Manitoban men for six years, those who had more social connections felt happier, were more able to live independently, and were even less likely to die during the study.

There's no magic number of friends, or number of times per week or per day to reach out by phone, e-mail, old-fashioned letter, or in person. You do need at least one friend other than your spouse—something that 25 percent of participants in a Duke University friendship study didn't have.

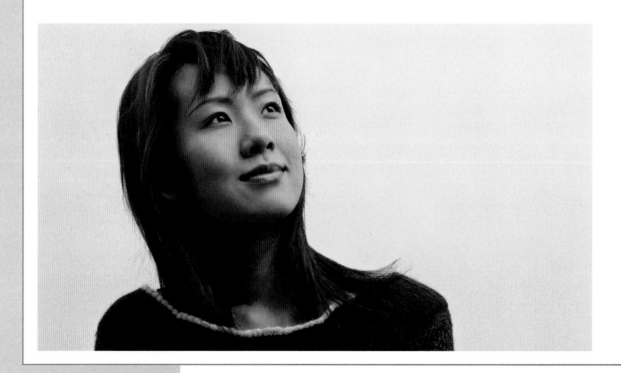

Can I Undo It? Yes!

All you need to do is get past the mental blocks that have prevented you from reaching out. For some, that isn't easy—shyness, insecurity, low self-confidence can all get in the way of making new friends or reviving old ties. But all these can be overcome, and the benefits of doing so will be immediate.

+ BENEFITS

More social interactions will have a less-than-subtle positive effect on your mood, making you much more happy, engaged, and confident. And with these emotions, every aspect of your health will benefit.

Repair Plan

Make a list. With whom from your past would you most enjoy being closer? The answer could be friends, former co-workers, family members, even people you have met just once or twice but with whom you were highly impressed. Put them in order, and commit to a plan to contact them in a slow but steady sequence.

Use the Internet to get started. Today, e-mail has become a wonderful way to reconnect with long-lost friends and colleagues. Write a short note saying hello, confirming the address, and asking if it's alright if you send a longer note. Who can turn down such an offer?

Work on your personal script. As you begin to reach out to social connections new or old, you are going to be asked a lot of questions about you, your recent past, and your plans for the future. Anticipate them and work on your answers ahead of time. This will greatly help your confidence and will help you focus on positive, attractive messages.

Turn a hobby into a social activity. Do you play the clarinet? Join the town band. Do you love the theater? Volunteer to take tickets at local productions ... or dare to audition for a role on stage. Have a special skill or collection? Find others with the same interests.

Do lots of little interactions. For example, if you see a neighbor, walk over and chat for a few minutes. Linger after church services, classes, or even work and chat with acquaintances. Engage local shop owners in a little conversation. Talk to shoppers at the grocery store who are exploring the same products as you are. You'll find that these little conversations are great fun and bolster your confidence.

Volunteer with a local organization that performs good works in your community. With age, each of us should be more willing to donate our wisdom, time, and skills to help our communities. The benefit will be great conversations and newfound relationships.

I'm angry, worried, or stressed more than I'm happy.

DAMAGE DONE

Substantial, and not merely for your mental health. Anger, stress, and worry release a cascade of stress hormones that increase your blood pressure and blood sugar, depress immunity, slow digestion, and make you feel downright mean. Nature intended stress to be a short-lived fight-or-flight response to a threat. But modern life can lead to chronic stress—and to far-reaching impacts on your health.

Studies at the University of California, San Francisco, show that excess cortisol—an important stress hormone—prompts your body to store extra fat around your abdomen and to overeat high-fat, sugary foods. Both raise your odds for heart disease and diabetes. Meanwhile, stress hormones make cells throughout your body less sensitive to insulin, leading to higher blood sugar levels. And in a three-year Harvard Medical School study of 516 people with coronary artery disease, those with the highest anxiety levels were 6 percent more likely to have a heart attack or die than people who said they felt peaceful most of the time.

In a Duke University study of 127 healthy men and women, those who scored highest on tests of anger and hostility had levels of c-Reactive Protein (CRP)—a marker of heart-threatening inflammation—two to three times higher than calmer study volunteers. The more negative their moods, the higher their CRP levels, and the greater their risk for future heart disease and stroke.

Can I Undo It? Yes.

You have to keep an open mind and do some work, though. Stress-reduction techniques have been proven to lower blood sugar, improve immunity, reduce depression, speed healing in people with psoriasis, ease chronic pain, lower blood sugar, and possibly protect your heart, too. In one Harvard Medical School study, people with heart disease who had been anxious but lowered their stress levels significantly cut their risk for a heart attack.

+ BENEFITS

More than you can count. A regained sense of joy and control is worth its weight in gold, and the physical health benefits will be substantial as well.

Repair Plan

Train yourself to stop getting stressed so easily. You've heard it often: Stress isn't created by people or situations; it's entirely caused by how you react to them. You can let an obnoxious child, boss, or sales clerk get to you, or you can take a deep breath and decide not to let yourself react strongly or emotionally. So next time you feel a stressful situation emerging, work hard at managing it and staying cool. In time, you'll succeed wonderfully!

Learn a formal stress-relief process. Among the most proven are yoga, meditation, and deep breathing. Consider these essential tools for health, not unlike aspirin for a headache.

Try progressive relaxation. Close your eyes, breathe calmly, and release tension in each part of your body beginning with your feet and working up to your neck and head.

Rediscover your optimism. No one is born a pessimist; it is a learned behavior. Regaining your sense of hope can go a long way toward stifling stress and regaining a sense of happiness.

If stress is taking a significant toll on your attitude and health, talk to a cognitive therapist. You'll learn how to see yourself and your thought process in a new, more objective light.

Eat healthy and exercise. A healthy lifestyle does wonders for your ability to manage stressful situations.

Enjoy a relaxing hobby. Knitting, building model airplanes, making pottery ... whatever you love and that you can immerse yourself in will calm you down.

Rediscover silliness. One of the secrets of achieving happiness is to acknowledge that in every grown man resides a young boy, and in every mature woman, a young girl. Our bodies may age, but our spirits needn't, and on some matters, shouldn't! So don't suppress your sense of fun and silliness. At any age, it's perfectly appropriate to laugh at comedians, have a pillow fight, make silly faces at each other, and get a little saucy with your intimates. If you have lost your sense of humor, you need to do what it takes to bring it back, even if it's just renting goofy movies. Treat it as a doctor's prescription for your health.

■ FOR MORE ON A HEALTHY ATTITUDE, SEE PAGE 237.

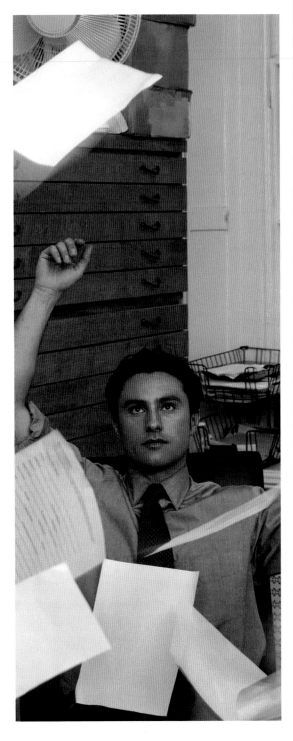

I rarely get a full night's sleep.

DAMAGE DONE

Skimping on rest can have far-reaching effects on your health, whether you're an insomniac who cannot sleep or someone who gives in to the temptation to use sleep time to catch up on work or TV. In one Yale University study of 1,100 men, those who got five to six hours of sleep a night doubled their risk for diabetes; a Harvard Medical School study found similar dangers for women, too. But that's not all. If you wake up feeling as though you've barely slept—and if your bed partner has told you that you snore—you may have obstructive sleep apnea, a breathing problem that raises your risk for high blood pressure, heart attack, and stroke.

Of course, not getting enough rest can also fog your thinking skills, slow your reaction time—raising your chances for traffic accidents—and leave you vulnerable to anxiety and depression.

Can I Undo It? Yes.

Just a night or two of refreshing sleep can lift your mood and clear your thinking. Just a few good nights begins to reverse metabolic changes that raise your odds of diabetes. And fixing sleep apnea can immediately lower blood pressure.

+ BENEFITS

Sleep is like a universal healer. Getting enough will provide you with numerous benefits like more energy, a better mood, and clearer thinking. Sleep can even lower your risk for apnea-related heart problems and diabetes.

Repair Plan

Sip some herbal tea after dinner. Avoid caffeinated coffee and teas, which block the brain chemical that makes you feel drowsy and fall asleep.

Do something soothing before bed. Don't work, watch high-energy shows on TV, or pay bills. Try a warm bath or a quiet hobby like knitting, reading, or listening to music. Create a pre-bedtime ritual that slows you down and calms both body and mind.

Turn off the computer. Working on that video display terminal (VDT) seems to affect the sleep/wake cycle and biological rhythms. So stay away from the computer as bedtime approaches.

Listen to your body. Sleepy? Turn out the light. Not sleepy? Get out of bed. The important lesson is to take your cues from your own body, and don't turn your bedroom into a place of worry over sleep.

Hide the clock. Don't let the glowing numbers—or constantly checking the time—keep you up.

Change beds. Women who sleep with snorers are three times more likely to have insomnia than those sleeping with nonsnorers (there are no studies on the effect of a snoring bed partner on men).

Talk with your doctor. He may decide you need a sleep apnea evaluation. An evaluation is especially important for snorers.

Get your sinuses and stomach checked. Allergies and heartburn are common yet frequently overlooked causes of sleep problems.

Do a med review with your doctor. At least eight classes of drugs, including antidepressants and blood pressure drugs, can keep you awake nights.

■ FOR MORE ON REMEDYING SLEEP TROUBLES, SEE PAGE 299.

I rarely exercise.

DAMAGE DONE

Less muscle strength and density. Lowered metabolism. Weight gain. Balance problems. Higher blood pressure. Higher levels of "bad" LDL cholesterol and lower levels of "good" HDL cholesterol. More depression, stress, and memory problems. And that's just the start of the damage caused by sedentary living.

All over the world, people are sitting more and moving less. A good name for it is sitting disease—a sedentary lifestyle that diminishes muscle mass and ages your cardiovascular system while it weakens your immunity and leaves you vulnerable to stress, low moods, and thinking problems associated with aging. If you change just one damaging habit, it should be this one!

Can I Undo It? Yes, at any age.

Studies of people in their eighties and nineties have found that adding walking and strength-training to their daily routines improves strength, balance, energy levels, and more. And that's just the beginning. Just six months of exercise can improve memory and thinking, boost self-esteem, lessen depression, ease stress, increase immunity, improve your sex life, cool off chronic inflammation, and strengthen your muscles so that you burn more calories.

+ BENEFITS

Moving more makes you less tired, less stressed, and less apt to have body aches and pains. You can count on being in a better mood and having a trimmer, stronger, more energetic body. Of course, exercising results in better heart health but it also helps strengthen your immunity and sharpen your memory skills.

Repair Plan

Live more actively. Walk a little faster. Take the stairs, not the elevator. Park in the farthest spot at the grocery store or mall. Stand while talking on the phone. But don't think that exercise can only be had during formal exercise sessions. Every moment of every day provides an opportunity to move in healthy, life-affirming ways. You'll find that high-energy living on its own can spark your energy and health.

Start slowly. Resolve to walk for 10 minutes a day. In a week or two, move up to 15 minutes if your feet, joints, legs, and lungs are feeling good when you walk. Keep slowly increasing your time and distance until you're walking 30 to 60 minutes every day.

Add strength-training. It builds muscle, increases circulation, and speeds your metabolism.

Find a buddy. Walking, swimming, or exercising with a friend is more fun—and you're more likely to stick with it if you have an exercise date with someone.

Have "active fun." Join in the badminton game at picnics. Ask a friend to join you for a walk in a nearby park instead of going for ice cream. Take the grandchildren to the local pool instead of to the movies. It bears repeating: Formal workouts are just one way to become active and stronger.

Wear comfortable clothes and supportive shoes. You don't need expensive athletic gear. Well-fitting walking shoes will protect your feet from injury, and pants (or shorts) and a shirt that breathes will keep you cool while you're active.

■ FOR MORE ON GETTING STARTED WITH EXERCISE, SEE PAGE 172.

I rarely go on vacation.

DAMAGE DONE

Yes, damage can be measured, including a higher risk for heart disease.

When researchers from the State University of New York at Oswego surveyed 12,000 men ages 35 to 57, they found that those who didn't take at least one week-long vacation per year boosted their risk of dying from heart disease by 30 percent during the course of the nine-year study.

Can I Undo It? Yes.

If you've been leading a high-stress lifestyle with few opportunities for relaxation, stay on top of your heart health.

How vacations help: Any stress reduction, even for a few days, gives your heart and blood pressure a break. In one small New Zealand study, researchers found that vacationers slept about an hour longer than they did at home and got three times more deep, rejuvenating sleep afterward than they were getting before their time off.

Even making relaxation a priority over the weekend can help. When Finnish researchers tracked the health habits of 800 women and men for 28 years, they found that those who didn't take a break from work-related stress over the weekend were three times more likely to have a fatal heart attack as those who got plenty of rest.

+ BENEFITS

This is your opportunity to spend time with and get reacquainted with your spouse, family, and/or friends. Sharing good times with people you like helps you feel less stressed. Get back in touch with the feeling of deep relaxation. In addition, you will enjoy overall better heart health.

Repair Plan

Don't work this weekend. Skip home repairs, major lawn and garden work (unless it's a hobby you really love), and any other stressful obligations. Pretend you're on vacation. Eat a leisurely breakfast. Go for a walk. Visit a local attraction that you like. Take in a concert. Dine out with friends. Then, plan to do the same on one day of every weekend from now on.

Plan a real vacation. Half the battle to taking vacations is committing to a time. So get out your calendar and pick a week (or more). Commit to it at work and among your family. Then get to the task of finding some great options, based on the budget you can afford. Merely looking for a perfect week-long sojourn can be relaxing and heart healthy!

Make sure your next trip is relaxing. Even if you take vacations, you may be missing out on the health benefits if you try to do too much or agree to do activities that others like but that you simply don't enjoy. Put activities you like on the agenda, including time for relaxation beside the pool, lake, or ocean ... or get a massage, spa treatment, or take a long walk in nature.

Move! See the sights on foot. Take advantage of outdoor attractions such as sculpture gardens, nature trails, lakeside paths, or a stretch of beautiful beach and take a long walk. Exercise releases feel-good endorphins: Using your feet makes for happy vacations.

Consider rural over urban. Vacations in cities are loud, exciting, and exhausting. Vacations in the country are quiet, peaceful, and recharging. For your health, the latter is what you need most. That doesn't mean choose a boring vacation—just one that gets you away from the hustle and bustle you face at home.

■ FOR MORE ON ACHIEVING BALANCE IN LIFE,
SEE PAGE 236.

I work the night shift or swing shift.

DAMAGE DONE

If you've ever spent a year or more on the night shift or a swing shift, you may be at higher risk for cancers of the breast and colon as well as cardiovascular disease, gastrointestinal problems, and sleep disorders. Experts say that the night shift's health damage rivals the problems caused by smoking a pack of cigarettes a day.

The culprits? Stress and altered melatonin levels. Normally, melatonin levels reach their peak during sleep. But if you're exposed to light at night, levels decline sharply. The cancer connection: This sleep hormone also seems to inhibit the growth of tumors. At low levels, researchers suspect, it may not be able to do its job. Surprisingly, a swing shift schedule may throw off things even more than a steady night job. In a study of 45 oil rig workers, researchers from Cardiff University in Wales found that guys whose work schedules changed every few days had lower, more erratic melatonin levels and higher levels of heart-threatening fatty acids in their bloodstreams than men assigned to steady night work. "Swing shift is a killer," one researcher noted.

And then there are the unhealthy habits that are linked to night-shift work. Because few restaurants are open in the middle of the night, eating habits tend toward fast food and vending machines. And because of the nighttime hours, late-night workers often skip on exercise.

Can I Undo It? Yes.

Altered melatonin levels seem to return to normal once nighttime or shift work ends. But the added cancer risk may not go away. Be sure to get all the cancer screenings you need.

+ BENEFITS

Being diligent about getting your sleep and taking care of yourself will give you more energy and less chance of gaining weight while you're working nights. Getting health screenings means you and your doctor will catch problems early, when they're most treatable.

Repair Plan

Establish a consistent sleep routine. Your body chemistry will adjust some to your nighttime work if you keep a regular schedule that includes plenty of rest. Go to bed soon after you return home, instead of trying to fit in errands and household chores. You can do them when you wake up.

Bring your own healthy meals to work. Eating healthy foods has no shortage of benefits, and one of them includes better sleep. A diet of sugar, caffeine, and fat—which is what you get from fast food and vending machines—not only hurts your health but also disrupts your natural energy/rest cycles.

Carry healthy drinks and lots of fruit or vegetable snacks. Having something healthy to crunch on or sip can help you avoid two of the biggest dangers of shift work: Drinking extra caffeine (as noted, it'll keep you awake when you finally have time to sleep!) and smoking cigarettes.

Take an exercise break. Walk around the building, use the company gym, or do sit-ups in the break room. You'll burn calories and feel more alert.

Don't skip screenings. Get mammograms, colonoscopies, blood pressure checks, and cholesterol tests as recommended by your doctor, even if you no longer work odd hours.

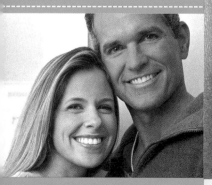

Living
Healthy Today

The best way to ensure you are healthy and energized 20 years from now is to become healthy and energized right now. Here's how to feel great today, tomorrow, and for the rest of your life.

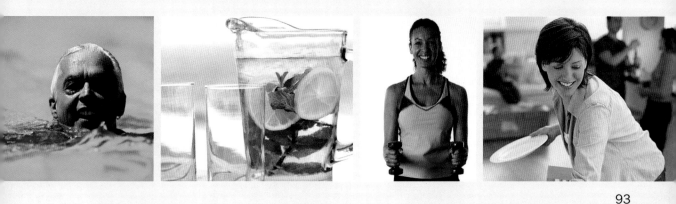

Am I Leading a healthy life?

Quiz ✳

You've just spent a lot of time exploring your past—the habits and lifestyle choices that have brought you to today. Now, it's time to talk about right now. What is your health like this very moment? Are you fit, well-fed, in good spirits, energized?

Here are 35 questions that probe all aspects of your well-being. Give yourself at least 30 minutes to take it. Some of the questions will ask you to get up and do things, so be dressed and prepared for activity, such as testing your balance and flexibility. Along the way, record your answers on the Scoring sheet on page 103.

The results likely will speak for themselves. But if you are the type who likes to keep score, the answer key provides a point system that will allow you to tally up and rank how well you are aging.

Answer the questions honestly! No one is judging you, and you're the only one who will know the results. This is for you to identify the areas in which your health needs work, and to let you understand thoroughly whether you are treating yourself the way you richly deserve.

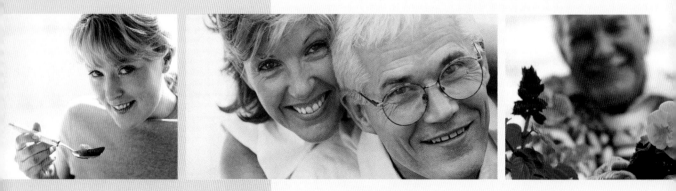

1 **Pinch the skin of the back of your hand for five seconds, then release. How long does it take the skin to snap back into position?**
   a. My skin is tight enough that I can't really pinch it
   b. Less than two seconds
   c. Three to four seconds
   d. Five to six seconds

2 **How long can you stand on one foot with your eyes closed?**
   a. One minute or longer
   b. 30 seconds to one minute
   c. Less than 30 seconds

3 **Bend over as far as you can without bending your knees. How far can your fingertips reach?**
   a. To my toes or the floor
   b. Within a few inches of my ankles
   c. Not much past my knees

4 **How much sleep did you average over the past five nights?**
   a. Less than six hours
   b. Six to eight hours
   c. More than eight hours

5 **Do you feel rested when you wake up in the morning?**
   a. Yes
   b. No

6 **How many servings of vegetables did you have yesterday?**
   a. One to two
   b. Three to four
   c. Five or more

7 **When was the last time you had a pleasant conversation with a friend?**
   a. Today or yesterday
   b. Three to seven days ago
   c. More than seven days ago

8 **How much of your free time yesterday did you spend in a chair or on a couch, watching television, using a computer, reading, talking, or just passing the time?**
   a. Less than four hours
   b. More than four hours

9 **Over the past seven days, have you spent more than four hours outdoors?**
   a. Yes
   b. No

10 The last time you were in a building or shopping center and had to go up or down one or two floors, did you take the stairs, escalator, or elevator?

a. Stairs

b. Escalator or elevator

11 If you took a poll among your friends or co-workers, how would they rate your attitude of late?

a. Happy, engaged, optimistic

b. Stable, even-keeled, guarded

c. Worried, frustrated, pessimistic

12 Did you floss your teeth yesterday?

a. Yes

b. No

13 The last time you flossed, did your gums bleed?

a. Yes

b. No

14 Think for a moment about the state of your overall health. How would rate it?

a. Great

b. Okay

c. Poor

15 Think about this past weekend. Were there things you wanted to do but couldn't or didn't because of physical or health-related limitations?

a. Yes

b. No

16 Think over the past week. Did you have any lapses in memory that you found annoying or troubling?

a. Yes

b. No

17 When you woke up this morning, were you in a good mood?

a. Yes

b. No

18 Over the past three days, did you engage in a hobby or activity that you really enjoy, liking cooking, hiking, or taking a class?

a. Yes

b. No

19 Do you have a person you could talk with tonight about your personal problems, concerns, or hopes?

a. Yes

b. No

20 Over the past week, how much exposure did you have to cigarette smoke, auto exhaust, fertilizers, or insecticides?

a. None that I can remember

b. A few exposures

c. Regular exposure

21 Do you know your cholesterol levels, roughly?

a. Yes, based on a blood test within the past six months

b. Yes, but based on a blood test more than six months ago

c. No

22 Over the past seven days, how many times have you eaten seafood?

a. Three or more times

b. Twice

c. Once

d. Not at all

23 Over the past three days, have you prayed or meditated?

a. Yes

b. No

24 As you are reading this question, do you have a cold, a headache, or any other noticeable pain, symptom, or health condition?

a. Yes

b. No

25 How many sodas or other pre-sweetened drinks did you have yesterday?

a. Three or more

b. One or two

c. None

26 Over the past two days, how many minutes would you say you felt totally relaxed?

a. None

b. Less than 30 minutes

c. More than 30 minutes

27 Did you eat breakfast this morning?

a. Yes, and it was very healthy

b. Yes, but it wasn't that healthy

c. No, skipped it

28 If a stranger did something very rude to you this morning, would you be angry and still talking about it tonight?

a. Yes

b. No

29 Sit in a strong, stable, armless chair. Hold the chair with each hand right next to your hips. Can you lift your body off the chair with just your arms?

   a. Yes

   b. No

30 As you read this, do you have a glass of water within arm's reach?

   a. Yes

   b. No

31 Since yesterday morning, how many servings of raw fruit have you eaten?

   a. None

   b. Two or three

   c. Four or more

32 Stand up and sit down rapidly, seven times. How difficult was that?

   a. I couldn't finish it

   b. It was challenging to my thighs and I'm breathing harder, but I did it

   c. Not very challenging at all

33 When was the last time you washed your hands?

   a. Within the past hour

   b. Within the past three hours

   c. It's been more than three hours

34 The last time you became really frustrated, what did you do?

   a. Ate some "comfort food"

   b. Got angry, maybe even lashed out verbally at someone

   c. Did something healthy to relieve the frustration, like walked or did something relaxing

35 Can you take your own pulse?

   a. Yes

   b. No

The Answers

___ **1 If you answered *a* or *b*, give yourself 1 point.** You are taking good care of your skin, and will look years younger as you age.

___ **2 If you answered *a*, give yourself 1 point.** This is a good test of your balance, and balance is a key factor in preventing falls. If you have trouble with this exercise, turn to page 262 for advice on improving your balance.

___ **3 If you answered *a*, give yourself 1 point.** But if the internet had yet to be invented the last time you touched your toes, then you're facing some serious issues with flexibility. Flexibility is important if you want to remain physically active, which is critical to overall health. See page 189 for exercises designed to keep you flexible.

___ **4 If you answered *b*, give yourself 2 points.** If you're having trouble falling asleep or staying asleep, turn to page 299 for tips on combating insomnia. And while answer *c* doesn't really signify a problem, some evidence suggests that people who sleep more than eight hours don't fare as well as they age. Sleeping too much could also be a sign of depression.

___ **5 If you answered *a*, give yourself 1 point.** Waking feeling rested is not only a sign that you had a good night's sleep but also an indicator of your overall health.

___ **6 If you answered *c*, give yourself 3 points.** With the exception of exercise, perhaps nothing is as important to your overall health and well-being as your diet. If you think of vegetables as the garnish on your plate, then you need to pay particular attention to the chapter, "Eat to Feel Good", beginning on page 108. Vegetables are without question the most important food for you to eat for disease prevention.

___ **7 If you answered *a*, give yourself 3 points.** As mentioned elsewhere in this book, there is strong evidence to support the importance of social relationships and healthy aging, says Rene J. McGovern, PhD, assistant professor of psychiatry at Case Western Reserve University in Cleveland. "The capacity to 'make new friends, yet keep the old' is important in maintaining connections," she says. "Basically, sharing your thoughts and feelings helps keep you healthy in mind, body, and spirit." You'll find tips on building your social networks throughout this book.

___ **8 If you answered *a*, give yourself 2 points.** Sedentary living is a serious health problem, and its antidote, physical activity, is literally the backbone of healthy aging. Without lots of movement, your muscles weaken and you put yourself at risk of frailty, not to mention a whole host of medical conditions including cardiovascular disease and Alzheimer's. Check out the chapter, "Move to Feel Good", beginning on page 172.

___ **9 If you answered *a*, give yourself 2 points.** Being outdoors is a strong indicator of whether you have active hobbies like sports, hiking, or gardening. "Not only is physical activity important but being able to enjoy the sheer pleasure of your body in movement and the joy of many productive and fun activities has been show to keep you vital and young," says Dr. McGovern. "It also keeps you socially connected and can recharge your spirit."

___10 **If you answered *a*, give yourself 1 point.** There's more to fitness than just formal exercise routines. Living life with high energy, which in large part means keeping your body moving, ensures that you get the blood circulation and oxygen you need, as well as stretching your muscles in every corner of your being, including your mind.

___11 **If you answered *a*, give yourself 2 points.** A cautious approach to life isn't bad—in fact, being risk adverse can help you live longer. But study after study shows that optimism and happiness are powerful healers and age-extenders. And, life is so much more fulfilling for positive thinkers. "An overly guarded, concerned, or worried approach to life limits opportunities for learning and personal growth," says Dr. McGovern. "Plus, people who are happy are more fun to be around, and those who are optimistic just seem to find the good in life."

___12 **If you answered *a*, give yourself 2 points.** Taking care of your teeth means more than a pretty smile; it could make a difference in your cardiovascular health as well. Adults should floss their teeth daily. You can learn more about what good dental health is all about on page 271.

___13 **If you answered *b*, give yourself 1 point.** Healthy teeth and gums are the proverbial "canary in the coal mine" when it comes to levels of inflammation in your body.

___14 **If you answered *a*, give yourself 4 points.** "Research finds that rating your health as fair or poor is a good predictor of future health, disability, and mortality," says aging expert Adam Davey, PhD, associate professor at Temple University. That means those who think their health isn't very good—even when it *is* fine—will eventually have their thoughts come true.

___15 **If you answered *b*, give yourself 3 points.** "Gerontologists differentiate between health problems and their effects on your lifestyle," says Dr. Davey. "As we age, for example, nearly everyone develops arthritis, but it only significantly limits activities for some." The less you allow your health problems to get in the way of your life, the better you will age.

___16 **If you answered *b*, give yourself 2 points.** This is a trick question. The mere fact that you had a lapse in memory tells you nothing about your brain's health or age. Memory problems are rarely a sign of aging; more commonly, they are a sign of a hectic, stress-filled lifestyle. See page 338 for more on protecting your memory as you age.

___17 **If you answered *a*, give yourself 4 points.** The simplest definition of aging well is waking up feeling refreshed and optimistic each day. "One of the early paradoxes that pioneers of gerontology set out to understand was why so many older adults reported being generally satisfied with their lives despite such obvious signs of poor quality of life, like illness, disability, relationship loss, etc.," says Dr. Davey. "As it turns out, some of us can make pretty good lemonade out of lemons, and the ability to make the best of our situation is one important component of successful aging."

___18 **If you answered *a*, give yourself 2 points.** "Maintaining active engagement in productive or key social roles is an important predictor of decreased disability and of a lower risk of death, even among centenarians," says Dr. Davey.

___19 **If you answered *a*, give yourself 3 points**. "In a very important study conducted back in the 1960s, researchers found that older people tended to do well as long as they had at least one close confidant relationship," says Dr. Davey.

___20 **If you answered *a*, give yourself 2 points.** "Environmental toxins have been found to limit the ability of our bodies, minds, and spirits to function optimally," says Dr. McGovern. "This can not only limit our health but, even more important, can limit our ability to think clearly and make healthy choices."

___21 **If you answered *a*, give yourself 2 points; if you answered *b*, give yourself 1 point.** You don't have to go to medical school, but understanding how things like high cholesterol and high blood pressure affect your overall health and when to have certain issues (like suddenly losing weight, losing your balance, or having unusual pain) medically evaluated can help you stave off problems before they can permanently affect your health.

___22 **If you answered *b*, give yourself 1 point; if you answered *a*, give yourself 1 point** (only if you made sure the seafood was raised and harvested from healthy waters—sadly, it's a proven fact that fish from open seas has high levels of toxins in their body). Fish is an excellent source of anti-inflammatory omega-3 fatty acids, which studies find can help maintain heart health and keep your brain young. They can also

help reduce the inflammation that contributes to the aches and pains many of us experience with age.

___23 **If you answered *a*, give yourself 2 points**. "Faith shares traits with optimism," says Dr. McGovern, "and, along with membership in a faith community, predicts longevity and fewer problems with mental health as you age."

___24 **If you answered *b*, give yourself 1 point.** On average, most people spend most of their lives healthy. If you're having repeat headaches, chronic pain, more than one cold or other infectious illness a season, then something is wrong. You need to reevaluate how you live your life, including taking a close look at your diet, exercise routine, and stress management.

___25 **If you answered *c*, give yourself 2 points.** There is just nothing to be gained from drinking soda or other presweetened drinks except weight. Stick to water, unsweetened iced tea (try green tea for a change), or the occasional glass of wine. If you do drink juices, dilute them with sparkling water.

___26 **If you answered *c*, give yourself 2 points.** The first person you need to take care of in your life is you, and that means finding time to relax, de-stress, or, as some like to call it, chillax (short for "chill and relax"). Doing so will stem the damaging effects of stress hormones, adding years of life to your heart, keeping your memory sharp, and even reducing your risk of conditions like insulin resistance and obesity.

___27 **If you answered *a*, give yourself 2 points.** You wouldn't drive a car with an empty gas tank, would you? So why would you start your day on empty? If you don't get some glucose into your brain, and some fat and protein into your stomach, you're going to find yourself sticking up the local convenience store for its stash of chocolate and chips. And that's not good for anything—particularly your waistline. Many studies show the huge health benefits of a small, healthy breakfast each day.

___28 **If you answered *b*, give yourself 1 point.** Learning to let go of frustrating things, rather than ruminating on them, protects you against mental health conditions like depression and anxiety, as well as the aging effects of stress-related chemicals.

___29 **If you answered *a*, give yourself 1 point.** You have good arm strength and also good abdominal or "core" strength, which is critical to reducing the risk of falls and back pain. Maintaining strength is crucial to remaining healthy and active in your future.

___30 **If you answered *a*, give yourself 1 point.** Staying hydrated becomes more difficult as you age because your thirst mechanism fades. And yet it also becomes more important for your overall health. If you always keep a bottle or glass of water nearby, you won't have to worry about it.

___31 **If you answered *c*, give yourself 2 points; if you answered *b*, give yourself 1 point.** Raw fruit provides valuable fiber and healthy glucose for cellular energy, not to mention disease-fighting antioxidants (even the best vitamins in the world can't compare). Consider fresh fruit a crucial part of a healthy, long life diet.

___32 **If you answered *c*, give yourself 2 points.** You're managing to stay in shape quite nicely! This test challenges your aerobic fitness—that is, how well your heart and lungs can deliver oxygen quickly to your muscles. It also tests your thigh and abdominal muscles.

___33 **If you answered *a* or *b*, give yourself 1 point.** Frequently washing your hands with hot, soapy water is the best way to avoid becoming infected with cold, flu, and other viruses or bacteria. Many people don't realize how often they touch their faces with their hands. And it's often your hands that pick up other people's germs from counters, doorknobs, or other often-touched surfaces.

___34 **If you answered *c*, give yourself 2 points.** While you can't necessarily eliminate or even reduce stressful events in your life, you *do* have control over how you let them affect you. Finding healthy ways to cope (and no, that leftover chocolate cake doesn't count) will add years to your life.

___35 **If you answered *a*, give yourself 1 point.** An overlooked but important part of good health is constantly monitoring yourself. If you know how to take your pulse, it's indicative that you have invested a little time and thought into knowing your body signals.

The Score Key

55–65:
Congratulations! You are doing most of the things you should to be healthy today—and many years from now. Be proud of yourself, but don't be complacent. With your healthy mindset, it should be easy to take on even more health-enhancing lifestyle choices that will make you even more likely to thrive for the rest of your life.

40–54:
You're not doing badly in terms of your aging potential, but there is definitely room for improvement. Look back at the questions and see if there are patterns to your answers. For example, did you do particularly poorly on the diet questions? Fitness questions? Attitude questions? Make a commitment to start there, and then revisit this quiz in a few months.

Below 40:
This quiz should be a wake-up call. It should have made clear, for example, that good health is not merely the absence of disease. It's time to ask yourself, "What do I want the next 20, 30, or 40 years to look like?" and then make the changes necessary to get there. If you keep going the way you're going, you're facing a host of age-related issues, ranging from frailty to memory loss to chronic health conditions, all of which will make your later years a burden, rather than a joy.

Am I Leading a Healthy Life?

Scoring Sheet

Answer all 35 questions first, then, score your results and tally all the points you've earned in the "Total points" box. Check your score against the key at left to see how you fair.

1. ....
2. ....
3. ....
4. ....
5. ....
6. ....
7. ....
8. ....
9. ....
10. ....
11. ....
12. ....
13. ....
14. ....
15. ....
16. ....
17. ....
18. ....

19. ....
20. ....
21. ....
22. ....
23. ....
24. ....
25. ....
26. ....
27. ....
28. ....
29. ....
30. ....
31. ....
32. ....
33. ....
34. ....
35. ....

Total points:

Ready, Set…Slow!

Surprise! Here's question 36 from the Are You Leading a Healthy Life quiz that you just completed:

36 **What is your reaction to the 35 questions you just answered?**

a. There are so many things I have to fix to get my health right, I don't know where to begin, or even whether to begin.

b. If those are the types of changes I need to make to achieve long health, that's easy! Let's get started!

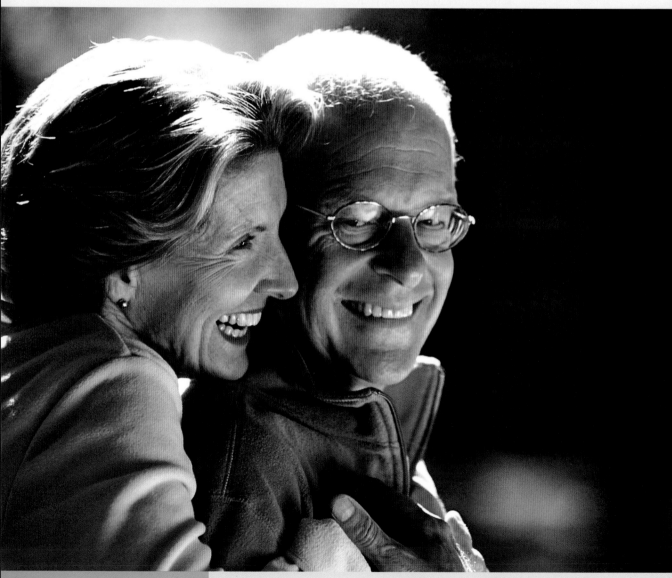

Hopefully, you picked *b,* but even if not, the message is the same for people of *both* viewpoints: Go slowly. Make one change at a time. Be patient and mindful of what your body's telling you.

The truth is that slow change can create a health revolution. When you make one change at a time in important areas affecting your health, you're setting yourself up for success. You won't feel overwhelmed. You'll have the time to fit a new habit into your life, no matter what else is going on. You'll see real benefits and build a foundation for making more changes successfully, too.

Starting with the next chapter, and for much of the rest of the book, you'll discover the exciting, research-proven core concepts of long life health—science-tested ways to eat, move, de-stress, and prevent disease that keep the world's longest-lived people vibrantly healthy for decades into old age. And the processes are broken down into lots of easy, small steps. Our hunch is that you'll want to try lots of them, and quickly.

Some experts would advocate that: overhauling your whole life with dozens of new rules to follow for what to eat, when and how to exercise, and required relaxation techniques. And honestly, for a few people, it works.

But when researchers at Baylor College of Medicine in Houston, compared the success rates of people who took an all-or-nothing approach to health (they stopped smoking, cut back on sodium, and started exercising, all at once) to that of people who adopted one healthy new habit at a time over an 18-month period, just 6 percent of study volunteers in the all-or-nothing group could maintain all of their new habits. In the same study, the "slow change" group was more successful at exercising (they added far more steps to their days) and lowered their cholesterol levels more than the all-or-nothing group.

For most of us, starting small is smart, practical, and most likely to help ensure that you

A Prescription to Move

Having trouble getting started with a more active lifestyle? Ask your doctor to write you an exercise "prescription"—a formal, detailed order from the doctor to get moving. A study published in the *American Journal of Preventive Medicine* found that when a doctor wrote an exercise prescription for people over age 65, they improved their fitness levels by 11 percent in six months and by 17 percent after a year. In contrast, another group that got no special Rx barely budged.

succeed. And, there's plenty of cutting-edge research on how our brains adapt to change that suggests it really does work best.

Experts who work with older people agree, too. "It takes time to figure out how to listen to your body when you're trying something new," says Mary Ann Wilson, RN, a nurse and fitness expert from Portland, Oregon, who hosts the television show *Sit and Get Fit.* "You want a new exercise routine, or anything new, to make you feel excited, not turned-off. You don't want to feel tired or sore or confused or ready to quit. People in the fifties to the upper nineties watch the show and come to my classes—and so do young people. They're surprised at how good it feels to do even a few short, sweet exercises—and what a difference they can make."

Small, it turns out, is big when it comes to changing your health habits.

The Power of One Small Change

Don't think little changes mean small health benefits. A little tweak—such as switching from white bread to whole-grain bread or ordering unsweetened iced tea instead of a soda or fitting 10 minutes of exercise into a busy day—can add up to big health bonuses. Consider:

- A brisk walk three times a week can reduce mild, moderate, and even severe depression, Duke University researchers have found.

- If you're a TV fan who watches the small screen several hours a day, cutting out just 1 hour could reduce your risk for a serious prediabetic condition called metabolic syndrome by 19 percent, say Tufts University researchers.

- Switching to whole-grain bread, brown rice, and whole-grain breakfast cereal could lower your risk for diabetes by up to 33 percent, say German scientists.

- Drinking two glasses of nonfat milk per day could cut your risk for insulin resistance by 62 percent and cut your risk for heart disease by 50 percent, say British researchers who followed 2,375 men for 20 years as part of the United Kingdom's landmark Caerphilly Prospective Study.

- Losing just 1 pound lightens the load on your knees by 4 pounds with every step—that translates to 4,800 fewer pounds of pressure every time you walk a mile.

"Making small, slow changes is a great way to dive into healthier eating," notes anesthesiologist and dietitian Christine Gerbstadt, MD, RD, a spokesperson for the American Dietetic Association. "I suggest that people add a new change each week, but not sooner. You'll start to see and feel the difference in four weeks or less. Your digestion will improve, and you may have more energy. And things you can't see will be improving, too—such as immunity, blood fats, and blood sugar."

And never believe it's too late to start. When researchers at the Medical University of South Carolina tracked health-negligent, middle-age adults who began eating five or more fruits and vegetables every day, exercised for a half-hour five days a week, and didn't smoke, they reduced their risk for heart disease by 35 percent. After four years, they even got their risk down to the same safe level as people who had always been active and eaten a healthy diet.

So where do you begin? Read the eating, exercise, and everyday living chapters ahead and choose changes that appeal to you most. Perhaps they sound fun (or delicious or as if they'd feel really good … hmmmm … yoga anyone?). Maybe they're smart ways to finally overcome a not-so-healthy habit that's been bothering you (hmmm …. Fruity iced tea in place of gallons of sweet drinks … grilled fish instead of a cheeseburger … a walk with your best friend instead of meeting for coffee and dessert, perhaps?) Try one change in each important area … then commit to sticking with it for the next four weeks.

Train Your Brain for Health

Forming a new habit—one you'll do automatically, as your "default" setting—takes at least two weeks of faithful repetition. The reason: You're rewiring your brain. Researchers have discovered that giving up bad habits such as overeating, watching TV instead of exercising, or anything else that may feel good but isn't so good for your health works against the brain's pleasure systems. Your brain may actually go into withdrawal when you swap bad habits for good habits, because you're no longer supplying the activity or foods that send surges of the feel-good chemical dopamine washing through your brain cells.

Outsmart withdrawal by substituting another feel-good food or activity—the kind you'll find throughout the coming pages. Experts suspect that sticking with a new, healthier pleasure long enough will teach your brain to release dopamine when you experience it—so that you actually look forward to that walk or slice of whole-wheat cinnamon toast in the morning.

"A lot of people stick to the old myth that change has to hurt to be good for you," notes Karl Knopf, EdD, professor of Adaptive/Older Adult Fitness at Foothill College in Los Altos Hills, California. "That's especially true when they think about exercise—it's gotta be painful. No pain, no gain. But the fact is, if it feels bad, it will be very difficult to stick with it. Exercise should make you feel good—feel beautiful. It should match your body type, your likes and dislikes, and your needs. When it does that, you'll be able to stick with it."

That's where mindfulness comes in. As you make changes, check in with yourself throughout the day. A change that's right for you will help you feel energized yet relaxed. You may feel a little tired if you've just taken a walk or performed a few strength-training moves, but you shouldn't feel achy or exhausted. You may feel a little lighter in the tummy if you're eating more moderate portions, but you shouldn't feel starved. And if you're trying to add more relaxation, more hobbies, and more socializing to your day, you should expect to feel excited and busy, but never overwhelmed.

Why? Change shouldn't become a source of stress. Research shows that when it does, stress hormones impel us to do whatever we've always done to calm down. That might mean eating a cupcake or smoking a cigarette, having a glass of wine or complaining. Stress, then, can interfere with efforts to change.

Remember this point: If you start with changes that are easy to make, and stick with them for a few weeks, you'll find that the next wave of changes is even easier. And suddenly, you are well down the path toward the long health you desire.

Four Traits of Successfully Healthy People

1. **They're patient.** It takes at least two weeks—and probably more like four to eight weeks—to turn a new strategy into something that's second nature. You have to stick with it long enough to face all the challenges you meet regularly in your life and find a way to fit it in, no matter what. "If you can do something for three weeks in a row, you've established a good habit," says Mary Ann Wilson, RN, a nurse and fitness expert from Portland, Oregon, who hosts the television show *Sit and Get Fit*. "You know you've created a strong habit when you miss whatever it is if you don't do it—if you find yourself saying, 'oh, gosh, no wonder I'm not having a good day, I've forgotten my exercise today!'"

2. **They take it seriously.** Buy the healthy foods you need. Set aside time for socializing. Schedule exercise. Don't leave change to chance. "Put exercise on your calendar, so you'll think about the best time of day for you," Wilson says. "Making it a regular part of your day is really a big help."

3. **They get support.** Researchers at the University of Missouri found that older women exercised an extra 37 minutes a week when they got friendly, weekly phone call reminders. You can get even better motivation by joining or creating an exercise group or finding an exercise buddy—someone with whom you can walk or work out, or just communicate by phone or via an online support group.

4. **They know that small changes lead to big things.** "One change begets others," says Karl Knopf, EdD, professor of Adaptive/Older Adult Fitness at Foothill College in Los Altos Hills, California. "You have to open the door, see the benefits, and feel the rewards. Then it propagates itself—you motivate yourself to make more changes."

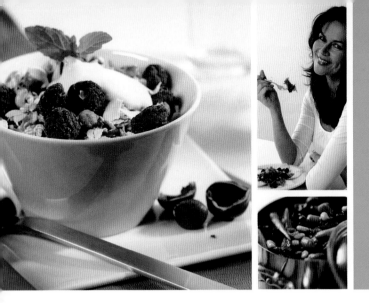

Eat to Feel Good

Imagine a place where joints ache less; minds and memories remain stronger; digestion problems are few; a good night's sleep is the norm; and energy levels stay shockingly youthful—even at age 90, and beyond.

Here, cancer is virtually unknown. People's arteries function as well at 85 as they did at 18—and their odds of having a heart attack or stroke are the lowest in the world.

Places like this do exist today—in Okinawa, on the sun-drenched Mediterranean island of Crete, and even in the modern 7th-Day Adventist households of America.

What do these people have in common? Primarily, a healthy attitude and an even healthier diet. The foods people eat every day in these Shangri-Las of longevity might amaze you. On a single day in Okinawa, the average person eats nearly a dozen helpings of fruit and vegetables, seven servings of noodles, rice, and grain, plus tofu, fish, seaweed, and green tea. Dairy foods and red meat are rarely seen—or eaten. At night, friends knock back a glass or two of a fiery alcoholic drink made with hot peppers.

The menu is similar on Crete, where poultry and fish replace soy foods as the primary protein and locals sip their own homemade red wines. The story is the same with 7th-Day Adventists, except they eat eggs and nuts for much of their protein. Many 7th-Day Adventists are vegetarians who also abstain from alcohol, tobacco, and coffee.

Notably absent from their diet: Salty, sweet, processed foods; buttery treats; juicy steaks; ever-flowing soda; and super-size portions.

The payoffs for a life free of cheese-drenched french fries, breakfast sweet rolls, and mega-gulp drinks? Healthy-eating 7th-Day Adventists live up to 9.5 years longer than other Americans, say researchers who tracked the diets and health histories of over 34,000 members of this Christian denomination. Okinawans have the longest life expectancies in the world—the average man lives to be 77, the average woman to 85. And more people on Okinawa have celebrated their 100th birthdays than people from anywhere else—35 in every 100,000. On Crete, the healthiest eaters were 25 percent less likely to die during a four-year study than their fellow countrymen who opted for more modern meals.

"We think diet plays an extremely important role in how long people in these parts of the world live and in how long they remain healthy, active, independent, and happy," says Bradley Willcox, MD, of the Pacific Health Research Institute in Honolulu and lead researcher of the Okinawa Longevity Study. "A low-calorie, low-fat, plant-based diet is the key to maximizing life expectancy and minimizing the risk for all of the debilitating health problems that come with aging."

In fact, what you put on your plate and in your mouth counts even more than whether or not you were born with longevity genes. "You could have Mercedes-Benz genes," says Dr. Willcox, "but if you never change the oil, you are not going to last as long as a Ford Escort that you take good care of."

You'd be surprised how much food many healthy people eat. Their secret: eating the right foods.

The ⑦ Choices of Long Life Eating

Here's the important point: You don't have to be born in one of these cultures to get their kitchen-table health benefits. Anyone, anywhere, anytime can eat for health and long life. If you really wish, you can start from this very moment forward, with your very next meal or snack. The benefits would be immediate.

"You'll feel more energetic, have better digestion, and even sleep better in just two to four weeks," says Christine Gerbstadt, RD, MD, a dietitian and practicing physician. "It's exciting how quickly you can feel the difference!"

That's just the start of the benefits, too. You'll have fewer colds as your immune system improves. Your body will naturally get to its proper weight. And you'll take bold steps to prevent the diseases that most plague our senior years. "Four out of the 10 leading causes of death in America—heart disease, stroke, diabetes, and cancer—have a huge diet component to them," notes Susan Moores, RD, an expert on nutrition for older people. "What we eat—and how we eat it—makes a big difference in our health."

The challenge is that if you ask 100 doctors the specifics of a healthy diet, you'll get 100 different answers. We're here to help. After taking a close look at the diets of the world's healthiest people, matching up those practices with the best scientific research, and then talking at length with many top experts on nutrition and health, what emerged were seven golden choices for eating for energy, disease prevention, and long life. We call them choices rather than guidelines, laws, or rules because we want *you* to be the one to decide that they are right for you. Only if you decide in your heart that they are worth doing will you take action!

Here they are in a nutshell; in the pages ahead, we'll get far more specific on how to make each choice super-easy to achieve.

Choice 1
Make more than half of your diet beans, fruits, and vegetables.

Human beings evolved on a diet that was at least 70 percent these three ingredients—and your body hasn't altered its nutritional expectations much over the past million years. And that's how most of us ate—until a few decades ago, when breakthroughs in convenience morphed our diet toward processed "food products" packaged in boxes, cans, wrappers, and freezer containers. It is no coincidence that these dietary changes have been paralleled by a massive rise in diseases linked to food, from heart disease to diabetes.

A mountain of research shows that making produce and legumes the centerpiece of meals and snacks—as they once were—is a powerful health insurance policy. There are several reasons, but one of the biggest is that plant matter is packed with compounds called phytochemicals that disarm free radicals. These are rogue oxygen molecules, created naturally in the body and also ingested with toxins and pollutants, that damage cells and raise the risk of cancer, heart disease, and many other health problems.

One Harvard School of Public Health study of 39,127 women found that those who ate more than 10 fruit and veggie servings per day had a 38 percent lower risk of heart attack than those who had less than 3 servings. Men who ate 9 servings a day cut stroke risk 39 percent. Just 5 servings a day lowers diabetes risk by 39 percent. A similar eating strategy cut levels of "bad-guy" LDL cholesterol 33 percent *in just two weeks*.

A more natural diet goes a long way toward protecting you from cancer as well. An extra helping or two of produce at each meal could cut your odds for stomach cancer by 21 percent, lung cancer by up to 32 percent, ovarian cancer by as much as 40 percent, and prostate cancer by 35 percent (even higher if you include lots of broccoli, cabbage, and brussels sprouts—and we'll show you how to make them taste great). Researchers aren't sure whether produce can protect against breast cancer, though one analysis found that cruciferous veggies like cabbage may help.

Choice 2
Eat more whole-grain foods.

Dietary fiber—also called bulk or roughage—is simply the parts of plant foods that your body cannot absorb or digest. Whole-grain foods are filled with it. Eat more fiber, and you'll fill up faster, making weight control a breeze. Fiber also eases constipation and diarrhea. In the long term, fiber can help control cholesterol, balance your blood sugar, and lower your risk of hemorrhoids, irritable bowel syndrome, and diverticular disease (the development of small pouches in the colon).

But whole grains deliver so much more than just fiber. When you add whole-grain breads and pastas, brown rice, and other grains to your diet, you're getting not only the chewy, high-fiber hulls (the bran) that cover the grain but also the nutrition-packed germ and endosperm found in each grain. This complete grain package is a rich source of niacin, thiamin, riboflavin, magnesium, phosphorus, iron, and zinc, as well as protein and a smidge of good fat. This extra nutrition may be one reason people who eat whole grains have a reduced risk of diabetes and heart disease.

Eat food from farms, not factories

Choice ③
Eat more "good" fats.

Learn the phrase "omega-3 fatty acids." This is the one type of fat in our diet that is truly terrific for our health. Omega-3s are found in foods such as fish, nuts, and olive or canola oil. They are the building blocks for hormone-like compounds that reduce chronic inflammation—a modern health problem fired up by too much belly fat, too little exercise, and a diet brimming with the wrong types of fats. New lab studies show that your body also uses good fats to make useful inflammation-fighting chemicals called resolvins.

Yet most of us eat far too few omega-3s these days, and far too many omega-6s—a fat found in high levels in corn, safflower, soybean, sunflower, and sesame oils. Omega-6 fats help your body produce compounds that *increase* inflammation. In prehistoric times, people ate omega-3s and omega-6s in nearly equal proportions; today, we consume as many as 30 times more omega-6s. Eating yummy foods like salmon, peanut butter, walnuts, and good-for-you oils can correct this balance. You'll slash your risk of heart attack and stroke and possibly cut your odds for arthritis pain and depression, too.

Choice ④
Eat calcium-rich foods.

Calcium's not just for bones anymore. While 99 percent of the calcium in your body is hard at work maintaining the strong, internal scaffolding that supports bones and teeth, the remaining 1 percent is a major player in keeping your cardiovascular system happy and your blood sugar control mechanisms healthy. A growing stack of research proves that calcium helps lower blood pressure, keeps arteries flexible, and assists your kidneys in flushing blood pressure–boosting sodium out of your body.

In concert with other minerals such as magnesium and potassium, calcium can also lower your risk of insulin resistance—a potent risk factor for heart disease, diabetes, and even some cancers—by up to 71 percent. It may also guard against memory loss and cut colon cancer risk by 36 percent.

All this said, there's a controversy brewing about just how much calcium we really need. While major health organizations in the United States still recommend high levels, some experts and health organizations in other countries suggest that less milk and less calcium may be sufficient to protect bones and more. Stay tuned—we'll sort it all out later on.

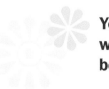
Yes, pork and beef fat taste wonderful. But for long life, the best fats come from plants and fish.

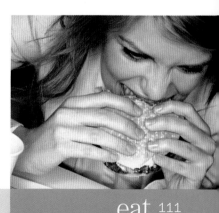

Choice 5
Enjoy lean protein.

Protein is your body's basic building material—used to make everything from muscles, bones, and the tissues of internal organs to hormones, enzymes, and even red blood cells. Putting lean protein on your plate delivers an immediate payoff: Meats, low-fat cheeses, eggs, and nuts linger longer in your stomach than bread, rice, fruit, or veggies, so you feel full longer. Protein also slows the absorption of sugar into your bloodstream, eliminating cravings that occur when sugar soars, then crashes after a carb-heavy meal.

Lean protein is also a rich source of the B vitamins that can help you feel more energetic, since the Bs help guide metabolic reactions throughout the body. You also get zinc, which builds strong immunity, and niacin, vital for clear thinking and efficient processing of blood sugar.

Protein's biggest bonus is preserving lean muscle mass. We all lose muscle mass at the rate of 3 to 5 percent per decade starting in our mid-twenties. By our fifties and sixties, we've lost plenty—and may be weaker, have poorer balance, and have slower metabolisms. Protein contains an amino acid called leucine that helps preserve more muscle mass, studies show.

Choice 6
Eat fewer calories.

Note that we didn't say eat less food. Fruits, veggies, and beans are filling and satisfying yet contain far fewer calories than fatty foods. That means you can usually eat them to your heart's content and still consume fewer calories.

But it's not inappropriate to face the hard question of whether you do eat too much food overall. Okinawans don't eat till their buttons burst. Instead, they practice a form of natural portion control called *hara hachi bu*, which literally means "80 percent full." In other words, they stop eating before they feel completely filled up.

"*Hara hachi bu* is sort of an insurance plan against feeling deprived or overeating," says Dr. Willcox. "It takes about 20 minutes for the body to signal the brain that there's no need for more food. *Hara hachi bu* gives the brain a chance to catch up." That restraint, plus a diet filled with low-calorie, high-satisfaction produce—and cooking techniques that use water (steaming and boiling) rather than frying or sautéing with oil—means that Okinawans eat about 1,800 calories a day, which is hundreds less than the typical Westerner scarfs down in a day.

Don't get us wrong—we don't advocate extreme calorie restriction. So far, no one's proven that drastically cutting calories extends human life (all those headline-grabbing studies show it works only in fruit flies and lab mice!). And when humans try it, super-low-cal eating seems only to lead to crankiness and potentially dangerous nutrient deficiencies.

But experts like Dr. Willcox believe that cutting back *a little*, without denying yourself the nutrients you need and the eating pleasure you desire, is an important reason Okinawans and others live to a vibrant old age. Why? Fewer calories mean lower body weight and less of the dangerous abdominal fat that raises risk for heart disease, stroke, diabetes, high blood pressure, and even some cancers—and perhaps even Alzheimer's disease. Living at a healthy weight also puts less stress on joints and may reduce the levels of cell-damaging free radicals in your body, too.

Meals should celebrate life.

Choice 7
Enjoy eating.

Sharing mealtime with family or friends, enjoying the smells and tastes of the foods before you, invoking feelings of gratitude and of being blessed—all of these make life worth living. Meals among the world's healthiest people are long, happy occasions, not something to rush through or gobble while watching TV. In Greece, the nation's official dietary guidelines include advice to "eat slowly, preferably at regular times of the day, and in a pleasant environment."

"Enjoying food is almost as important as the nutrients in the food itself," says Moores. "And meals need not be fancy to be cherished and savored." It's more an attitude of life-enhancing reverence and celebration. Small wonder that one way Greeks identify someone as a friend is by saying "we have shared bread together."

Beyond Food

Ahh, then there's the reality of the modern diet: Huge helpings of meat, mountains of grains stripped of their key nutrients, and processed food galore, filled with factory-engineered sweeteners, flavors, colors, and preservatives. Not only does the modern diet give you lots of what you don't need, it also shortchanges you on what you *do* need.

Many of the classic signs of aging—including fatigue, aches and pains, memory lapses, fuzzy thinking, balance problems, and more—may actually be symptoms of unrecognized yet easily reversible nutritional shortfalls, says Jeffrey Blumberg, PhD, of the Jean Mayer USDA Human Nutrition Research Center on Aging at Tufts University in Boston. Just because you feel that you're aging, Dr. Blumberg says emphatically, that doesn't mean it's because you really *are* aging. It's more how you are eating.

What do we mean by nutritional shortfalls? Consider B_{12}, a vitamin crucial for maintaining healthy nerves and red blood cells. As you grow older, your stomach produces less hydrochloric acid, and as a result, your body absorbs less B_{12} from food. Taking an acid-suppressing drug to protect against stomach ulcers (as millions of older people do) may cut absorption even further, experts suspect.

The result: One-fourth of Americans age 50 are low in B_{12}; by age 75, the number rises to 40 percent. Most don't know it, but they may be experiencing troubling signs of low B_{12}, such as memory lapses, tiredness, joint pain, and tingling hands and feet. Healthy foods are a big part of the answer, but so is a multivitamin, since the form of B_{12} in supplements is easier for your body to absorb than the form found in foods.

Then there's vitamin D: In your seventies, your skin synthesizes 60 percent *less* D than it did when you were a child, Harvard Medical

5 Foods to Protect Your Arteries

These amazing foods can: reduce your risk of atherosclerosis ● whittle your cholesterol ● lower your blood pressure ● cool inflammation ● neutralize damaging free radicals ● reduce your chances of developing metabolic syndrome by keeping blood sugar lower and steadier ● keep your heart pumping at a healthy beat

1 **Roasted almonds—with the skins.** A single fistful of almonds packs a whopping 9 grams of monounsaturated fat to help slash bad cholesterol and boost good cholesterol. Simply choosing almonds instead of a doughnut, chips, or pretzels for two snacks a day could cut "bad" cholesterol by nearly 10 percent. Natural vitamin E in the almond's "meat" plus flavonoids in this nut's papery skin help halt the development of artery-clogging plaque.

2 **Avocados.** In a study from Mexico's Instituto Mexicano del Seguro Social, women and men who ate one avocado per day for a week had a reduction in total cholesterol of 17 percent. The amazing details: While their levels of unhealthy LDL and triglycerides fell, good HDL levels actually rose— thanks, perhaps to the avocado's high levels of "good" monounsaturated fat. This fatty fruit is also full of cholesterol-cutting beta-sitosterol.

3 **Tomatoes—fresh, sundried, and in sauce.** Eating seven or more servings per week cut risk of cardiovascular disease by 30 percent in a recent study of more than 35,000 women conducted by doctors at Boston's Brigham and Women's Hospital. The heart-smart factor? It could be the antioxidant lycopene or the tomato's stellar levels of vitamin C, potassium, and fiber. Cooking tomatoes for 30 minutes or longer raises levels of available lycopene. And 1/4 cup of sun-dried tomatoes has more blood pressure–lowering potassium than a medium banana.

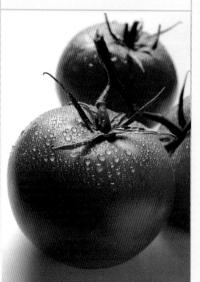

4 **Canned salmon.** Among omega-3–rich fatty fish, salmon is king: One serving contains about 1.8 grams of eicosapentaenoic acid (EPA) and docosahexaenoic acid (DHA), important omega-3s that help cut your risk of deadly out-of-rhythm heartbeats; reduce bad cholesterol; cool inflammation; and may even discourage atherosclerosis and the formation of blood clots.

5 **Old-fashioned oatmeal.** Betaglucan, the soluble fiber found in oats, acts like a sponge, trapping cholesterol-rich bile acids in the intestines and eliminating them. The result is lower "bad" LDL because there's less cholesterol to be absorbed into the bloodstream. A big bowl of oatmeal per day (about 1 1/2 cups) could cut cholesterol an extra 2 to 3 percent, suggests a study published in the *Journal of the American Medical Association*.

School researchers have found. (Staying indoors or wearing sunblock cuts it even further.) Small wonder, then, that about one-fourth of people over age 60 have low vitamin D levels; as a result, they may be at higher risk for brittle bones, muscle weakness, and a stunning variety of cancers.

Again, healthy foods to the rescue, in the form of low-fat milk, seafood, and greens. But that multivitamin is also the perfect form of insurance.

Or take a look at the curious case of calcium. "For some reason, people think they don't need calcium as much when they're older," says Moores. "They think it's only important early in life, during the bone-building years of your childhood, teens, and early twenties. But the fact is, women and men need even more calcium after age 50 than before because absorption drops with age." A whopping 9 out of 10 older people don't get enough calcium from food, and plenty don't take calcium supplements. But research confirms that inexpensive calcium pills can bridge the gap for women and may help men, though some experts warn that extra calcium could raise prostate cancer risk.

In addition, many prescription medicines and over-the-counter remedies can also create nutritional shortfalls by blocking absorption or speeding up the excretion of vitamins and minerals. Among the big culprits are acid-suppressing drugs (such as Pepcid, Prilosec, Prevacid, Tagamet, and Zantac) that target heartburn and other gastrointestinal problems. But antibiotics, antidepressants, cholesterol-lowering statin drugs, diabetes drugs, diuretics, pain relievers, laxatives, and tranquilizers all can cut levels of many vitamins and minerals, research shows.

The combination of a less-than-healthy diet and nutrient-draining medications may help explain why two landmark studies, the Framingham Heart Study and the Baltimore Longitudinal Study on Aging, found that older people often face these health-threatening nutritional shortages as well.

- Thirty percent of people ages 67 and older don't get sufficient folic acid, a vitamin that may play a role in heart health.

- Twenty percent are low in B_6—a vitamin that plays a role in sleep, appetite, and mood.

- In addition, most older women and men may not get enough magnesium—important for healthy blood pressure, and zinc—important for wound healing, immunity, and maintaining your sense of smell and taste.

For all these reasons, we are convinced that a trio of daily supplements—a multivitamin, a calcium supplement, and fish-oil capsules—offer sufficient benefits to justify making them part of your daily routine. Studies prove that these can fill real nutritional gaps—sometimes, as is the case with B_{12} and vitamin D, even better than food or sunshine.

We'll cover these three supplements in greater detail later in this chapter. But let us reiterate our key point: For long life and ongoing health, it's mostly about food. Diet expert Moores says it well: "Supplements may help fill in gaps, but the best way to get the nutrition you need is from the foods you eat. There are nutrients in food, thousands of nutrients, we don't even know about yet. They're buddies that work together in our bodies to keep us healthy—something pills can't do. That's the beauty of food."

And so, without further ado, here are the seven choices of Long Life Eating and hundreds of tips and tricks to make each an easy part of your daily meal routine.

Is Your Diet Making You Old?

Quiz ✳

Pick the answers to these 11 questions that best reflect your current eating patterns.

1 **My usual breakfast is:**

a. Oatmeal or high-fiber cereal with low-fat milk and some fruit.

b. Sausage or bacon, an egg, and a muffin.

c. A cup of coffee and maybe a slice of white toast.

2 **My favorite fruits:**

a. Change with the seasons: I love berries, peaches, watermelon, apples, mangoes, and more!

b. Are the occasional apple, orange, or banana.

c. Are the cherries in chocolate-cherry ice cream.

3 **On a typical day, I eat this many vegetables:**

a. Loads—a salad or soup with lunch, several helpings at dinner, and even a helping as a snack.

b. Two—a salad or side dish with dinner and maybe some lettuce or tomatoes at lunch.

c. One—assuming french fries and ketchup count.

4 **Whole grains are a _____ part of meals in my house:**

a. Big. We eat whole-grain bread and brown rice, and have tried other grains, too.

b. Small. I get brown breads sometimes or wheat crackers.

c. Nonexistent. I prefer the comforting, smooth texture of white bread, white rice, and white noodles.

5 **My beverage of choice is:**

a. Water.

b. Coffee or hot tea.

c. Soda, fruit punch, or bottled tea.

6 **When I eat chicken, I:**

   a. Usually have it sliced (without skin) into vegetables, salads, or other dishes.

   b. Have it grilled, with the bone and skin.

   c. Have it battered and fried.

7 **My regimen for supplements is:**

   a. Consistent—I take a multivitamin every day, plus one or two other smart choices.

   b. Inconsistent—I've got lots of vitamins in my kitchen cabinet, and once in a while, I might even take one.

   c. Nonexistent—vitamins are not a part of my life.

8 **When it comes to dairy foods, I:**

   a. Make sure I have several low-fat servings a day.

   b. Have an occasional container of yogurt, cup of milk, or piece of cheese.

   c. Add milk to my coffee—that's about it.

9 **When I grocery shop, my cart is mostly filled with:**

   a. Unprocessed foods, such as fruits, vegetables, eggs, orange juice, and raw meat.

   b. A mix of fresh foods, packaged foods, and frozen meals.

   c. Boxes, cans, jars, and precooked meals.

10 **My typical dinner is:**

   a. Slow and social. I eat with my family or, when possible, with relatives or friends.

   b. Quiet. I often watch TV or read while dining.

   c. Expedient. I just grab whatever's at hand and don't make a formal sit-down meal of it.

11 **If I were hungry at 3 p.m., I probably would:**

   a. Have a piece of fruit or a fistful of nuts.

   b. Tell myself that dinner is just a few hours away.

   c. Have a candy bar, cookie, bag of chips, or scoop of ice cream.

YOUR SCORE

If you circled mostly (a.)

answers: Your meals—and your way of eating—are in line with the age-defying traditions of long-lived, healthy people in places like Crete and Okinawa. You can take your nutrition-packed good habits to new heights by trying new fruits and vegetables, adding more types of whole grains to your cooking repertoire, snacking on good fat–rich nuts, and savoring mealtimes even more.

If you circled mostly (b.)

answers: You're modestly healthy, but you're not doing much to prevent disease or add healthy years to your life. Your diet's too low in fruits, veggies, whole grains, and bone-building calcium. And it's also too high in sugars, refined carbs, and artery-clogging fats. As a result, you may be feeling tired and moody, and have digestive problems. Choosing to eat well could help you feel better in just a few short weeks—and lay the foundation for years of better health ahead.

If you circled mostly (c.)

answers: Not only have you put yourself at greater risk for many serious diseases, but you are eating in a way that saps you of energy, reduces brainpower, and makes you susceptible to colds, flu, and other everyday challenges. The seven choices of Long Life Eating should become a top priority! Start by making small changes such as adding a multivitamin and calcium supplements to your daily routine, substituting fruit for sweets, and starting meals with a salad. You'll soon discover that healthy eating is filling, flavorful, and downright pleasurable. And you'll feel better immediately.

Choice ① Make more than half of your diet beans, fruits, and vegetables.

Want to slash your risk for everyday health problems like migraine headaches, colds and flu, and slow-healing wounds, as well as big medical problems like heart disease, cancer, and dimming vision? Skip the drugstore—and drive straight to your local farmer's market instead.

"Eating lots of fruit, vegetables, and legumes—foods high in antioxidants and other phytochemicals—is the cornerstone of the diets of healthy, long-lived populations around the world," says Dr. Willcox. "It's one reason their rates for heart disease and many cancers are so low. When we compared the Okinawan diet to the typical Japanese diet, we found that Okinawans ate so much of these foods that they had three times the recommended levels of vitamin C, almost double the vitamin E, and their antioxidant intake was really high, too. So were calcium, magnesium, and phosphorus—important for bone health and high blood pressure prevention. It's the power of good carbohydrates."

A glass of Concord grape juice at breakfast, a big spinach-and-white-bean salad at lunch, and a fruit salad after dinner provide immediate gratification, too. In one Australian study of 453 women and men ages 70 and older, those who ate the most healthy foods had the fewest signs of wrinkles! Treating yourself to the hundreds of important disease-fighting compounds found only in plant foods boosts immunity, speeds wound healing, and cuts your odds for everyday annoyances such as easy bruising, frequent nosebleeds, yeast infections, hemorrhoids, gout, and attacks of asthma brought on by physical activity.

At work are thousands of beneficial compounds collectively known as phytochemicals. Among the best known are antioxidants, which protect cells from damage by free radicals (notice how often these rogue oxygen molecules get mentioned?) As we've discussed, free radicals damage cell membranes as well as the DNA that encodes the cell's operating instructions. Free radical damage has been linked to many major diseases. What neutralizes them best? Antioxidants found in plant-based foods.

Other important phytochemicals include:

- Carotenoids that help cells communicate better (possibly cutting cancer risk)
- Lutein, zeaxanthin, and other compounds that act almost like sunglasses to protect your eyes from vision-robbing sun damage
- Flavonoids that can attack invading viruses and bacteria
- Building blocks for vitamin A that improve immunity by promoting the growth of the thymus gland, bolstering the functioning of white blood cells, and keeping the delicate tissues inside your mouth and nose strong to deter disease-causing invaders better.

Fruits and vegetables aren't the only plant foods loaded with phytochemicals. Dark chocolate, green and white tea, and wine are tops, too. When 130 chocoholics got kicked out of a recent Johns Hopkins University study on aspirin/heart disease because they couldn't give up their favorite fun food, researchers decided to study them as a separate group—and found that chocolate-eaters had lower blood-clotting rates. Their conclusion: An ounce of dark chocolate a day may be good for your heart.

"Eating a little bit of chocolate or having a drink of hot cocoa as part of a regular diet is probably good for personal health, so long as people don't eat too much of it and too much of the kind with lots of butter and sugar," says Diane Becker, MPH, ScD, a professor at Johns Hopkins University School of Medicine and the Bloomberg School of Public Health. Pair it with the right red wine (read on for our own Long Life wine list) or a steaming cup of tea for even more phytochemical prowess.

True Superfoods

Low in calories, high in satisfaction, and downright delicious (who can say no to a perfectly ripe peach in summer or a steaming bowl of bean soup on a snowy winter evening?), fruits, vegetables, and legumes deserve a starring role on your plate. Eat them to your heart's content, suggests Dr. Willcox, one of the lead researchers for the Okinawa Longevity Study. "I never limit produce or legumes," he says. "When I'm hungry, I'll have some ripe pineapple or strawberries. I don't count my servings of legumes, either. They're higher in calories but so satisfying that you really can't overdo it, as long as you watch the added fat."

This is a very important point, worth reiterating. As long as you don't use lots of oil or high-calorie add-ins, you can healthily eat as much fruit, vegetables, and beans as you wish. No limit! (The exceptions are people who have diabetes or are prone to big blood sugar swings; then sweet fruit should be eaten in greater moderation.)

Beans in particular are antioxidant superstars. When researchers analyzed the antioxidant concentrations in more than 100 foods, small red beans came in first, followed by red kidney beans and pinto beans in second and third place, respectively. And as you'll discover later on, beans are packed with fiber and are a terrific source of protein. No single food can help you fulfill the Long Life Eating guidelines as well as beans.

But let's not undersell vegetables! You can't go wrong if you shop in season. Just-ripe fruits and veggies have the highest levels of vitamins and antioxidants; levels decline as produce sits on the shelf. And don't assume that raw is better than cooked. Some phytochemicals are actually more available for absorption when veggies are processed, such as the prostate-protecting lycopene in tomato sauce and the carotenoids in lightly steamed spinach and carrots.

Don't shy away from convenience produce, either, says dietitian and physician Dr. Gerbstadt. "Prepackaged, single-serving bags of baby carrots or raisins are one serving, and they're ready to go," she says. "Other options include half-cup servings of fruit in juice, available in the canned fruit section. Even fruit roll-ups count if they're all fruit. So do all-fruit pops—just look for brands that are 99 percent fruit and have very little sugar; I've seen some with just 4 grams per pop."

LONG LIFE EATING GOAL: At least 5 servings per week

Have main-dish beans on Tuesdays and Thursdays. For those who don't eat beans that often, it's hard to think up many interesting meals in which beans are the star. But a glance at a bean cookbook will be a revelation. Beans are the successful centerpiece of many stews, soups, cassoulets, whole-meal salads, and even sandwich spreads. Find a few recipes and give them a try!

Always have beans on hand. Your pantry should contain a large assortment of canned beans ready for cooking (rinse twice to remove added sodium) and plenty more dried beans for overnight soaking and cooking. Both are healthy, but dried beans have more crunch and texture and aren't salted and flavored like many canned beans. We suggest using dried beans when you're cooking a bean dish from scratch (change the water before simmering to remove indigestible sugars that cause bloating and embarrassing personal gas!). Use canned beans when you want to toss some into other types of dishes.

Add beans to everyday dishes. Beans go well in rice dishes and even better in soups. They work fine in pasta sauces and add texture to roasts. Every time you cook a dish, ask yourself, "Can I add some beans to this?"

Make dips and spreads. No need to keep their original form. Blend beans with herbs, garlic, olive oil, or other flavorings and use as dips for vegetables or spreads for sandwiches or hors d'oeuvres.

Mix plain canned beans with baked beans. The tasty sauce in canned baked beans is full of sugar and calories. Keep the taste and lose some of the sugar by mixing in small red beans or kidney beans. Serve at lunch with a low-fat sandwich or hot dog.

Make this marvelous lunch. Just toss together black beans, baby spinach, mandarin orange sections, and spicy vinaigrette. Add other high-antioxidant veggies left over from last night's dinner, such as steamed broccoli or beet slices.

Use beans as a garnish. Keep chickpeas (garbanzo beans) in a sealed bowl in the refrigerator and put it on the table at every meal. Get in the habit of adding a few to your salads, your vegetables, or your pasta. Or just nibble on them as you would if a bowl of olives or almonds were on the table.

Great Combinations

Not sure which bean's best? Try these flavor suggestions.

Black beans: Great with brown rice and in Mexican dishes.

Black-eyed peas: Good in casseroles and curries or paired with ham and rice in Southern-style entrées.

Chickpeas (garbanzo beans): Toss into minestrone or mash with garlic and a touch of sesame seed paste (tahini) for classic hummus dip.

Fava or broad beans: Add to stews or serve alone as a side dish.

Lima beans: Use for succotash or mix with canned baked beans.

Navy beans: Stir into Boston baked beans.

Pinto beans: Pair with rice.

Red beans and kidney beans: Good in three-bean salads, chili, and spicy Cajun dishes.

White beans (cannellini): Delicious in chicken broth–based soups.

LONG LIFE EATING GOAL: 3 to 5 servings per day

Have a piece of fruit with breakfast every day. Toast and an apple. A roll and a banana. A bowl of cereal and berries. Yogurt with cantaloupe. Fruit is the perfect breakfast food. Make it a mandatory part of your day's start.

Have citrus as your midmorning snack. Most of us have a midmorning nosh. Make your choice an orange! One serving a day of citrus cuts the risk of mouth cancer—the seventh most common cancer—by 67 percent, according to an Italian analysis of 16 studies. Like variety? Try a different citrus fruit every week, from blood oranges to sweet-tart Mineolas, juicy clementines to luscious navel oranges, tart white or yellow grapefruit to sweet red grapefruit.

Eat fruit for dessert six nights a week. When scientists for the giant US cereal company General Mills measured antioxidants in fruit, the winning choices read like the perfect shopping list: blackberries, raspberries, blueberries, strawberries, red plums, black plums, red grapes, red apples, green grapes, nectarines, bananas, kiwi, pineapple. Why not eat a bunch of them at once? Having a brimming fruit salad after dinner most nights of the week equals at least two produce servings and a huge variety of good-for-you phytochemicals. Cut fruit will keep for six to nine days with minimal loss of vitamin C, carotenoids, or other phytonutrients, say researchers who tested mangos, strawberries, watermelon, pineapple chunks, kiwi slices, and cantaloupe cubes. Just store it in a covered container. Fruit salad too hard to make? Then make dessert a handful of strawberries, or a peach, or banana slices topped with orange juice. Fruit is the perfect way to end a nice meal.

Always keep frozen fruit on hand. It's a perfect summertime Sunday project: Visit a farmer's market or pick-your-own fruit farm, get a large quantity of your favorite berries or tree fruit, take it home, clean it all, and pack it up for the freezer. Then you'll have year-round local produce, perfect for blender drinks, pies, sauces, salads, and toppings for that special healthy dessert treat. Don't want to do the work yourself? Most food stores sell frozen fruit. Prices are best in season, though, so don't wait until winter to stock up.

Stock up on canned fruit, too. It's nearly as nutritious as fresh, and you'll avoid "Uh-oh, I've suddenly got 10 overripe bananas" syndrome. We love mandarin oranges packed in juice, low-sugar peach slices, pineapple tidbits, and unsweetened cherries. Have a half cup over oatmeal or high-fiber cereal at breakfast; spoon some onto yogurt and top with a dusting of good fat–rich crushed walnuts at lunch; or heat with your favorite warm spices (cinnamon, cloves, allspice, ginger, nutmeg), thicken with a little cornstarch, and serve with chicken or ham. We love single-serving, pull-top canned fruit, too. Toss a can into your tote bag along with a plastic spoon, and you've got a healthy snack.

Shop European-style. That is, stop at a fruit market every few days, buy small amounts of what looks the very best, and eat it within a day or two. This is so much more pleasant than buying large bags of the same ol' stuff at the chain grocery store every two weeks. And even if the fruit costs more at the small market, you'll probably save money by eating everything you buy. Sadly, when you buy infrequently, you tend to throw out more than you realize due to spoilage.

Fruit continued

Stock your kitchen gadget drawer with an apple slicer, a mango slicer, and a sharp box grater. With one push, an apple slicer divides your favorite Granny Smith, Golden Delicious or McIntosh into delectable slices and separates the pesky core. It does double duty as a pear corer, too. Build your repertoire of fruit uses with a mango slicer to easily turn balky mangos into sweet, ready-to-enjoy sections and a sharp box grater for grating apples into muffin batter and onto oatmeal.

Freeze the bananas. "Peel and wrap each one in plastic wrap, then freeze," Dr. Gerbstadt suggests. "Frozen bananas are a delicious, sweet snack. Better than a Popsicle!"

Savor a glass of *real* juice every day. Many packaged fruit drinks are laden with sweeteners and flavored artificially. But enjoying a glass of real orange juice (from a carton or from concentrate) or pure Concord grape juice every day is a healthy pleasure with a big payoff, experts say. One Vanderbilt University study found that people who enjoyed three glasses of fruit (or vegetable) juice a week had a 76 percent lower risk of Alzheimer's disease than those who had less than one glass per day. Or try pomegranate juice. Lab studies suggest it can cut the risk of brain degeneration and fight cancers of the breast, prostate, and skin. Bonus points: Choose orange juice fortified with bone-building calcium and vitamin D.

Let fruit and vegetables—not cake and soda—provide sweetness in your diet.

Choice **1**

Serve yourself a double portion—every time.
It's the simplest way to get more vegetables into your diet. At first, it'll seem odd to have your lunch or dinner plate be so full of green, but in time, it will be a welcome habit. Make sure you haven't "de-healthed" your vegetables with excessive butter, oil, or fat. Otherwise, your calorie count will surge. Also, don't double up on high-starch vegetables like corn and potatoes, since they're higher in calories.

Flavor your vegetables the tasty, healthy way.
Steamed or raw vegetables are boring. But you needn't smother them in butter or sauté them with bacon—as most restaurants do—to deliver great flavor. There are many ways to make vegetables delicious without pushing up their calorie counts.

- Drizzle with a little honey.

- Grate on a light sprinkling of cheese.

- Toss with olive oil, lemon, salt, and pepper.

- Mix with a small amount of soy sauce and sesame oil.

- Sprinkle with a vegetable-friendly herb like savory, rosemary, or basil.

- Grill with just a light coating of olive oil, salt, and pepper.

- Add a jolt of pepper heat with a few drops of a favorite hot sauce.

- Stir-fry with a little oil and curry powder.

Add microwaved baby carrots and frozen peas or chopped green beans every time you heat up soup. Microwaving the carrots allows you to add them to the soup fully cooked; otherwise, they need simmering time to soften. "And you get more vitamin A from cooked carrots, too," Dr. Gerbstadt says. Frozen vegetables need only to be heated through, so you can add them directly to the simmering soup. In a few minutes, you'll have a hearty lunch or a light supper.

Use veggies in place of pasta. Most sauces that work well on pasta work well on vegetables, too. Serve spaghetti sauce over steamed green beans or strands of luscious spaghetti squash. Make lasagna with strips of eggplant or zucchini in place of noodles. Make "cauliflower and cheese" in place of "macaroni and cheese."

Get into a raw-vegetable habit. Tomatoes, cucumbers, carrots, celery, radishes, broccoli, and bell peppers are just a few examples of vegetables that are outstanding to eat raw. Try to get in the habit of a daily raw-vegetable snack—

The Soy Truth
Experts no longer believe that soy's a magic bullet against heart disease, cancer, or menopausal hot flashes. But soy foods such as edamame (young green soybeans), tofu, and tempeh are low-fat meat substitutes that pack high levels of flavonoids and other antioxidants, says Dr. Bradley Willcox of the Pacific Health Research Institute in Honolulu. "Soy contains at least five different classes of flavonoids, from catechins to isoflavones, that have interesting physiological effects that other types of beans may not have to the same degree. Soy is a major part of the diet on Okinawa but certainly isn't in the Mediterranean diet. People in that part of the world eat different types of beans. It's just one option."

Choice ①

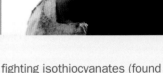

It's the craziest conundrum in the garden patch: Many of the healthiest vegetables taste unappetizingly bitter because of natural chemicals that give them their healing oomph.

Human taste buds are wired to detect minute amounts of bitterness in food, a trait that stopped cave dwellers from dining on poisonous wild plants. But thanks to a genetic quirk (and up to a sixfold higher concentration of taste buds), one in four adults is a "super-taster." These people are particularly sensitive to bitter chemicals—even if they're good for you. As a result, these people frequently skip proven heart-protecting, cancer-defying foods like beets, broccoli, brussels sprouts, cabbage, eggplant, kale, and spinach—all of which earned high marks on official lists of high-antioxidant vegetables.

Beets. Mix grated raw beets with lemon juice, golden raisins, and celery. Or roast with balsamic vinegar. In animal studies, the pigment responsible for the beet's purplish-red hue, called betacyanin, disarmed cancer-triggering toxins. The earthy taste of beets comes from geosmin, a type of chemical that also has cancer-fighting powers.

Broccoli. Mash steamed florets with potatoes or shred peeled broccoli stems and sauté with garlic and a dash of olive oil. One antioxidant that makes broccoli bitter, called sulforaphane, whisks cancer-promoting substances out of the body. Another, dubbed indole-3-carbinol by scientists, discouraged tumor growth in lab studies and reversed suspicious precancerous changes inside cervical cells in women.

Brussels sprouts. Roast 'em with onion chunks, then toss with rice vinegar. These broccoli cousins have plenty of bitter sulforaphane as well as compounds called isothiocyanates, which detoxify cancer-causing substances in the body before they can do their dirty work. In one Dutch study, guys who ate brussels sprouts daily for three weeks had 28 percent less genetic damage (gene damage is a root cause of cancer) than those who didn't eat sprouts.

Cabbage. Cook red cabbage, chopped apples (leave the skin on for more antioxidant power!), and raisins in apple juice; season with ground cloves. Eating cabbage a few times a week can cut your risk of cancer of the breast, prostate, lungs, and colon. In one study of 300 Chinese women, those with the highest blood levels of cancer-fighting isothiocyanates (found in cabbage) had a 45 percent lower risk of breast cancer than those with the lowest levels.

Eggplant. Brush with olive oil, sprinkle with oregano, and grill or broil. All types of eggplant are rich in bitter chlorogenic acid, which protects against the buildup of heart-threatening plaque in artery walls (and fights cancer, too!), say USDA scientists in Beltsville, Maryland. In lab studies, eggplant lowered cholesterol and helped artery walls relax, which can cut your risk of high blood pressure.

Kale. Braise in cider to offset bitterness. Kale has compounds called glucosinolates that seem to fight cancer by activating liver enzymes that help disarm carcinogens.

Spinach: Eat it fresh and raw. Create a salad dressed with pureed raspberries (defrost frozen raspberries first), balsamic vinegar, and a dash of canola or olive oil. Possibly the healthiest veggie in the world—thanks to high levels of vitamins A, B_6, C, and K and riboflavin, plus generous amounts of manganese, folate, magnesium, iron, and calcium—spinach also contains the antioxidant lutein, which protects the retinas in your eyes from damage or vision loss.

if you eat them unadorned, you can eat as many as you wish! Also, put out a plate of raw vegetables at every dinner. You and your loved ones will naturally nibble them throughout the meal.

Start every dinner with a salad. That's at least one serving—and if you fill your bowl with your favorite salad veggies, you'll start the meal with a smile. Be choosy. If you dislike iceberg lettuce, try a beautiful salad green mix or baby spinach. Add juicy produce like tomatoes, sliced red bell peppers, or even strawberries or raspberries. For more flavor, sprinkle chopped fresh herbs such as basil and cilantro on top. Drizzle with a teaspoon of olive oil and a teaspoon of lemon juice.

Sip vegetable juice with your afternoon snack. A glass of low-sodium, low-sugar vegetable juice counts as a full serving of vegetables. Tomato-based juices are high in the antioxidant lycopene.

Ask for a plain vegetable in place of potatoes or noodles when you eat in a restaurant. Choose one that's not fried or served in a creamy or oil-based sauce. If nothing fits that description, ask for a green salad instead.

Instead of cheese, add a thick layer of vegetables to your sandwich. We like dark green lettuce, fresh herbs, sliced tomatoes, and onion. But leftover vegetables from last night's dinner can be delicious, too: How about a turkey sandwich with grilled zucchini?

Turn cold cooked vegetables into a side salad. Don't let leftover green beans, peas, carrots, beets, asparagus, corn, or other vegetables go to waste. Simply serve with lunch as a cold salad, topped with a spritz of lemon juice and a dash of coarsely ground black pepper.

Use shredded vegetables in cooking. Finely shredded carrots, cabbage, lettuce, squash, and other vegetables add wonderful texture to many dishes that might not otherwise include such healthy ingredients. Add to soups, pasta sauces, and even rice dishes. Or use the vegetables as a bed for your chicken or fish. Smart habit: Keep a tightly sealed container of shredded vegetables in your refrigerator with the goal of using it up over the next three to four days. If you have a lot left after a few days, just sauté it with a bit of olive oil, lemon juice, and herbs for a terrific side dish.

The Two-Color Rule

It's simple: Always have fruits and veggies of two different colors on your plate. This holds for breakfast, lunch, and dinner. Start breakfast with a berry/citrus salad or have red and black berries with yogurt. Have red and orange bell peppers on your lunchtime salad. Heap your plate with purple-skinned eggplant and yellow/orange winter squash at dinner.
Why is this sensible? First, you'll automatically have two servings of produce. Second, they'll flood your body with a wider variety of beneficial antioxidants and other phytochemicals. Third, brightly colored fruits and vegetables are often more nutritious than subtler-colored versions. Two examples: Red-leaf lettuce has three times more antioxidants than green-leaf lettuce, and yellow and orange bell peppers have more than red or green peppers, experts report.

Choice **1**

Antioxidant Superfoods

LONG LIFE EATING GOAL: Up to: 1 ounce of quality dark chocolate a day, 1 alcoholic drink a day for women, 2 for men, 4 cups of green or white tea a day

Pair chocolate with citrus. Ascorbic acid in oranges, lemons, tangerines, and other citrus fruits may release more of the healthy antioxidants locked in cocoa, University of California researchers report. Try making a chocolate dip by heating one can (14 ounces) fat-free sweetened condensed milk and 7 ounces semisweet chocolate baking chips on low heat until the chocolate melts. Use as a dip for peeled, segmented clementines, tangerines, or sweet-tart Mineola oranges (serves eight).

Blend equal parts nuts, dried fruit, and mini chocolate chips for a delicious, high-antioxidant snack mix. Use dark chocolate, of course—it packs more antioxidants than milk chocolate. Include dates, raisins, and prunes, the dried fruits with the highest antioxidant levels, as well as pecans, walnuts, hazelnuts, pistachios, or almonds—all high-antioxidant nuts. Parcel out 2-tablespoon portions into tiny zipper-seal bags and freeze. Drop one in your purse or briefcase for a fun snack when you're out and about.

End the day with a cup of cocoa. Mix 8 ounces fat-free milk, a teaspoon or two of sugar or no-calorie sweetener, and 1 tablespoon dark cocoa powder in a cup. Microwave until hot, dust with cinnamon, and sip! When Dutch researchers studied the diets and health of 470 older men for 15 years, they found that higher cocoa intake was associated with lower blood pressure and a whopping 50 percent drop in risk of dying from heart disease.

Have a cup of green, black, white, or jasmine tea at midmorning and midafternoon. "Older, healthy people in Okinawa drank plenty of jasmine tea, which is rich in antioxidant catechins," Dr. Willcox notes. But skip the milk. A British study found that in your teacup, milk proteins bind to some beneficial compounds and could prevent absorption. A Swedish study of 61,000 women found that a cup of black tea a day lowered ovarian cancer risk by 24 percent.

Try instant green tea. One packet of instant green tea packs 40 milligrams of antioxidants—about half what you'd get from a cup of fresh-brewed tea. Bottled teas (get a diet or no-sugar-added variety) claim to have up to 55 milligrams per serving.

Or grab low-sugar, bottled cold tea. Cold tea is packed with antioxidants, too. Just look for one that's low in sugar (otherwise, bottled iced tea can be as high in calories as a cola!).

Toast your health with red wine. Take advantage of high concentrations of artery-scouring compounds found in these red varieties: Zinfandel, Syrah, Pinot Noir, and Cabernet Sauvignon, suggest University of California, Davis, researchers. (Tannat, a red wine variety that's big in southwestern France and Uruguay, is also super-high in tannins!) Or ask your wine salesperson for a wine that has been given extended contact with tannin-rich skins, seeds, and stems.

Of course, the most important thing to know about sipping wine for its health benefits is when to stop. Studies show that the safest limit is one 5-ounce glass a day for women and two 5-ounce glasses a day for men.

20 Top Antioxidants

Mother Nature tucked a medicine chest full of disease- fighting antioxidants into fruits, vegetables, grains, and even spices. These beneficial compounds fight damage to cells from rogue molecules called free radicals—and can help reduce your risk of heart disease, cancer, and dozens of age-related health problems.

Until recently, experts didn't know which foods had the highest levels. When researchers from the USDA's Arkansas Children's Nutrition Center in Little Rock tested the antioxidant power of more than 100 different foods, they got a surprise: Beans and berries are best.

1 Small red beans
2 Wild blueberries
3 Red kidney beans
4 Pinto beans
5 Cultivated blueberries
6 Cranberries
7 Artichoke hearts
8 Blackberries
9 Prunes
10 Raspberries

11 Strawberries
12 Red Delicious apples
13 Granny Smith apples
14 Pecans
15 Sweet cherries
16 Black plums
17 Russet potatoes
18 Black beans
19 Plums
20 Gala apples

Choice 2 Eat more whole-grain foods.

Once, high-fiber eating was perfectly natural because we ate mostly unprocessed foods. Then the rise of the processed food industry stripped our diet of fiber. What happened next was even worse. Once the need for fiber was recognized, manufacturers introduced a new crop of high-fiber health foods that made for less-than-pleasant eating—"bran" cereals that made you feel as if you were chewing on pebbles, gritty whole-wheat pasta, and health bars with the texture of sawdust. So health-conscious people took to the alternative, which wasn't very appealing either: mixing gluey fiber supplements with water, then downing it as quickly as possible.

No wonder the concept of "high-fiber" foods creates apprehension in many people. But fear not. Today, food store shelves are crammed with dozens of high-fiber cereals and whole-wheat breads that taste absolutely great and have wonderful texture. Delicious whole-grain pastas, brown rice, and more exotic grains are as commonplace as elbow macaroni. Despite this bounty, however, most of us manage to get just 12 grams of fiber a day—far short of the 20 to 30 grams recommended by health experts.

Fiber becomes more important with each passing birthday, simply because with age, food moves more slowly through the digestive system. Partly, it's a natural slowdown, but often, getting less physical activity and drinking less fluid play a role, too. How fiber helps: It makes your stools bulkier, which stimulates your digestive tract to keep things moving. (Of course, it's also important to drink plenty of water as you increase your fiber intake!)

Supplements work, but nothing beats the fiber in real food. "I'm a huge proponent of getting the fiber you need from fruits, vegetables, and especially whole grains," says Moores. "You can get fiber from a supplement, and it will help with constipation. But you'll be missing out on all the other wonderful nutrients you get in whole grains—the vitamin E, good fats, protein, and antioxidants that help protect against heart disease and diabetes and even cancer. You lose all that when you have white bread and white rice and white pasta, then make up the difference with a pill or a powder."

How much fiber do you need? The National Academy of Sciences recommends 21 grams a day for women 51 and older and 30 grams for men ages 51 and older. Your Long Life Eating goal: At least three whole-grain servings a day. That, plus a plate heaped with fruits and veggies, will help you meet or your fiber quota.

Getting fiber from a wide variety of sources yields the most health benefits, say French researchers who analyzed the diets and health of 6,000 people. They found that whole grains worked best for weight control, lowering blood pressure, and reducing levels of heart-threatening homocysteine in the bloodstream; fruits controlled tummy fat and cut blood pressure (thanks in part to all the fiber in the tiny seeds packed into berries); vegetables lowered blood pressure and homocysteine; and fiber in nuts had the strongest effects on weight control, tummy fat, and controlling blood sugar.

Switching to whole grains is one of the easiest eating upgrades you can make. After all, you probably already eat bread, rice, and noodles, so there's no need to add or subtract anything from your diet. Just reach for a different type. But if you're new to high-fiber eating, make your switch gradually—over the course of a month or so, suggests Dr. Gerbstadt.

"If you ratchet up your fiber all at once, you could have a lot of bloating, gas, even cramping," she says. "The first week, switch to whole-wheat bread and aim for four daily servings of vegetables and fruit. The second week, have six produce servings and add brown rice. The third week, go to nine servings of fruit and vegetables and give whole-grain pasta a try. During this time, eat more beans, too. They're a great source of fiber."

High-Fiber Superfoods

We've already extolled the virtues of beans as antioxidant powerhouses, but their fiber content is among the best of any food. In fact, 15 of the top 20 foods on the US government's chart of best fiber sources are beans!

Beans contain both kinds of fiber: insoluble, which helps your gastrointestinal system eliminate waste products more quickly, and soluble, which forms a gel in your intestines that helps lower levels of "bad" LDL cholesterol by whisking it out of your body. Research shows that eating a cup of beans per day can lower cholesterol by up to 10 percent in just six weeks. In fact, no natural, ready-to-eat food has more fiber. And all that fiber, plus the protein, means beans register low on the glycemic index, a measure of food's impact on blood sugar.

Beans aren't the type of food you eat several times a day, though. More likely, you'll turn to breads and pasta for much of your fiber intake. But beware: Just 20 percent of the bread, crackers, and pasta sold in America are whole grain. Sadly, many bread manufacturers try to dupe buyers into believing their products are whole grain even when they're made primarily from refined flour. Don't fall for promotional lines that shout "100 percent wheat," "Multigrain," "Stone ground," or "Made with whole grains." These misleading descriptions (and others, such as "unbleached wheat flour," "cracked wheat," or "stoned wheat") aren't guarantees that you're buying a high-fiber bread made primarily with real whole grains. Rely on the full ingredients list on the packaging.

Another bread pitfall: Some dark, hearty-looking loaves, such as rye, pumpernickel, and brown breads sprinkled with oats and seeds, aren't high in fiber either. Rather, they are made in large part of refined white flour and made to look dark by the addition of ingredients such as molasses.

Not a bread eater? Then how about whole-grain cereal or oatmeal? Both are health superfoods. Betaglucan, the soluble fiber found in oats, acts like a sponge, trapping cholesterol-rich bile acids in the intestines and eliminating them. The result is lower LDL cholesterol because there's less cholesterol to be absorbed into the bloodstream. Having a big bowl of oatmeal per day (about 1 1/2 cups) could cut cholesterol by an extra 2 to 3 percent, suggests a study published in the *Journal of the American Medical Association.*

Healthy, filling, and ready to eat, whole-grain cereal is a perfect convenience health food you can eat straight from the box (in fact, it makes a terrific snack!). A Harvard study found that participants who ate whole-grain cereal every day were 17 percent less likely to die over the next several years from any cause and 20 percent less likely to die from cardiovascular disease than those who rarely or never ate whole-grain cereal. And there's a weight-control bonus. A recent survey found that women who have cereal several times a week weigh 9 pounds less than those who pass up a bowl of flakes.

Want whole-grain options for other parts of the day? Then add brown rice and other fiber-rich grains like barley or couscous to your dinner plate.

What's wrong with white rice? Milling and polishing rip off more than the chewy coating on rice; they also steal fiber and nutrients that make brown rice a delicious, satisfying, disease-battling superfood. Compared to white, brown rice packs four times more insoluble fiber as well as good amounts of niacin, vitamin B_6, magnesium, manganese, phosphorus, selenium, and vitamin E. Best of all, it's easy to find in supermarkets these days—even in quicker-cooking forms for nights when you just don't have 45 minutes to wait for dinner to cook.

Toast Your Health with Water!

Sparkling or still, bottled or straight from the tap, good, old-fashioned water could cut your risk of a deadly heart attack by as much as 54 percent—and at the same time ease constipation, boost flagging energy, and perhaps even lower your risk of cancers of the breast, prostate, and large intestine, research suggests.

In a study of 20,000 women and men, researchers from California's Loma Linda University found that those who downed at least five glasses of water every day had a significantly lower risk of heart attacks than those who wet their whistles with coffee, orange juice, and other beverages. Why? Water is absorbed readily into the bloodstream, keeping blood diluted and less likely to form heart-threatening clots. Other liquids, the researchers say, require digestion, a process that draws fluid out of the bloodstream, thickening the blood and increasing clot risk.

Are you getting enough water? After age 60, don't rely on feelings of thirst to tell, says registered dietitian Susan Moores, RD. "Your sense of thirst diminishes," she notes. "You may also be drinking less water so you don't have to deal with a urination problem such as stress incontinence in women or prostate problems in men."

The best way to know if you're fully hydrated? "Look at your urine—if it's pale and has only a faint odor, you're most likely getting enough," Moores suggests. "If it's dark, scanty, or has a strong odor, you probably need to drink more water and other fluids."

What you need:

about six glasses a day.

The standard advice to get eight glasses a day is now considered by many experts to be overstated, she says. "And remember that tea counts, too. So do coffee and juice, but try to get a lot of plain water as well. If you're eating a lot of juicy fruits and vegetables, you'll get fluid from them, too. A cup of cubed watermelon contains a half cup of water!"

Say a permanent good-bye to white bread.
Don't give yourself or your loved ones a choice. When your current bag of white bread is finished, don't buy another one. Use whole-wheat bread in all the same ways you'd use white. For French toast, with eggs, for a sandwich, and with dinner, whole-wheat bread can replace all the white bread you've used in the past. It's that simple. Even if you love crusty French loaves or baguettes, there are whole-grain alternatives that have a lovely texture and mix well with Mediterranean foods.

Create a bakery habit. You and your family deserve individually made, freshly baked bread. So why settle for a loaf made on an assembly line at a distant bread factory? Make it a habit: Stop at a good-quality bakery, say hello to the proprietor, and pick up healthy, whole-grain bread. Eat it over the next two days, then head back for a new loaf. Make it a never-ending cycle.

If you buy packaged bread, study the label.
Look for whole-wheat flour as the first ingredient, then check the nutrition facts label for the fiber content. Your goal: buy a loaf with at least 3 grams of fiber per slice.

Another clue: Look for products that display this health claim: "Diets rich in whole-grain foods and other plant foods and low in total fat, saturated fat, and cholesterol may reduce the risk for heart disease and certain cancers." Products displaying this health claim must contain at least 51 percent whole grain by weight.

What if the fiber's high, but the bread's not made from whole grain? Put it back and keep looking. Many high-fiber, "light" breads contain mostly refined white flour to which manufactur-

ers have added highly processed cottonseed, oat, or soy fiber. While the fiber can help with digestion (and prevent constipation), the loaf won't have the phytochemicals and nutrients of real whole-grain versions.

Try double-fiber whole-grain bread. Just as tender as regular whole-wheat bread, two slices of double-fiber bread can net you a whopping 10 grams of fiber.

Crunch it. Look for whole-grain crackers that supply at least 3 grams of fiber per serving. Choose a lower-fat, low-sodium variety, such as Scandinavian-style flatbreads that taste great with bean dip or nut butter or as a bread substitute for open-faced sandwiches. Five or six crackers count as one grain serving.

Make your own. Replace the white flour in bread, muffin, and quick-bread recipes with whole-wheat flour. Start with half whole wheat and half white. If you totally replace white with wheat, use 7/8 cup whole wheat for every cup of white you remove, since wheat flour has a heavier texture. In bread recipes, use a tablespoon to transfer the whole-wheat flour to the measuring cup instead of scooping or dumping; this introduces extra air into the flour, which makes loaves lighter. You can also replace some of the liquid in baked goods recipes with orange juice to temper the sharper, tannic-acid taste of wheat flour. Or try "white whole-wheat flour," which is milled from hard, white, winter-wheat berries rather than the hard, red, spring-wheat berries of traditional whole-wheat flours. It has a fiber and nutrient profile similar to that of standard whole-wheat flour.

Whole-Grain Cereal

LONG LIFE EATING GOAL: Have for breakfast at least 3 times per week.

Make cereal your breakfast default. That means starting each morning with a bowl of cereal, milk, and fruit. You can't get much healthier than that. Just find a cereal—or several—that you'll be happy to face first thing in the a.m. We're happy to report that there are dozens upon dozens of choices crowding supermarket shelves. Be sure yours fits our "superfood" criteria for cereal: It should be made with whole grains, contain at least 4 grams of fiber, and have only modest amounts of added sugar or corn syrup.

"The first item on the ingredients list should be a whole grain, such as whole wheat or whole oats," says Moores. "Look at the sugar content, too. Remember that 4 grams of sugar equals 1 teaspoon. So if you see 12 grams of sugar, the cereal's got the equivalent of 3 teaspoons—that's 1 tablespoon—of sugar. Lower is better; 4 to 5 grams is great to strive for."

Moores recommends a moderate fiber level, from 3 to 6 grams. "Higher-fiber cereals contain more bran—the high-fiber, low-nutrition outer covering of the grain. It serves one purpose—pushing things through your colon more effectively. High-bran cereals don't include the germ or the endosperm of the grain, and that's where all the great fats and vitamins and phytonutrients are. If you eat whole grains, beans, and fruit and vegetables throughout the day, you won't need a high-fiber cereal. But if you'd rather make a huge dent in your fiber quota first thing in the morning, remember to include other true whole grains throughout the day to make up the missing nutrients."

Use cereal as a topping. Keep a small box of high-fiber cereal in the cupboard to use as a crunchy topping on yogurt, oatmeal, fruit salads, and green salads, Moores suggests. "It almost acts as a fiber supplement."

Be sure to finish the milk. The B vitamins added to cereals leach into milk quickly. Be sure to spoon up the milk at the bottom of the bowl to get the cereal's complete nutritional offerings.

New to higher-fiber cereal? Mix it half and half with an old favorite. You'll get loads more fiber than before, yet at the same time ease the transition to a new breakfast habit. The next week, fill your bowl with two-thirds higher-fiber brand and one-third old favorite. The week after, try sprinkling a little of your old standby over your new favorite cereal as a topping.

Put oatmeal on your breakfast table at least twice a week—more often in chilly weather. To eat more, start with old-fashioned oats and add a little brown sugar or maple syrup (or both!), dried or fresh fruit, chopped nuts, and fat-free milk. You'll get about 4 grams of fiber per cup.

Try this quick cooking method for old-fashioned oats. Bring a saucepan of water to a rolling boil, add the oats, and bring the water back to a boil. Turn off the heat, cover the pan, and take a shower. In 10 minutes, the oats will be ready to eat.

Or try long-cooking Irish oatmeal. This delicious, stick-to-your-ribs porridge takes 45 minutes to cook, unless you know this chef's secret: The night before, bring the oats and water to a boil, cover, and turn off the heat. In the morning, simply simmer for 5 to 10 minutes, until the oats are as tender as you like.

Serve no-worry brown rice in place of potatoes tonight. Yes, classic brown rice does require 45 minutes of cooking time, so you have to plan ahead a little. Make the cooking process easier by investing in a rice cooker (toss in rice and water and turn it on—no need to worry about a burned pot!) or cook a big batch of brown rice on the weekend and freeze meal-size portions in zipper-seal freezer bags. Reheat in the microwave on weeknights.

Stock instant, boil-in-bag or quick-cooking parboiled brown rice, too. These grains are cooked, then dried. Yes, they lose some texture along the way, but they retain most or even all of brown rice's fiber and nutrients. Their stellar quality: They cook in 5 to 20 minutes, making this convenience food great as a once-in-awhile fallback. You can also cook up quick brown rice to use in place of the ubiquitous tub of white that comes with Chinese takeout.

Replace white rice in recipes with brown. It works as well—or better—in chicken-and-rice dishes, stuffed cabbage, soups, and casseroles. You'll love pudding made with brown rice, too, for its nutty flavor and chunky yet tender texture.

Shop for another great grain this week. Other whole grains you may find in your grocery store or health food shop include amaranth, barley, kasha (buckwheat groats), couscous, millet, quinoa, wheat berries, and wild rice. Each has a unique flavor and texture. Try a new one each week. Give it the sniff test before purchasing to be sure the oils in the germ don't have a stale, rancid odor. Refrigerate or freeze grains to retain freshness.

Keep a supply of fast-cooking favorites on hand. We love pearled barley for its creamy texture, its 6 grams of fiber per cup (including cholesterol-lowering soluble fiber), and its fast cooking time: just 30 minutes. It's a delicious side dish replacement for rice and gives soups and stews a soft, thick texture. Bulgur is just whole wheat that's been steamed, dried, and cracked. Think of it as a whole-grain convenience food; it cooks in 20 minutes. Traditionally used for Middle Eastern tabbouleh (a salad with bulgur, tomatoes, cucumber, and parsley), it also makes a delicious side dish. Couscous is really a tiny-grained pasta made from wheat flour. The catch: Some is refined, some is whole wheat. Your assignment: Look for whole-wheat couscous in the supermarket or natural foods store. It's the fastest-cooking whole-grain product of them all: Just add boiling water and cover, and in 5 minutes, it's ready to serve. Switching to whole-wheat couscous means getting 7 grams of fiber per serving, compared to just 2 grams in regular couscous.

Stir it in. Add a half cup of cooked bulgur, wheat berries, brown or wild rice, or barley (not pearled) to stuffings, soups, stews, salads, or casseroles. Add a cooked whole grain or whole-grain bread crumbs to ground meat or poultry for extra body. Make risottos, pilafs, and other rice-type dishes using grains such as barley, brown basmati rice, bulgur, millet, quinoa, kasha, or sorghum.

Popcorn counts! Use your air popper for a high-fiber, low-fat snack. Each cup of air-popped popcorn has 1.2 grams of fiber (and just 31 calories)—and who can eat just 1 cup?

Choice ❷

Food is not the only cause of chronic inflammation in your body, and it isn't the only cure, but it certainly plays an important role. Research shows that even a regular-size fast-food breakfast (egg and sausage on an English muffin plus fried potatoes) quickly floods the bloodstream with inflammatory compounds and keeps levels high for the next three hours. If you have a fast-food meal for lunch as well, you start the cycle all over again, keeping inflammation fired up indefinitely.

An equally dangerous eating problem is that most modern humans no longer eat a healthy combination of two important fats—omega-3 fatty acids and omega-6 fatty acids. We need both for healthy brain function. But while two important omega-3s—eicosapentaenoic acid (EPA) and docosahexaenoic acid (DHA)—reduce inflammation and prevent chronic health problems like heart disease and arthritis, omega-6s tend to *increase* inflammation. The modern dilemma: While early humans ate a good balance of these two fats—about 4 to 5 times more omega-6s than omega-3s—today we eat 11 to 30 times more omega-6s.

Why? In part because we eat lots of processed foods, often dripping with corn, sunflower, and soybean oil, all top sources of omega-6s. We eat grain-fed beef and poultry instead of free-range meats (grass-fed animals have more omega-3s in their fat stores). Just as dangerous is skimping on good fats—the omega-3 fatty acids found in cold-water fish such as salmon as well as in canola oil, olive oil, and nuts—which can also promote inflammation.

The Long Life Eating solution? Rebalance your fat portfolio by eating more fish, more nuts, and more good-for-you oils. The immediate benefits: Getting more good fats could help ease arthritis pain, relieve asthma, lessen symptoms of eczema and psoriasis, and even cut your risk of depression. When Ohio State University psychologists compared levels of depression and levels of omega-3s and omega-6s in the bloodstreams of 43 older women and men, they found that those who were the most depressed had 18 times more omega-6s than omega-3s. Those who weren't depressed had 13 times more.

The long-term benefits? Good fats may cut your risk of dangerous heart arrhythmias (out-of-sync heartbeats that can lead to a heart attack), high blood pressure, stroke, cancer, diabetes, and even Alzheimer's disease.

Anti-Inflammatory Superfoods: Fish, Nuts and Seeds, and Oils

Fats = bad. Carbohydrates = good. Not too many years ago, those were the basic rules of healthy eating. How simplistic they were! In the previous section, we showed that the story isn't nearly that simple for carbs. While whole grains are terrific for you, refined grains cause sharp blood sugar swings and are stripped of important nutrients.

Our understanding of fats has changed similarly. In the past 20 years, we have learned that certain fats are indeed among the most unhealthful foods you can eat, but other fats are among the most healthful. Don't worry, though—it's still pretty easy to separate the good fats from the bad. Here's the basic breakdown.

Bad fats: Fats from pork, beef, and other land animals and "trans fats" artificially created in factories.

Good fats: Fats from plants, such as those in nuts, olives, and beans, and fats from most fish.

How good are good fats? Well, good enough that you should go out of your way to have plenty in your daily diet. We've already discussed one big reason: Healthy fats reduce inflammation in your body, greatly reducing your risk of many major diseases. Another reason is that they help shore up levels of "good" HDL cholesterol, which becomes more and more important as a heart protector as we age. Maintaining healthy HDL levels, in fact, may become more important than keeping "bad" LDL low after about age 60.

Get started today by putting good-fat superfoods on your plate. And while you're enjoying these anti-inflammatory powerhouses, don't forget about fruits and veggies. They contain a natural form of salicylic acid, the same inflammation-cooling compound found in aspirin. Meanwhile, spice up your cooking with delicious anti-inflammatory add-ins like ginger and turmeric.

Here are the good-fat superfoods.

- No other food comes close to delivering the high-quality, high-concentration omega-3s you'll find in **salmon, sardines, herring, mackerel and other fatty, cold-water fish.** They're the richest sources of the two most powerful omega-3s, EPA and DHA. Fish is so powerful that even just three servings a month could cut your risk of stroke by 40 percent; two meals a week could slash your heart attack odds by 59 percent. Yet most of us manage just 4 ounces of fish per month!

  Often, scary reports of environmental toxins like methylmercury, PCBs (polychlorinated

biphenyls), and DDT (dichlorodiphenyl-trichloroethane) lurking in fish scare us away. (Women in one Harvard Medical School study cut their fish consumption 17 percent after a mercury warning was released in 2001.)

You can eat fish without fear, says the National Academy of Sciences. Just choose a variety of fish so you're not exposed to one potential source of toxins over and over again. That could mean salmon salad sandwiches on Tuesday and flounder on Saturday night, or tuna salad on Wednesday and a sardine snack on Friday.

- Crunchy, tasty treasures, **nuts and seeds** are rich sources of heart-healthy monounsaturated and polyunsaturated fats and even, in a few cases, of plant-based omega-3s that may play a special role in preventing cancer and heart disease. With nuts, a little is good, but more isn't better. All that fat makes them high in calories: a palmful of nuts has about 200 calories. For a 100-calorie snack, all you need are 8 walnut halves, 16 to 20 almonds, 10 to 12 cashews, 10 pecans, 7 or 8 macadamia nuts, 15 hazelnuts, or 1 tablespoon of peanut butter.

"I always measure out my nut serving, such as a small handful or about 15 pieces, and then cap the jar and put it away before I start eating," says Dr. Gerbstadt. "It's too easy to start munching and before you know it, be halfway through a jar of peanuts."

- Move over sunflower, soybean, and corn oil. The good fats found in **olive, canola, and grapeseed oil** have proven health benefits and can help you establish a healthier, more natural balance between omega-6 and omega-3 fatty acids. Researchers believe that the higher omega-3 content of Mediterranean and Okinawan diets contributes to many more healthy years of life.

LONG LIFE EATING GOAL: At least 2 servings per week

Have no-mess baked fish for dinner on Friday— and a double-good-fat fish sandwich for lunch on Wednesday. Just place a fish fillet on a large sheet of foil and top with your choice of flavorful additions (we like sun-dried tomatoes and chopped garlic with salmon and slices of fresh lemon over flounder) plus a splash of water, wine, or fruit juice. Bake at 350°F until cooked through, usually about 20 minutes.

On Wednesdays, mix canned salmon or tuna with a bit of canola-oil mayo and grated carrots and apples. Enjoy on double-fiber bread with a leafy green side salad.

Want fresh? Don't shy away from farm-raised varieties. Despite the scary headlines about PCB contamination and environmental problems caused by fish farming, farm-raised salmon has no more toxins than a piece of chicken, experts say. And it "contains the same amount of omega-3 fatty acids as wild fish," notes Alice Lichtenstein, DSc, who heads the Cardiovascular Nutrition Laboratory at Tufts University in Boston.

Even the ecologically savvy Environmental Defense Fund recommends the following farmed fish and seafood because they're low in contaminants and raised in an ecologically responsible manner: catfish, caviar, clams, mussels, oysters, scallops, shrimp, and striped bass.

Stocking up? Look beyond the fish counter. "It's a misconception that frozen and canned fish isn't as healthy as fresh, wild fish," says Jeannie Moloo, RD, PhD, a registered dietitian in private practice. "Frozen tilapia, sole, orange roughy, and mahi-mahi are great choices—just let your fillets thaw in the refrigerator during the day, then broil with lemon or poach lightly."

And don't overlook canned fish. There's even affordable wild salmon hiding in the canned foods aisle, Dr. Moloo says. "Canned red or pink salmon is wild salmon—full of omega-3s and low in contaminants. It makes great salmon salad, salmon cakes, even a salmon loaf." Canned pink salmon has 1.7 grams of omega-3s in a 3.5-ounce serving; canned sockeye (red) salmon's got 1.3 grams. Use it to make salmon salad, salmon loaf, or salmon burgers.

Reach for light tuna instead of white or albacore. Light is skipjack, a short-lived fish that has two-thirds less mercury than long-lived albacore.

Love shrimp? Don't wait for company to come over. Shrimp cocktail and peel-and-eat shrimp are fun ways to work more low-fat protein into your week. And don't fall for the high-cholesterol shrimp scare. Shrimp's quirky cholesterol count—about 200 milligrams in 12 large ones, about the same as the amount in one large egg—could make you pass up this low-cal delicacy. But for most of us, shrimp should get the green light. In a definitive Rockefeller University study, shrimp raised "bad" LDL cholesterol by 7 percent, but it also boosted "good" HDL cholesterol even higher and decreased heart-threatening blood fats called triglycerides by 13 percent. The bottom line is that it is heart–friendly. In fact, you may want to have shrimp salad instead of smoked salmon on your next bagel. Smoked salmon is high in sodium, and the smoking process may cut beneficial omega-3s by as much as 75 percent.

Snack on bite-size inflammation coolers. Peckish? Have a small serving of sardines, herring, or smoked sable. They're all packed with good fats.

Nuts and Seeds

LONG LIFE EATING GOAL: At least 3 snack-size servings per week

Sprinkle chopped peanuts on your brown rice tonight. Or spread a tablespoon of peanut butter on a slice of whole-wheat toast for breakfast (top with banana slices for natural sweetness). In five big population studies, nut consumption cut heart risk by up to 35 percent. Peanuts pack an extra nutritional bonus that may explain why: They've got beta-sitosterol, which blocks cholesterol absorption and, in lab studies, discouraged growth of tumors of the breast, colon, and prostate. Peanuts can also help you feel full and satisfied longer. In a Pennsylvania State University study, peanut eaters weighed less than peanut avoiders.

Scatter sunflower seeds on top of muffins or hot cereal; add to a green salad. Sunflower seeds also provide linoleic acid, an essential fatty acid your body cannot produce and must obtain from food. In studies, women who got the most had a 23 percent lower risk of heart disease. Store in the freezer, since their fats turn rancid fast.

Munch 22 almonds tonight. "Bad" LDL levels dropped 6 percent and "good" HDL levels rose 6 percent in a University of California study of people who ate almonds and used almond oil in place of half the regular fats in their diets.

Instead of a candy bar for a snack, carry nuts in a metal breath-mint box. (Wash it out first!) One of those cute little tins is the perfect size to hold 22 almonds—a full snack-size ounce—and it couldn't be more portable.

Add a dusting of ground walnuts or flaxseed to your cereal, veggies, or salad every day. Both contain impressive amounts of another beneficial omega-3 oil, called alpha-linolenic acid. Getting some into your diet is a good idea, nutritionists say; plenty of studies show that eating walnuts or flaxseed can help cut heart disease risk.

Coat fish with sesame seeds before baking. A quarter cup packs 144 milligrams of phytosterols—super-healthy chemicals that block cholesterol absorption.

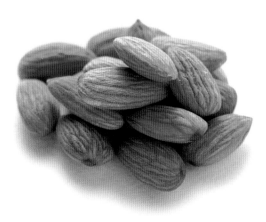

Choice **3**

Healthy Oils

LONG LIFE EATING GOAL: 1 to 2 tablespoons per day

Flavor with olive oil. One of the richest sources of monounsaturated fats, olive oil seems to cool the inflammation that leads to heart disease, diabetes, cancer, and worsening arthritis. In one Spanish study of 755 Canary Islands women, those who had 1/3 ounce a day were the least likely to get breast cancer.

Watch the calories, though. A tablespoon of olive oil—or virtually any oil—packs 120 calories, so use a light hand. Drizzle 1 to 2 teaspoons on veggies like squash, asparagus, and green beans instead of butter. Buy an oil mister and spritz your pans with it instead of spray-on oil. Get only what you'll use in the next two months and store it in a cool, dark spot. Old olive oil goes rancid and tastes like soggy cardboard.

Splurge on extra-virgin. This is the fruity, full-bodied good stuff to use in situations where taste is important, such as in salad dressings; it also has the most antioxidants. In a Spanish study comparing the effects of extra-virgin olive oil with olive oil that had all of its antioxidant phenols filtered out, the arteries of people who had the extra-virgin oil expanded and contracted easily in response to changes in blood flow—a trait that cuts heart attack risk.

Use canola oil when you don't want an assertive flavor. Replace butter in baking recipes with canola oil, using a ratio of 3/4 tablespoon of oil for each tablespoon of butter called for in the recipe. Also, switching from corn or sunflower oil to canola oil in muffins, cakes, and sautéed dishes is one of the most powerful "good fat" strategies you can deploy.

It's smart to keep canola as well as olive oil in your pantry; each has its nutritional and culinary charms. Canola is lower in saturated fat and has more polyunsaturated fat, which lowers "bad" LDL cholesterol more effectively than monounsaturated fats do.

Try grapeseed and flaxseed oil. Grapeseed oil, also rich in healthy fats, is perfect for high-temperature cooking. Flaxseed oil, which breaks down in high heat, is best used at room temperature as a salad dressing. Dress leafy greens with flaxseed oil by shaking up a smart vinaigrette with flaxseed oil, balsamic vinegar, and your favorite herbs and spices. Then store the extra in the fridge: Heat destroys the essential fatty acids in this fragile, light-tasting oil. Think oil's too much of a luxury on your salad? It's time to rethink fat-free dressing. New research shows that none of the cancer-fighting alpha- or beta-carotene antioxidants found in salad greens are absorbed unless oils are present. (You could add nuts or avocado instead.)

Olive oil is one of nature's greatest gifts: Its extraordinary flavor is matched only by its healthiness.

Once, the equation for avoiding brittle bones was simple: Get more calcium. After all, your bones do need it—and when your body doesn't have enough for other functions, it draws more from your skeleton. Not getting enough calcium is one important reason that one in every two women and one in eight men over age 50 will have an osteoporosis-related bone fracture at some point in their lives. Brittle bones account for 700,000 spine fractures, 300,000 hip fractures, 250,000 wrist fractures, and 300,000 other bone breaks each year in the United States.

But there's new thinking on calcium and bone health. Experts the world over now believe that the best bone-protecting equation begins with adequate calcium but doesn't stop there. You also need vitamin D, magnesium, and potassium to help your body absorb and use calcium, and you need regular bone-protecting resistance moves to build or maintain bone density. Some experts say this changes the calcium equation—that in fact, we need *less* than the standard 1,200 milligrams a day recommended by some major health organizations.

We took this new thinking into consideration. Calcium's still important, and not just for your bones. There's plenty of evidence that getting enough can also help control your blood pressure, lower your odds of developing a prediabetic condition called insulin resistance, and even help prevent memory loss and colon cancer. But do you need 1,200 milligrams a day, or closer to the 700 milligrams a day recommended by British health authorities? We think you and your doctor should decide. In the

meantime, it's hard to argue against getting two servings of low-fat dairy foods a day as part of your diet. Combine that with the smaller amounts of calcium in other foods you eat, and you'll get about 900 milligrams. If you want to reach 1,200 milligrams, add one calcium supplement a day. If your doctor suggests a lower daily amount, adjust accordingly.

You may have heard that calcium is a weight-loss miracle mineral. The truth is, research on the issue is conflicting and controversial. This much does seem to be true: If you don't drink milk or get adequate calcium from other sources now, adding fat-free milk or other fat-free dairy products to your diet may help. In one study from the University of Tennessee Nutrition Institute, 32 obese women and men who cut 500 calories a day from their meal plans lost more weight when they added 800 milligrams of supplemental calcium daily, and they lost even more weight and fat when they took supplements containing 1,200 to 1,300 milligrams of calcium. In a second study, 34 obese people on weight-loss diets lost more pounds and more fat if they had three daily servings of yogurt than if they had one.

Calcium Superfoods: Milk and Beyond

Fat-free milk, low-fat cheese, and fat-free yogurt are among the richest sources of calcium on the shelf at your local food store. Each serving provides about 350 milligrams of calcium along with minerals and vitamins you need to absorb and use it. If you love milk, that's great news. It's just another reason to pour some over your morning cereal, end the day with a steaming mug of cocoa, or enjoy cheese and whole-grain crackers for a midafternoon snack.

What if you don't like milk, though, or simply can't drink it? Plenty of people feel bloated and uncomfortable after eating dairy foods, because their bodies are missing the enzyme needed to digest the milk sugar lactose. If you're lactose intolerant or just prefer not to consume much dairy, we've got loads of calcium-rich alternatives, from leafy green salads to nuts to fortified soy milk and orange juice and even yogurt.

It's true—many people whose systems are intolerant of milk can have yogurt without any problem. Why? Enzymes in yogurt convert milk sugars into a digestible form. "If milk makes you uncomfortable, yogurt may be a good alternative," Moores notes.

As a food, yogurt is a multitasking marvel: It works as a breakfast food, a frozen dessert, or a dip; you can also use it as a base for smoothie drinks and salad dressings and as a sauce for chicken or seafood. It's packed with calcium and protein as well as magnesium, riboflavin, and vitamins B_6 and B_{12}—plus beneficial "probiotic" bacteria that improve digestion and boost immunity.

Be sure to read about calcium supplements later in this chapter. Nutrition experts agree that they're one of the smartest supplements women—and possibly men—can take.

problem ? solver

I Just Don't Feel Like Eating

Sarah Lerner's appetite isn't what it used to be. Often, breakfast is a container of yogurt or a slice of bread. Lunch is maybe a bowl of soup or a piece of fruit or even just a handful of cookies. Sometimes she eats a big dinner, but other times, she just doesn't feel much like eating. And food just doesn't taste as appetizing anymore. As a result, she's lost 5 pounds in the past few months.

"Sarah's not alone," says registered dietitian and practicing physician Christine Gerbstadt, RD, MD, a spokesperson for the American Dietetic Association. In one recent survey, 30 percent of older people admitted that they skip meals on a regular basis because they just don't feel like eating.

"The first thing to do for loss of appetite is to see your doctor," she says. "It can be a subtle sign of an underlying medical problem or even of depression. If health problems are ruled out, think about making mealtimes more social. We tend to eat more when we're out with other people—and socializing makes meals a pleasure again. Eating with others doesn't have to be expensive. You could meet a friend at a park and eat brown-bag lunches together or invite someone over for lunch or dinner. You could even go out yourself to a place where there are more people. It doesn't have to be a senior citizens program, either. Go to a local college cafeteria or the food court at the mall—and make healthy choices, of course."

"If food itself seems unappealing, experiment with spices," suggests registered dietitian Lola O'Rourke, MS, RD. "Spices are a great way to go—you get extra antioxidants with no added calories."

LONG LIFE EATING GOAL: 1 to 2 servings per day

Close your eyes and move to a lower number. If you're drinking whole-fat milk, switch to 2%. If you're drinking 2%, move to 1%, and if you're drinking 1%, well, you get the idea. Here's an easy way to make the switch: Buy a small container of the next percent down, shut your eyes, and sip. Experts at the Center for Science in the Public Interest say that when thousands of consumers put on sunglasses so they couldn't tell what kind of milk they were drinking, 9 out of 10 said that they liked the taste of either 1% or fat-free milk better than that of higher-fat milks. Why it's worth it: Each glass of fat-free milk you drink instead of whole milk saves you 5 grams of saturated fat, one-quarter of your recommended daily total.

Sip delicious "hot vanilla" or hot chocolate on a drizzly, cold morning. Mix 1 cup fat-free or low-fat milk, two packets sugar substitute (or 2 teaspoons sugar or honey if you prefer), and your choice of 1/4 teaspoon real vanilla extract or 2 teaspoons unsweetened cocoa in a small saucepan or microwavable cup. Heat for about a minute.

Cook with milk instead of water. Instant hot cereals and low-sodium instant or canned soups mix easily with milk, which lends extra body and flavor to these quick comfort foods.

Make milk your drive-through beverage. Most fast-food restaurants sell the low-fat variety in cartons or single-serving bottles.

Order a skim-milk cappuccino. Skip high-calorie coffee drinks at your favorite coffee shop. Skim milk makes cappuccino extra-foamy and fun to sip. Sprinkle with your choice of cocoa powder, cinnamon, or nutmeg—or all three!

Make it sweet. Mix sugar-free instant pudding with low-fat or fat-free milk and serve with berries. It's a great snack, dessert, or breakfast surprise.

Hide it in plain sight. Use canned fat-free evaporated milk in place of milk in baked goods, soups, or sauces. A cup contains 742 milligrams of calcium—more than double the amount in low-fat milk.

Whip it up. Use an eggbeater or electric mixer to whip partially frozen fat-free evaporated milk for a high-calcium dessert topping with one-tenth the calories of regular whipped cream.

Make a healthy dairy pasta topping. Puree fat-free or low-fat cottage cheese and fat-free evaporated milk with lemon juice and rosemary for a light pasta sauce.

Stay comfy. "Lactose intolerance increases with age," notes Moores. "Even if you could drink milk before, you may be finding that it makes you feel uncomfortably full, gassy, or even crampy." Try Lactaid or other brands of milk with predigested lactose. Before meals, you can also take over-the-counter pills that supply the missing digestive enzyme.

Chose guilt-free cheese ... When the full-fat cheese in your refrigerator is all gone, resolve to never buy it again—and scout the dairy case for new fat-free and reduced-fat cheeses. (They're worth a second look. As with whole-grain pasta, current supermarket offerings are lightyears better in terms of taste and texture than the first-generation low-fat cheeses on the market 15 years ago.) Full-fat cheese is one of the top three sources of artery-clogging saturated fat in our diets. Go lower fat, and you can keep the flavor *and* spare your heart.

... Then savor it in small doses. Grate a little over chili or spaghetti or veggies. Have one slice on your sandwich. Have an individually wrapped piece of low-fat string cheese with whole-wheat crackers as a snack. "If you don't have to worry about your weight or your cholesterol level, a little cheese is very pleasurable and can make all kinds of foods taste even better," Moores notes. "If you are overweight or have high cholesterol, think twice. Cheese is high in saturated fat, and its richness makes it easy to overeat." Each ounce of full-fat cheese has 4 to 6 grams of saturated fat. What's an ounce? A quarter cup of shredded cheese, 1 1/3 slices of American cheese, or the amount you'd find melted on a slice of a medium pizza. Going low-fat (or fat-free) and reducing your portions could save you a significant 5 grams of heart-threatening saturated fat per day.

Order pizza and other cheesy dishes with half the cheese and twice the sauce and vegetables. Americans eat 13 pounds of mozzarella and other Italian-style cheeses each year—nearly one-third of our total intake of 31 pounds of cheese per person. You can cut this in half and never notice the difference.

Lighten up your Italian cooking. Get light mozzarella instead of part skim. Light has half as much fat as regular mozzarella, while part skim cuts saturated fat by only 1 gram per ounce.

Use milk or yogurt as a secret ingredient in soups, desserts, and sauces.

LONG LIFE EATING GOAL: 5 servings per week

Buy one large container of plain yogurt at a time rather than lots of preflavored small ones. If only store-bought strawberry yogurt were just yogurt with slices of fresh strawberry. Instead, it's yogurt with sweetener, more sweetener, and a little bit of fruit. All those refined sweeteners double the calories of the yogurt without any extra nutrition. Instead, buy plain yogurt and use it creatively throughout the week in your cooking. If you want to flavor some with fruit for breakfast, add a teaspoon of your favorite jelly or jam and some slices of real fruit, then mix it together. It will be equally delicious but far less calorie heavy than the store-bought version.

Make a breakfast smoothie a few times a week. It's easy! Blend 8 ounces plain, low-fat, or fat-free yogurt with a banana, a handful of fresh or frozen berries, a splash of orange juice, and a few ice cubes until smooth. An amazing breakfast in a glass! Once you master this basic approach, you can start experimenting with other fruit juices and fresh fruits.

Serve raw fruits and vegetables with a yogurt-based dip. Mix curry seasoning and honey into plain low-fat yogurt for a sweet and spicy dip for carrots. Or add chopped fresh basil and lemon to yogurt for a Mediterranean flavor that's great with sliced cucumber and zucchini.

Have a yogurt parfait at snack time or for dessert. Layer low-fat or fat-free yogurt, berries, mandarin oranges, and granola or chopped almonds in a pretty wine glass or dessert bowl. It makes a treat worthy of royalty.

Buy frozen yogurt pops. Buy the brand with the least sugar and saturated fat and keep them in the freezer. Don't you feel like a kid? Or freeze a carton of frozen yogurt, then whirl in the food processor with frozen or fresh fruit for a delicious dessert.

Skip yogurts with built-in toppings. Chocolate chips, party sprinkles, granola—many yogurts come with their own fancy mix-ins in a special cup on the lid. Skip these; they only add extra fat and sugar, raising the calorie count of that little tub of yogurt to way over 200.

Check the calcium count on cultured soy yogurts. Dairy-free soy yogurts have only the teeniest smidgeon of saturated fat. If you're trying to avoid milk products or just want to get more soy into your diet, consider these soy-gurts only after you check the calcium content. Many are lower than their made-from-milk cousins. Many are also lower in magnesium, protein, and B vitamins.

Make your own cheese. It's easier than you think, and you get a low-calorie, cheeselike spread that can be sweetened with honey or spiced up with pressed garlic and herbs as a sandwich spread. Simply line a strainer with paper towels, dump in plain yogurt, and set over a bowl or pot. Cover and refrigerate overnight. In the morning, you'll have a wheylike liquid in the bowl and thick yogurt cheese in the strainer, ready for your culinary spin.

Use yogurt as a topping. For example, spoon a dollop onto thick black bean or split-pea soup, then sprinkle with black pepper or herbs. You'll never know it's not sour cream.

Check out fortified OJ and soy milk. Some contain as much calcium as a glass of fat-free milk, but be sure to read the label so you know how much you're getting. "Don't shortchange yourself by thinking your juice or milk has more calcium than it really does," Moores says. Shake soy milk well before pouring; the calcium added to it can settle to the bottom.

Go for "green calcium." Yes, there is calcium in some vegetables. And your body can absorb the calcium in veggies even better than it can calcium in milk. The levels aren't quite as high as in dairy foods, though. You'd have to eat 1 1/2 cups of cooked kale, 2 1/4 cups of cooked broccoli, or 8 cups of cooked spinach to equal the calcium in a glass of fat-free milk. That means to reach a daily quota of 1,200 milligrams of calcium, you'd need to eat 6 cups of kale, 9 cups of broccoli, or 32 cups of cooked spinach. Think of calcium-rich veggies as a nice add-on that can help you reach your goal and provide a range of minerals and vitamins that help calcium keep bones strong. The best vegetable sources of calcium are collards, kale, broccoli, spinach, bok choy, and almonds.

Eat more rhubarb. It takes a creative cook to figure out how to get more rhubarb into your diet, but it's worth it. A cup of cooked rhubarb has 348 milligrams of calcium, making it one of nature's top sources of the mineral. Only the stalks of a rhubarb plant are edible, and they are quite tart. That's why rhubarb is primarily paired with sweet fruits in breads, cakes, pies, and ice cream.

Nibble on dried figs. A serving of 10 dried figs provides 269 milligrams of calcium, a wonderfully large amount.

Some tofu counts, too. Tofu made with calcium sulfate (check for it on the ingredients label) supplies a respectable 204 milligrams of calcium in a half-cup serving.

Eat more beans. As we've said, beans are an anti-aging superfood, and here's one more reason: They're good sources of calcium. A 1-cup serving of boiled white beans has a substantial 161 milligrams.

And have nuts and seeds, too. Calcium can be found in healthy amounts in Brazil nuts, hazelnuts, chestnuts, filberts, sesame seeds, tahini (sesame seed paste), sunflower seeds, and pumpkin seeds. A good idea: Keep a canister of your favorite seeds on your kitchen table and add a teaspoon as a topping to cereals, vegetables, salads, and soups.

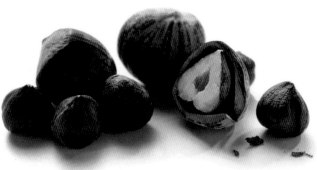

Choice **4**

A juicy baked chicken breast. Beef stew studded with chunks of rich, lean meat. Turkey burgers with all the fixin's. These protein-packed dishes aren't just mouthwatering; they can help you maintain strong muscles and strong immunity, keep you feeling full longer after you eat, and deliver key vitamins and minerals that become even more important for good health as the years pass.

You don't need more protein after age 55. Your challenge: Eating *enough* without getting too much heart-threatening saturated fat. "For many older people, getting all you need may be more challenging," says registered dietitian Lola O'Rourke, MS, RD. "You may not feel like taking the time to roast a chicken or grill a hamburger. You may have more difficulty chewing a steak. Or you may be relying on types of protein like fast-food burgers and fried chicken that are also full of saturated fats and trans fats."

The solution to this protein puzzle is a delicious new eating strategy—similar to the way healthy older people in Okinawa and Crete eat: Put more protein like poultry or lean beef on the table, add fish, and mix in plenty of other healthy foods that fill in protein gaps, such as dairy products, nuts, beans, and even some vegetables. Our modern twist? Use healthy convenience foods like skinless, boneless chicken breasts and make easy substitutions such as grabbing skinless ground turkey instead of ground beef the next time you're hankering for a burger.

At the beginning of this chapter, we mentioned the key reasons protein is so important to your diet. It provides essential body-building materials that are used to create muscle cells, bone cells, blood cells, and more. And no matter what your age, your body is still generating new cells all the time. Protein also slows absorption of blood sugar, helping to keep hunger and food cravings at bay.

Plus, lean protein is a rich source of the B vitamins that can help you feel more energetic. Why? The Bs help guide metabolic reactions throughout the body. And they can help protect against heart disease by controlling levels of a compound in the bloodstream called homocysteine.

With lean protein, you also get healthy doses of multitalented zinc, a mineral important for maintaining strong immunity—it plays a role in the production of infection-fighting white blood cells. In one study of women and men over age 70, those who ate the most protein had significantly stronger bones over four years than those who ate the least. Another bonus: brain-protecting niacin. When Chicago researchers checked 3,718 people ages 65 and older, then tested their cognitive skills for six years, they found that those who got the most niacin from food were 70 percent less likely to develop Alzheimer's. Vitamin B_6 and niacin can also help your body process blood sugar more efficiently.

So why does meat get such a bad rap in terms of health? Two reasons. First, protein and fat are closely bound together in most cuts of meat, and animal fat is among the most troublesome parts of your diet. That's why we keep using the word "lean" in front of protein; it's important that you choose meats that are as low as possible in visible fat. Second, we tend to eat huge helpings of meat. Steakhouses love to taunt you with the size of their burgers or steaks or racks of ribs. Often, what they provide is as much as eight times more than a healthy serving. When it comes to beef, pork, or lamb, many people have a hard time showing moderation.

So how much protein do you need? Experts suggest 4.5 grams for every 10 pounds of body weight. Translation: If you weigh 150 pounds, you need 67 grams. That's just what you'd get if your day's menu looked like this:

- Cereal with a cup of fat-free milk for breakfast
- A tuna sandwich on whole-wheat bread for lunch
- A medium-size skinless chicken breast for dinner
- A cup of hot cocoa made with fat-free milk before bed

As you can see, that's not a whole lot of meat. Yet for some reason, as women age, they tend to eat less and less protein. Roughly 10 to 20 percent of women over age 55 get less than 30 grams of protein a day—even if they're eating plenty of food.

Protein Superfoods: Chicken, Turkey, and Lean Beef

What's not to love about chicken? A roasted, skinless breast has just 120 to 140 calories, and it's packed with all the protein satisfaction you could ask for with less than half the fat of a trimmed T-bone steak. It's versatile—starring in everything from chicken soup at lunch to a plump, roast bird for Sunday dinner. In a hurry? You can find it ready to eat virtually everywhere—like the grilled chicken sandwiches available at most fast-food drive-thrus (minus the mayonnaise).

And turkey? This grand bird is not just for special occasions anymore. A 4-ounce serving of turkey breast provides 60 percent of the protein you need each day without the fat you'd get in many cuts of pork or beef. And these days, you don't have to buy a 22-pound bird to enjoy a mouthwatering turkey dinner. Small cuts of boneless turkey are readily available in many markets.

As far as red meats go, there are more healthy choices than you might realize. Lean beef cuts like top sirloin, tenderloin, and top loin are surprisingly low in fat—and the fat they contain isn't all the artery-clogging kind. Half the fatty acids in a 3-ounce serving of lean beef are monounsaturated fatty acids, the same heart-healthy kind found in olive oil that research shows may have cholesterol-lowering abilities.

What's more, a third of the saturated fat in beef is a unique fatty acid called stearic acid, which has been found to have a neutral or cholesterol-lowering effect. A 3-ounce serving of beef is an excellent source of five essential nutrients: protein, zinc, vitamin B_{12}, selenium, and phosphorus, and a good source of four more: niacin, vitamin B_6, iron, and riboflavin.

The story is similar with pork: The tenderloin is super lean, luscious, and perfectly healthy in moderate portions.

Meat Meets Greens

Here are two intriguing reasons why you should always eat green vegetables with meat.

1. A mysterious component of beef—known to scientists simply as **"the meat factor"**—helps your body absorb more of the iron in vegetables.

2. **Cruciferous vegetables** such as broccoli and brussels sprouts help your body disarm unhealthy carcinogenic compounds called heterocyclic amines that are produced when meat is grilled or charbroiled.

LONG LIFE EATING GOAL: 1 serving per day

Grab fast, low-fat chicken. Grocery stores typically stock skinless, boneless breasts; thighs; and fast-cooking breast-meat strips called chicken tenders. Don't let price stop you from stocking up on them. As these healthier, quicker-to-prepare alternatives to whole birds grow in popularity, their prices are falling fast. And 100 percent of what you buy ends up in your meal, as opposed to the waste of a whole chicken.

Buy a roasted chicken. Many food stores today offer roasted chickens for sale. Go ahead and buy one! When you get home, strip off the skin, remove the meat from the bones, and drain off the sauce. That way, you get rid of the fat and the excessively high sodium levels of the store-applied marinade. What's left is deliciously healthy, lean chicken meat, ready for instant eating. Serve it up on its own, shred it into soup or onto salad, or add to vegetables.

Make a 10-minute chicken-and-veggie meal. Grab a pack of boneless, skinless tenders and some precut vegetables, such as squash, broccoli, green and red bell peppers, and onions. Dump them all in a pan with a spritz of olive or canola oil and some low-sodium broth, bring to a boil, then reduce to a simmer. Season with garlic, ginger, basil, tarragon, or just a sprinkle of salt and pepper. Cook until the chicken's done and the veggies are as crunchy—or soft—as you prefer. Voilà! It's dinner!

Create a marinade habit. Marinades make your poultry amazingly tender, moist, and flavorful. The day before you intend to cook, place the raw chicken in a sealable container, pour on a marinade, cover, and refrigerate until cooking time the next evening. Almost any liquid can be the base: orange juice, buttermilk, a vinaigrette, even a cup of yogurt. Add your favorite herbs and spices for flavor. If you want even greater convenience, use a store-bought low-fat marinade. Then cook your favorite way. One important rule: Discard marinades once you've removed the chicken.

Leftovers? You've got lunch! Leftover cooked chicken will keep for three days in the fridge. Put some in a whole-wheat tortilla; sprinkle with chopped tomatoes, diced avocado, onions, and grated low-fat cheese; and broil for a healthy burrito. Or combine chopped chicken with a dollop of canola-oil mayo, tarragon, and grapes for elegant chicken salad.

Make chicken chili. Add chunks of cooked chicken to white-bean chili to bump up the protein content.

Buy skinless ground turkey breast instead of ground beef. Use it as you would ground beef in chili, meat loaf, and burger recipes.

Grill or bake a turkey breast instead of a whole chicken. Slice, then refrigerate or freeze leftovers for use later in turkey burritos or turkey salad (toss diced turkey with low-fat mayo, chopped apples, walnuts, celery, and grapes).

Make an autumn turkey salad. Place cubed turkey, sliced cooked sweet potato, cranberries, and walnuts on a bed of spinach and drizzle with your favorite olive-oil dressing.

Keep turkey in the freezer for quick meals. Put skinless, boneless turkey cutlets in zipper-seal bags and freeze. Thaw in the microwave, then sauté in a skillet with a dash of olive oil.

Choice **5**

Lean Beef and Other Meats

LONG LIFE EATING GOAL: 1 serving per day

Look for "lean" or "extra-lean" on the label. These cuts have 4.5 grams or less of saturated fat and 5 to 10 grams of total fat per serving. Or look for these lean cuts: bottom, eye, or top round; round tip; top sirloin; top loin; or tenderloin.

Use lean meat as an *ingredient*, not a main course. This may be the best trick of all when it comes to getting meat portions correct. Rather than thinking of meat as something to be served by itself, make it part of other dishes. Here are several smart ways.

- Add thinly sliced beef to your sautéed vegetables or wok stir-fries.

- Top a crunchy, robust salad with beef slices.

- Make kebabs with lean meat cubes and vegetables.

- Add small chunks of cooked pork and sautéed vegetables to cooked brown rice for a one-dish meal.

- Add lean ground beef to spaghetti sauce.

- Make bean, vegetable, and meat combinations, such as chili or cassoulet. Just be sure to add the meat to the beans after it's been cooked and drained; otherwise, the beans will absorb the fat.

Serve your beef sliced. Typically, steaks and pork chops are served whole, and that makes for a giant portion, far beyond the healthy amount. The solution: Slice the steak in the kitchen and fan out slices on the dinner plates. This looks great and really reduces the portion sizes.

Garnish your steak. Even better, sauté thinly sliced onions, peppers, tomatoes, and garlic cloves and spoon a healthy portion over the steak slices. This will make the meat portion seem even larger and more inviting—without extra meat.

Rinse your cooked ground beef. After you brown the beef, drain it, then rinse it with water. That's the best way to remove as much fat as possible.

Cook roasts separate from vegetables. Roasting makes fat melt away from meat. That's good. If potatoes, carrots, turnips, or other vegetables are in the pan, they'll absorb the fat you're trying to avoid. That's bad. A better approach: Cook the meat, decant the fat, and *then* cook the vegetables in the remaining broth.

Use the "see it, lose it" rule. If you see fat on your food, remove it. For example:

- If there's fat on the meat, trim it off.

- If there's skin on the chicken, remove it.

- If there's liquefied fat on top of the stew or soup, skim it off.

- If there's a pool of grease underneath your meat, sop it up with a paper napkin.

Put meat-based soups or stews in the refrigerator overnight. In the morning, it'll be super-easy to remove the hardened fat on top.

Use bacon as a flavoring, not a serving. One piece of crumbled bacon goes a long way toward adding that wonderful smoky flavor to healthier dishes.

Choice 6 Eat fewer calories.

When your meals are mostly vegetables and fruits, along with moderate portions of beans, whole grains, lean protein, and good fats, you're harnessing an important longevity secret: More food but fewer calories.

The key is choosing the right foods in the right portions. You don't have to be stingy with the amount you eat or ever feel deprived or count a single calorie if you make the first five choices of Long Life Eating—namely, by feasting on fruits and veggies and enjoying moderate amounts of other healthy foods like yogurt, salmon, olive oil, cheese, and chocolate. On Okinawa, this strategy (minus the chocolate!) allows people to eat *more* food by weight than people in other parts of Japan yet consume several hundred fewer calories per day because their choices are naturally lean.

This is an important point: You can eat heaping platefuls of veggies and fruit for fewer calories than are in a small bag of potato chips! And the vegetables and fruit pack several huge health bonuses. First is what they contain that packaged snacks don't: oodles of antioxidants, vitamins, and fiber. Second is what they *don't* contain that packaged foods do: fat, refined carbohydrates, and artificial additives that play a role in memory loss, fatigue, and so many killer diseases.

We've made these points before, back in the *The Seven Keys to Aging Well* chapter. There we told you about two exciting keys to longevity: not obsessing about the bathroom scale and choosing foods that you can eat to your heart's content without overdoing the calories. In this section, we'll show you how to achieve these goals—and

enjoy every luscious bite of this natural, never-say-diet approach to achieving a healthy weight. The bonus? Eating this way brings extra pleasure to your table because you never have to worry about eating the wrong things or "cheating" on the latest weight-loss scheme.

Best of all, it's a great, natural, feel-good way to step off the crazy, unhealthy weight-loss roller coaster. Too many weight-loss gimmicks and gurus want you to believe that temporary deprivation and restriction are the keys to slimming down. They've demonized some foods as the cause of the world's obesity epidemic and often market highly processed alternatives (such as food-replacement shakes, bars, and frozen meals) as the alternative. The truth is, when you rebalance your plate and choose from a wide variety of healthy foods (and treat yourself to the ones you love most), you've found a way to eat that will help your body settle at its natural, healthy weight; give you the energy you need to be more active; and promote lifelong health.

Should you worry about your weight at all? It depends. If excess weight is hurting your health, energy, or mobility, then discuss weight loss with your family doctor (and if she agrees that weight loss is a good idea, plan to lose pounds slowly!). But if you're just hoping to fit into a smaller bathing suit next summer, reconsider. For many people, "vanity" weight loss provides limited health benefits, and a growing stack of intriguing research suggests that after age 55 or 60, vanity weight loss is *detrimental* to your health. In one 12-year study of 1,801 people over age 71, women who lost weight increased their risk of dying by

38 percent, and men increased their odds by 76 percent. (Of course, your best option if you'd still like to be trimmer and more fit is exercise!)

Whether or not weight loss is your goal, you can't go wrong with our Long Life approach to healthy eating. It's as simple as choosing a big fruit salad over a slice of chocolate-mousse pie. Having a large piece of skinless chicken instead of a small cheeseburger. Or choosing a double portion of grilled veggies instead of a handful of french fries. It's delicious and satisfying—and it means never going hungry!

We've already extolled the nutritional wonders of healthy foods, from sweet cherries to hot red peppers, whole-wheat bread to succulent lean beef. Now we can reveal their added Long Life health bonus: Each time you choose one of these natural wonders instead of a more processed food, you save a significant number of calories while you flood your body with important vitamins, minerals, antioxidants, fiber, anti-inflammatory compounds, and satisfying components like proteins and fats.

Some examples: A hot-fudge sundae with two scoops of ice cream plus fudge sauce, whipped cream, a cherry, and nuts could contain 700 calories—or more. A generous bowl of fresh raspberries, strawberries, and chunks of ripe mango and pineapple might have 150 calories. A cheeseburger on a bun made from refined flour might have 600 calories. But a grilled skinless chicken breast and a whole-wheat roll has just 300 calories. And if you add a side of green beans and a lettuce-and-tomato salad with olive-oil vinaigrette, you've got a whole meal for less than the calories in a single cheeseburger!

problem ? solver

I'd Rather Open a Can Than Cook from Scratch

John Reynolds, a widower, lives alone and never did like to cook. He likes frozen dinners and hearty canned stews, hot dogs and beans, and ice cream for dessert. He'd like to eat more fruits, vegetables, and even whole grains, but all that preparation seems discouraging. What can he do?

"John can really improve his diet without even tying on an apron if he scours the supermarket for healthy convenience foods," says registered dietitian and practicing physician Christine Gerbstadt, RD, MD, a spokesperson for the American Dietetic Association. "You can eat well without having to chop, dice, and fuss. Look for prepackaged fruit—like the little ring-top or plastic single-serving containers in the canned fruit aisle. Just go for the ones packed in juice or light syrup. That's a serving of fruit right there. Buy single-serving bags of baby carrots or prechopped vegetables from the salad bar or the produce aisle. You can microwave them and add them to a low-sodium bean soup for a high-fiber, high-nutrition meal that nets you several vegetable servings.

"Canned beans are perfect for John—he already likes hot dogs and beans. Try plain beans instead—they're hearty and don't have the sugary sauce on them. Just rinse well and enjoy as a side dish with seasonings or some tomato sauce. Canned vegetables and soups are wonderful comfort foods—healthy, hearty, and satisfying.

"I would also suggest that if a friend or relative offers to cook for him once in a while, he could freeze single-portion servings of soup, stew, or a casserole and have homemade convenience food—just microwave and eat."

More Food but Fewer Calories

LONG LIFE EATING GOAL: Fruit or vegetables making up at least half of what you eat

Have unsweetened cereal for breakfast. You can enjoy a bigger serving of healthy whole grains for fewer calories. The reason: Sugar is very high in calories yet has virtually no bulk. Add chopped fruit for flavor and sweetness.

Start every lunch with salad. A big, fresh salad brimming with veggies or fruit fills you up, fits in several veggie servings, and tastes great. Start with a generous bed of lettuce and top with chopped tomatoes, grated or sliced carrots, cucumber rounds, sliced green or red bell pepper, and any of these: shredded zucchini, sliced raw mushrooms, onions, fresh herbs (basil is heavenly), celery, fennel, or shredded cabbage. Top with fat-free dressing, a dash of low-fat dressing (about one capful), or a tablespoon of olive oil–based vinaigrette.

Add a first course of vegetable soup to dinner every night. Research from Pennsylvania State University suggests that your body's satisfaction sensors are activated when a food is bulked up with water. Think of a bowl of low-fat, low-sodium chicken broth brimming with carrots, tomatoes, onions, and green beans. For the quickest soup, heat a can of low-sodium vegetable soup, then add your favorite frozen veggies and spices.

Serve your food "plated." That's restaurant talk for putting food on the plates in the kitchen rather than putting serving bowls of food on the table (that's typically called family style). The only serving bowl you should allow on the dining room table is the one holding the vegetables. That way, there's no temptation to take another piece of meat or an extra helping of noodles.

Keep chopped fruit at the front of the eye-level shelf in your refrigerator. Studies show that cut fruit retains important nutrients for nearly a week. And it's easy and delicious to open the refrigerator door and indulge in chunks of watermelon, wedges of melon, pineapple slices, grapes, and strawberries.

Eat a bulky, high-fiber food when you're hungry. Would you rather have 19 tiny peanuts or a whole juicy apple adorned with a teaspoon of peanut butter? Both snacks are healthy, and each has about 110 calories. But the apple's size makes it a much more satisfying and appealing choice.

Don't underestimate the power of bulk. In a study at the University of Sydney in Australia, potatoes were the most satisfying of the 38 foods that volunteers sampled—in large part, researchers suspect, because the portion was four times larger than for fatty foods with the same number of calories. The same strategy makes air-popped popcorn, cherry tomatoes, a big bowl of salad greens (with a dash of dressing), and other high-fiber foods a good choice if you need to fill up.

Designate healthy, low-calorie "free foods." Sometimes we all just want to snack—and snack and snack some more. Keep some low-calorie, nutritious foods that you enjoy on hand, such as apples, frozen berries, carrots, sliced red bell peppers, and air-popped popcorn. Allow yourself to eat as much as you want.

Switch to zero-calorie beverages. Water, iced tea, hot tea, and seltzer with a dash of lemon juice are all great choices. Getting away from sweetened drinks can save you hundreds of empty calories every day.

Make fruit your usual dessert. To make it special, spend some time in the produce section of your food market. Look beyond your usual choices for something new or indulgent. If you usually skip berries or pomegranates or melons because of the price, for instance, consider buying them. If you usually buy just one type of fruit, buy two or three and plan to make a pretty fruit plate or salad. After all, you're not spending money on cookies and cakes. Why not treat yourself to the best Mother Nature has to offer? (And check out the choices in the canned-fruit aisle and the frozen food case. Often, the best-quality berries are frozen. Just thaw gently in the microwave.)

Reverse dessert priorities. Usually, people adorn calorie-dense, nutrition-light desserts like cakes and cookies with a few berries. Next time you plan a nice dessert, do the opposite: Make the bulk of your dessert berries or fruit sorbet and adorn it with a small cookie or a square of high-quality dark chocolate.

Create a stack. Fine restaurants often present appetizers and entrées in a stack, rather than spread around the plate. It looks dramatic, and makes it less obvious how much of each dish you're getting. So try this at home. The next time you serve up, say, steak, mashed potatoes, and sautéed spinach, create a stack from the three. Make your bottom stack a large serving of vegetables (in this case, spinach spread into a nice circle on the middle of the plate). Put a modest-size, nicely sculpted disk of mashed potatoes on the spinach. On top, put four lovely slices of the beef. Then add sauce, herbs, or other final touches and serve for a dinner that's yummy, beautiful, and filled with the right proportions.

Have salad for a snack. Many people snack not out of hunger, but to satisfy a desire for flavor or texture. That's why so many snack foods are salty and crunchy! You can satisfy that desire for texture just as easily, and far more healthfully, with a salad. Use head lettuce, carrots, cabbage, celery, and bell peppers to give your mouth the robust texture it desires. If you go light on the dressing, you can eat a whole bowl of salad before you get to the calorie count of a handful of pretzels or potato chips.

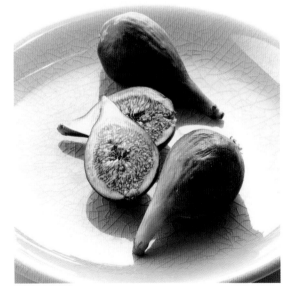

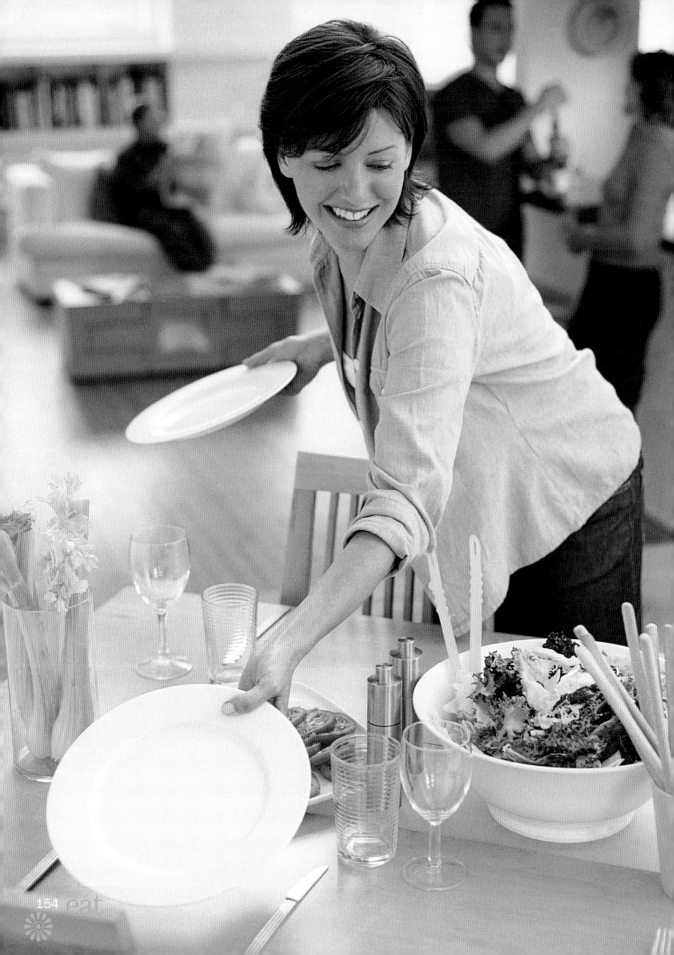

LONG LIFE EATING GOAL: Eat small amounts of food six times a day, every day.

Practice *hara hachi bu*. This Okinawan eating practice translates to "80 percent" and means that traditional Okinawans stop eating when they're 80 percent full. This is a great way to avoid overeating because it gives your brain time to notice what's in your tummy and send an "I'm full" signal. Instead of reaching for seconds, put your fork down and clear the table as soon as you feel the first slight twinges of fullness. (Return to the table for more conversation or take cups of tea into the living room with your dining companions to extend the pleasure of your meal.) "When you start to feel full, your stomach really has become full," Dr. Willcox says, "but physiologically, there's about a 20-minute delay before the stomach tells the brain."

Downsize your dinnerware. In recent years, many dinnerware manufacturers have increased the size of the plates and bowls they sell to keep pace with the larger portions to which we've grown accustomed. If you tend to overeat, serve meals on salad plates instead of dinner plates.

Never skip breakfast. The first meal of the day revs up your metabolism and fills your belly with the fuel you need for energy. A good breakfast prevents excessive eating later in the day. If you're not a natural breakfast lover, wait an hour after you wake up. Or try an unconventional meal, such as a sandwich or bowl of soup.

Practice the three-hour rule. Don't let more than three hours pass between your meals and snacks. Eating regularly keeps you from becoming ravenous or experiencing the effects of low blood sugar: Feeling lightheaded and low on energy. Moderate-size meals and snacks can also help you avoid overeating because it's comforting to know that there's another chance to eat coming soon.

Make lunch the big meal of the day. In traditional European societies, the midday meal is the star. Not only do people take time to linger together over the food, but they also eat more of it than they do at dinner—giving their bodies more time for digestion and more fuel for the rest of the day. Eating a bigger lunch can also help you avoid the late-afternoon slump that can lead to overeating and to poor food choices such as sweets and snack foods.

Set a new second-helpings rule. Allow yourself second helpings of only fruit and vegetables, not of grains, fats, or meats.

Eat 90 percent of your meals at home. You're more likely to eat high-fat, high-calorie, highly processed foods away from home than in your own kitchen or dining room. And you'll avoid the temptation of large restaurant portions, too.

Eat slowly and calmly. Set aside at least a half hour to eat each meal of the day. Make the food last for that whole length of time by eating slowly and stopping frequently to enjoy the conversation of your companions, the view out the window, or the music on the radio. This slow-eating strategy gives your brain the opportunity to notice how much you've already eaten and send a signal that you're done.

Practice the grounded-fork rule. To help slow your eating, force yourself to put down your fork after every bite and do not pick it up until you've swallowed what you've just put in your mouth.

Choice **7** Enjoy eating.

Welcome to the last choice of Long Life Eating: enjoyment. Seems a little redundant, doesn't it? We've mentioned taste and flavor countless times throughout this chapter, and we've repeatedly made the point that healthy eating is a celebration, full of pleasure and ritual. So why this particular topic again?

Simple. Many people don't eat for enjoyment or nourishment. They eat because they're nervous or bored or frustrated or because at 3:30 p.m., it's just second nature to take a break and have a candy bar. Or they eat because they feel they have to—Mom would be insulted, after all, if you didn't have seconds.

Other reasons why we eat are more positive, even if misguided. We show affection with food ("I love you so much, here are *two* boxes of chocolate!"). We celebrate with food. We assuage our guilt with food ("I'm really sorry. I brought you a cake as a peace offering.") We reveal our heritage and tradition with food. In this modern world, eating is habit, ritual, therapy, and relaxation. All this is well intended, but at what cost to our health?

Sometimes the problem is merely hectic living. Do you eat so fast you can't remember what you've just consumed, mindlessly nibble while watching TV, or find yourself gobbling fast-food meals in the car while you drive? While all of us eat on the run occasionally, if you make a practice of eating quickly and without pleasure, you will miss out on the profound life- and health-enhancing joys of the table.

In cultures where people live long, healthy lives, meals are events. In Japan, for example,

"Okinawans look for meaning in food and in meals," notes Dr. Willcox. Instead of throwing a box of grocery-store cookies on the table when guests arrive, Okinawans respectfully serve tea. Gathering around the table is a social time as much as a time for food. There's more conversation, more time between bites of rice or fish or vegetables. When this type of meal is over, you leave the table with a full belly and a full heart.

Eating slowly—and savoring the colors, textures, temperatures, and flavors of the foods before you—enhances digestion, discourages overeating, and promotes relaxation. Sharing a meal or snack with friends is a stress-reducing opportunity to reconnect. Now take the pleasure a step or two further. Shop unhurriedly for fresh ingredients and enjoy the sensual experience of washing, chopping, and cooking them to create a wonderful experience for yourself and others.

Each of us has deeply embedded habits and prejudices regarding food. Our message: Reconsider the role of food in your daily life. Are you eating merely out of habit? Is food providing solace for insecurities or frustrations? How many times a day do you gobble down food mindlessly, without the flavor even registering?

Be a mindful eater. Don't focus just on the right foods but also on the right *reasons* to eat—for nourishment, health, social ritual, and of course, enjoyment. A bag of potato chips may sound like the right medicine for a tough day, but we suggest hugs or a walk instead—followed by a healthy sit-down meal with someone you love.

Celebrate Food

LONG LIFE EATING GOAL: Laughter, conversation, and relaxation at as many meals as possible.

Give thanks. Privately or as a group, give thanks for the fact that you're here and able to enjoy the company and the food. It need not be a prayer if you're uncomfortable with that. Come up with your own ritual. It could be a toast or everyone saying hello or a quick moment of silence or even holding hands. Whatever you are comfortable with is the best choice of all.

Really taste the food and enjoy the moment. Put your utensils down between bites. Use the time to chew and swallow. Note the flavors, colors, and textures of the meal as well as the look of the table and the ambience around it. Look out the window and enjoy the view. Think about ways the food fits into the scenery: Are you having oatmeal because it's a cold, snowy day out, just as you did as a child? Are you having a light, no-cook supper that features juicy fruits on a sweltering summer evening, just what you enjoyed on a vacation to a tropical place years ago?

Make conversation. Take turns sharing a positive experience you had during the day, then discuss a challenge you faced and overcame—or are still confronting. Talk about the food and about enjoyable subjects from local or world news. Save complaints and controversies for another time. The table should be a happy place!

Turn off the TV and put away cell phones, pagers, and laptops. Make mealtime inviolable. Friends, phone solicitors, and colleagues can reach you later.

Invite a friend or meet somewhere for a meal. Make a meal even more social by sharing it with someone who's not in your household.

Don't feel like cooking? Meet at a café or local cafeteria or bring brown-bag lunches to a table at a park. The important part is being together.

Savor every nuance of your meal. Think of a traditional Japanese tea ceremony, in which every sense has a role to play: You listen and observe as the tea is poured, feel the hot cup in your hand, smell and taste the tea. To focus your mind and slow things further, bring a meal to the table course by course and leave time between courses for relaxation and conversation.

Eat seasonally. Enjoying local seasonal produce can make a meal more meaningful by linking your plate to the place where you live. Visit a farmer's market for seasonal vegetables or meats. As you prepare and eat them, think about how they grew in the same sun and rain you've experienced over the past few months.

Treat family like company. Fresh flowers, a nice table setting, garnishes on the plates—you and your family deserve such niceties every day! Resolve to never eat at a messy table.

Break Bad Food Habits

LONG LIFE EATING GOAL: Never use food to cope with life's challenges.

Figure out your stress-eating triggers. Experts estimate that 75 percent of overeating is due to emotions. Do you eat when you're angry? Bored? Lonely? At a party when you're feeling nervous? Pay attention to the situations that prompt you to reach for extra helpings or snacks. Identifying your overeating triggers is the first step in fixing emotional eating problems.

Fix emotional eating. Once you've discovered which emotions are behind your bad eating habits, you can fix the situation. If you're feeling angry, try putting on some music and dancing. Worried? Turn off the news and read a joke book or turn on a comedy station. Sad? Read something inspirational, meditate or pray, or call a friend. Lonely? Call or write to a friend or take a walk to a place where there are people, such as the library. Just be mindful that food can't soothe or solve your troubles; at best, it will mask them for a short time. That's not a benefit at all.

Chat more, eat less. Never stand by the chips and mindlessly eat while you talk with other guests at a party. Instead of letting conversation lead you into mindless eating, let socializing be the centerpiece of your experience by staying far from the buffet. When you arrive at a picnic or backyard barbecue, grab a low-calorie drink and scope out a great seat at a table filled with friends, family, or friendly strangers. This is your home base. Then approach the buffet table or grill with a purpose: Grab a plate, add carefully chosen foods, and carry it back to your spot at the center of the real fun.

Write in your journal. Paying attention to your feelings by writing them down is a powerful way to make yourself feel valued—and feel better—without resorting to sour-cream-and-onion chips. Keep a feelings journal and pay attention to situations that lead to overeating. That way, you'll learn how to spot dangerous situations sooner and take preventive steps.

Have more fun. When life is busy and your to-do list is long, it's easy to turn to food as quick entertainment and solace. In fact, you may be missing out on other healthy pleasures that would be more satisfying. When was the last time you enjoyed your favorite activities, such as going to concerts or dog shows, gardening or museum hopping, roller-skating or antiquing? Make time for fun, and you may find you don't need that "fun pack" of cookies after all.

Tune in to your true hunger level. Before you take a bite, stop and rate your hunger on a scale of 1 to 10—with 1 meaning famished and 10 being totally stuffed, the way you'd feel after a big Thanksgiving dinner. The time to eat is when you're at about 3. The time to stop eating? When you're at 5 to 7—feeling comfortably satisfied but not overly full. If you're reaching for food when you're not at 3, pull back and remind yourself that it will be snack time, or mealtime, soon.

Get moving! Physical activity cuts stress and pumps feel-good endorphins throughout your body while burning calories. Make a new commitment to getting a half hour of activity most days of the week. Great options include walking, exercising to aerobics videos and DVDs, taking a class or doing strength training at a gym, or simply choosing active fun like hiking, bowling, swimming, or skating.

Healthier Snacks

LONG LIFE EATING GOAL: Replace junk food in your diet with healthy alternatives.

Eat between meals. Yes, you read that correctly. We believe you should eat every three hours or so to avoid severe hunger that leads to low blood sugar and overeating.

Snack on fiber-rich produce plus protein. When snack time does roll around, treat yourself right with a satisfying mini-feast of fruit or veggies plus protein. Have a handful of cherry tomatoes plus a piece of low-fat string cheese in the morning instead of a muffin. Try apple slices with peanut butter or a few slices of chicken or turkey on a slice of whole-wheat bread in the afternoon. Target your morning snack to be about 80 calories and your afternoon snack to be about 150 calories. You can also have a serving of whole grains, such as a slice of whole-wheat bread, instead of the protein or in place of fruit for an afternoon snack.

Good protein choices include one hard-boiled egg, 1 tablespoon peanut butter, 1/2 ounce nuts (such as 12 almonds, 8 cashews, 8 pecan halves, 26 shelled pistachios, or 6 walnut halves), 2 slices of roasted chicken (about a quarter of a breast), and 1/2 cup yogurt.

Easy veggie choices include cherry tomatoes, baby carrots, sliced bell peppers, cucumbers, and chopped broccoli.

Fruit choices include a piece of any whole fresh fruit or 1/2 cup chopped or sliced fruit.

Plan for a treat. Strive for balance on a big day out, such as at an amusement park or fair. You don't want to drive home regretting what you ate, but you also don't want to spend your special outing feeling deprived while everyone else slurps their lemonade and tosses back handfuls of kettle corn. Your smart strategy: In advance, decide on one moderate-calorie treat per day.

Take your own snacks. Head off a moment of hungry weakness by packing ready-to-eat veggies, fruit (in a protective plastic container), a zipper-seal bag containing nuts or a handful of whole-grain crackers and low-fat cheese, or half of a peanut butter sandwich on whole wheat.

Invest in a water-bottle carrier. These slings allow you to easily carry a bottle of water. Having water with you at all times will help you resist sodas and other sweetened drinks and keep you hydrated. Often, when we think we're hungry between meals, we're actually thirsty.

Keep an emergency snack in your purse or car. A healthy cereal bar—look for one with less than 200 calories and at least 3 grams of fiber— could help you avoid overeating or choosing high-calorie snacks if you find yourself away from home for longer than you expected.

Use snacks to fill nutritional gaps. If you notice sometime after lunch that you haven't eaten much fruit, for example, or haven't had any dairy products, plan your next snack to strategically fill the gap.

Sit down when you snack. Put your snack on a plate or in a bowl and sit at the table to eat it. Have a glass of water or a cup of tea at the same time. This will make the "mini-meal" last longer and feel more substantial.

Say no to vending machines. For the rest of your life. Convince yourself that bags of salty, greasy snacks and bars of sugary processed candy have no place in your life. After a month or two of successful avoidance, you'll forget that stuff ever appealed to you.

Foods That Harm

When you eat for long life and lasting health, there's no room in your diet for these three health-robbing, aging-accelerating food additives: sodium, sweeteners, and bad fats.

Packed into processed foods, drive-through lunches, and manufactured treats (from commercial baked goods to soft-serve custards), these ingredients seem to have an addictive power over us—and long-term health consequences such as high blood pressure, high blood sugar, and a higher risk of heart disease and stroke.

Small wonder that top nutrition experts call them everything from "the biggest food-processing disasters in history" to "Frankenfoods" (referring, of course, to Dr. Frankenstein's manufactured monster). No wonder either that the American Medical Association, the foremost organization of doctors in the United States, has asked that the government remove one of them—sodium—from its list of "safe" food additives.

Breaking free of these health robbers can be a real effort. Sodium and sweeteners heighten the flavor of foods—especially low-flavor or tasteless processed foods like french fries. And saturated fats and trans fats lend a pleasing crunch to crackers and cookies and keep other baked goods moist and tender. But it can be done. When Purdue University researchers checked in with volunteers who followed a low-sodium meal plan for 12 weeks, the participants rated lower-salt foods just as appealing as regular foods.

"It can take a while to retrain your taste buds," Moores notes. "But you'll notice that you enjoy the flavors of fresh, whole foods more and that you feel better. Moving away from processed foods full of these additives requires patience and perseverance, but it's worthwhile." The other key: Eating outside the box—or wrapper. Opting for unprocessed foods, in their natural state (think fresh fruit, veggies, whole grains, and freshly brewed tea) automatically means you'll get less of these bad guys.

Here's what you need to know.

Sodium

Too much sodium raises your odds of developing high blood pressure—one reason that 90 percent of all 55-year-olds with normal blood pressure will eventually have hypertension. And it may not matter if you're "salt-sensitive" or not. Too much sodium prompts your body to hold on to more fluid (to "dilute" the extra saltiness!); this increases blood volume, forcing your heart to pump harder with every beat and putting extra stress on blood vessel walls. Small wonder people with high blood pressure are at high risk of heart attacks and strokes! But that's not all. A high-sodium diet can thin your bones, boost your risk of gastric cancer, and worsen lung function in people with exercise-induced asthma—a condition that plagues 9 out of 10 people with asthma, studies show.

The biggest youth robbers: Condiments, processed meats and cheeses, canned beans and vegetables (we'll show you how to slash the sodium in these otherwise healthy foods), salad dressings, and pickles. Here's how to get rid of the extra saltiness.

Automatically toss all "flavor packets" and "spice mixes" that come with cook-at-home grain dishes. They're mostly salt. Instead, invest in several sodium-free spice blends or make your own. Three we love: ground black pepper mixed with a dash of sodium-free dried lemon peel; oregano, ground cumin, and a shake of red pepper flakes; and basil, marjoram, and thyme. You can save about 500 milligrams of sodium per serving.

Always buy natural—or better yet, reduced-sodium—cheese. A slice of pasteurized, processed Swiss cheese packs 435 milligrams of

Learn to crave healthy foods.

sodium; a slice of real Swiss cheese contains 54 milligrams; and a low-sodium slice has just 4 milligrams. Same goes for grated Parmesan: A tablespoon of pregrated regular Parmesan has 76 milligrams, while the low-sodium version has 3 milligrams. Choosing low-sodium cheese is a great strategy because it's so flavorful you won't miss the salt.

Never eat canned beans or vegetables unless you've rinsed them twice. Canned veggies and beans may contain one-fifth of your daily sodium allotment, up to 500 milligrams per half cup! Drain off the liquid, dump the beans or veggies into a colander or strainer and rinse thoroughly, then rinse again. A good "shower" can remove nearly half the sodium, say University of Michigan experts. In one study, a three-minute rinse cut sodium in canned tuna by 80 percent.

Make your own salad dressing. Bottled salad dressings can contain up to 620 milligrams of sodium in a single 2-tablespoon serving—and reduced-fat dressings often have more salt to offset the loss of flavor. Make your own dressing with 1/2 cup olive oil, 1/4 cup balsamic or cider vinegar or lemon juice, and your choice of herbs and spices (we love crushed garlic, black pepper, and oregano), then refrigerate. A 2-tablespoon serving packs less than 3 milligrams of sodium!

Eat real meat instead of lunchmeats, hot dogs, bacon, and sausage. A single slice of deli ham packs 350 milligrams of sodium; one strip of bacon, 192 milligrams; and deviled ham for one sandwich, 700 milligrams. Pretty much any meat product that's processed in a factory or cured or smoked for flavor is off the charts when it comes to sodium. Make sandwiches instead with unsalted slices of turkey breast or lean beef.

How Bad Are We?

Let's be honest: You can't—and shouldn't—completely remove sodium, sweeteners, and saturated and trans fats from your diet. But we have a long way to go just to get to acceptable levels. Here's how much we typically eat in a day and how much experts say is safe.

INGREDIENT	SAFE AMOUNT	WHAT MOST OF US GET
Sodium	1,500–2,300 mg	4,000 mg
Sweeteners	10–12 tsp	34 tsp
Saturated fat	13–20 g	50–60 g
Trans fats	2 g or less (0 is best!)	5.8 g

Eat cucumbers, not pickles. A single dill pickle can pack up to 830 milligrams of sodium! Instead, slice a cucumber and serve with plain yogurt sprinkled with fresh or dried dill and some lemon juice or dried grated lemon rind.

Toss the blood pressure time bomb condiments! Garlic and onion salts pack 1,480 milligrams of sodium per teaspoon; soy sauce, 500 to 2,000 milligrams per tablespoon; and bouillon cubes, 1,200 milligrams per tiny cube. Throw them out—now. Safe alternatives include onion flakes, garlic powder, and low-sodium soup stock. Don't bother with reduced- or low-sodium soy sauce, as it packs 300 to 830 milligrams per tablespoon.

Shake less sodium in the kitchen—and at the table. Use kosher salt in recipes—it's coarser, so it doesn't pack as tightly in a measuring spoon. And put light salt or a salt substitute in your saltshaker. Just train yourself not to use more; some substitutes still contain salt, and using more simply raises levels again.

The "Bad" Fats

Trans fats do not appear in nature. They were invented in a laboratory to be a healthy alternative to artery-clogging saturated fats. But in a classic case of consumer science gone awry, trans fats are now estimated to cause 50,000 deaths a year by promoting heart disease and cancer as well as dementia and diabetes. Dubbed "the worst kind of fat" by detractors, these Franken-fats are even worse than the artery-clogging saturated fats in butter, well-marbled steaks, and ice cream. Both raise levels of heart-threatening LDL cholesterol. But trans fats also hike up dangerous blood chemicals like triglycerides and lipoprotein (a), depress levels of "good guy" HDL cholesterol, and even make cells more resistant to insulin—a step toward diabetes. They also fire up low-level inflammation—a chronically "on alert" immune response linked with heart disease, stroke, cancer, and diabetes.

Unfortunately, it took a long time before scientists discovered the damage that trans fats cause. In the meantime, food manufacturers had already made trans fats key ingredients. Today, they're in at least 42,000 food products—keeping stick margarines solid at room temperature, making packaged cakes moist, and keeping boxed cookies and chips crunchy. But a growing stack of research confirms that trans fats are health robbers—and in response, more and more trans fat–free processed foods are becoming available. (Keep reading labels, though. Now that food manufacturers must list trans fats on food labels, some may revert to saturated fat–rich palm or coconut oil, experts warn. Those aren't healthy alternatives!)

Here's how to steer clear of bad fats—and fill your fat quota with the good stuff every day.

Permanently ban factory-made cookies, crackers, and other baked goods from your diet. Instead, snack on individually wrapped dark chocolates, crunchy nuts, or raisins. Some experts estimate that up to 95 percent of prepared cookies and 100 percent of crackers may contain trans fats. More trans fat–free options appear every day, but these snack foods provide tons of age-accelerating saturated fat, sweeteners, refined carbohydrates, and calories. (One famous brand of chocolate chip cookies packs 300 calories per serving and as much fat as a 12-ounce sirloin steak!) But don't give up treats. An ounce of dark chocolate provides heart-healthy antioxidants. A small handful of nuts (about 19 nuts, the amount that would fit into a breath-mint box) or a small box of raisins provides lots of flavor and chewing satisfaction as well as a wealth of fiber and antioxidants, and, for the nuts, good fats that protect arteries.

Say "no thanks" to commercially fried foods. Get a grilled chicken sandwich instead of the crispy fried version, and have a salad in place of french fries. Experts at the Harvard School of Public Health warn that commercial fryers are still filled with trans fat–rich oils. And even restaurants that claim their foods are trans fat–free probably aren't using good fats—the fryers are usually filled with blends containing high amounts of omega-6 fatty acids, a type of fat we already consume way too much of.

Bake—and spread—good fats. If you've been eating stick margarine instead of butter, the news about trans fats may find you rethinking your spread of choice. Don't throw in the towel and return to butter. Instead of trans fat–heavy stick margarine (or some brands of tub margarine), look for one with no saturated or trans fats, such as brands made with yogurt or olive oil. The best provide heart-healthy monounsaturated fats and even a smidge of omega-3 fatty acids.

Unmask hidden trans fats. A product can claim "0 trans fats" and still have up to 0.5 gram

Fall in love with olive oil.

per serving. So if you have four cookies instead of two, you could eat 1 gram of these nasty fats without realizing it. To ferret out hidden trans fats, check the ingredients list for "partially hydrogenated," "fractionated," and even "shortening." The higher on the list these terms appear, the more fat is in the food.

Check your favorites online. Many food chains—from fast-food joints to upscale coffee bars to casual-dining spots—list the trans fat content of their menu items on their Web sites. If you've got a favorite, check it out. Example: The pumpkin scone at one famous coffee bar weighs in with a shocking 6 grams of trans fats!

Drink coffee, not fat. Love special coffee drinks? Order a latte or cappuccino with fat-free milk and a shot of low-sugar flavor syrup, then sprinkle cinnamon, cocoa powder, and vanilla over the foam. You'll get a serving of bone-building, calcium-rich milk and avoid saturated-fat sticker shock: A mocha drink, for example, can pack nearly 500 calories and 16 grams of fat, much of it saturated.

Replace butter in recipes and sautéing with good-for-you oils. Use canola for baking—a good rule of thumb is 3/4 tablespoon of oil for every 1 tablespoon of butter called for. Keep an oil spritzer loaded with olive oil near the stove and spray pans before cooking—you'll get flavor but keep calories down.

Have a fancy fruit salad deluxe instead of premium ice cream. Fancy ice creams can contain as much fat as a fast-food double cheeseburger. Switching to an all-fruit sorbet is a better choice but will still flood your body with loads of extra sugar in most cases. The best choice: Indulge in an over-the-top fruit salad. Layer frozen raspberries, sliced mango, super-sweet fresh pineapple (buy it precut in the produce department), mandarin oranges

The Anticancer Diet

Here are some of the ways to cut your cancer risk, based on recent studies.

Say "yes" to onions, apples, berries, kale, and broccoli.
Eating lots of antioxidants called flavonols—found in these foods—cut pancreatic cancer risk by 23 percent. Among smokers, a flavonol-rich diet lowered risk by 59 percent, report researchers from the Cancer Research Center of Hawaii who studied 183,518 women and men.

Go to the limit with fruits and veggies.
Study participants who got 12 produce servings per day lowered their risk of various cancers by 29 percent as compared to women and men who ate just 3 daily servings, a recent study of 500,000 men and women age 50 and older has found. Merely adding 1 or 2 produce servings a day could lower your risk by 6 percent.

Choose the red wine.
Red-wine drinkers cut their risk of colorectal cancer by 68 percent in a recent study from the State University of New York at Stony Brook. In contrast, white-wine aficionados did not. Researchers suspect that an antioxidant in red wines called resveratrol may offer powerful protection against colon cancer.

Have fish more often.
Men who ate fish five times a week or more had a 40 percent lower risk of developing colorectal cancer compared to those who ate fish less than once a week, say Harvard Medical School researchers who are tracked the health of 22,071 guys.

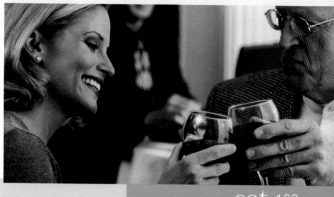

packed in juice, and whatever else you love. It's colorful, sweet, and fun to eat—and gives you a bonus of age-defying antioxidants and fiber.

Corn Syrup, Sugar, and Other Sweeteners

Also demonized as a sinister "Frankenfood"—even as "the Devil's candy" and "the crack of sweeteners"—thick, goopy, high-fructose corn syrup is hiding in a stunning variety of foods, from soft drinks and ice cream to soups and salad dressings. Until recently, scientists suspected that this popular sweetener's unique chemistry actually fueled feelings of hunger instead of satisfying them, and they blamed it for the American obesity epidemic.

The truth, it seems, is that corn syrup isn't a demon—at least, not any more so than table sugar. New research has debunked claims that corn syrup alters levels of appetite-suppressing and appetite-raising hormones.

But sweeteners aren't off the hook. Whether it's sugar, corn syrup, honey, or a fancy organic sweetener, downing too much can pack on extra pounds (especially because many sweet foods are also high in fat) and raise your blood sugar, increasing your risk of diabetes, heart disease, and stroke. And we're eating more sweetener than ever: 100 pounds per person in the United States in 2005, up from 75 pounds each in 1975. To blame: super-size beverages, decadent desserts, giant candy bars, and cookies as big as salad plates.

We're addicted to sugar. The more we eat, the more we want. Why? A big shot of refined sugar makes blood sugar skyrocket, then plummet as the hormone insulin ushers the sugar into cells throughout your body. Sometimes it can fall to a lower level than before you drank that giant cola or ate those 35 jelly beans. As a result, you feel tired, hungry, and cranky—and crave more sugar. But these tips can help you break the sugar habit and get off the roller coaster for good.

Replace soft drinks with healthier sips. As we've discussed, one of the best things you can do for your health is to gradually replace soda, sweetened teas, fruit drinks, and other sweetened beverages with water, unsweetened tea, club soda, or diluted fruit juice. To start, try mixing fountain drinks half and half with the diet version. Pour an ounce of grape or orange juice into seltzer water for a low-sugar spritzer. Add a squeeze of lemon or lime juice to filtered water. Visit the herbal tea section of your grocery store and bring home new flavors to drink hot or cold. Treat yourself to one glass of real fruit juice—without added sugar or sweeteners—each day. Go beyond orange: We love Concord grape, tangerine, and pomegranate. Yes, real juice has calories (between 100 and 140 per 8-ounce glass), but it counts toward your daily fruit serv-

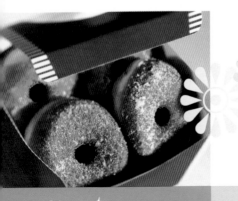

Processed-food manufacturers— not Mother Nature—train us to love sweetness.

ings, and the full-bodied flavor and natural sweetness is intensely pleasurable.

Buy 100 percent fruit juice. Many juices at the food store are enhanced with sweeteners, to the point where there are nearly as many grams of sugar per serving as in a cola. So don't assume the juice you buy is all juice. Read the label; if it contains corn syrup or other sweeteners, put it back and find a brand that's all juice.

Look at other labels as well. It's worth checking almost every packaged food you buy, be it cookies, kielbasa, or spaghetti sauce. If a sweetener is among the first five ingredients, it's probably sweeter than you want for your health.

Sprinkle strategically. No need to banish your sugar bowl. Dusting your high-fiber breakfast cereal with a little sugar or stirring a teaspoon into homemade hot chocolate (made with fat-free milk and cocoa powder) is a great way to make it easier to enjoy high-fiber cereal or an extra serving of bone-friendly fat-free milk. Just limit sugar add-ins to one or two a day.

Make your own candy alternative: grown-up gorp. Mix equal parts of your favorite nuts, raisins, dried cranberries, and high-fiber cereal and store in a zipper-seal bag. Allow yourself one handful per day when your sweet tooth clamors for a treat.

Have fruit for dessert six days a week, then indulge on the seventh. Sometimes the best way to give something up is to have a little once in a while. You won't fall off the wagon when you pass the bakery stand at the mall on Wednesday if you know you can have two home-made chocolate chip cookies on Saturday night.

Rediscover the tang of plain yogurt. Mixed with fresh fruit and topped with a dusting of nuts, plain yogurt has half the sugar of sweetened vanilla yogurt and 60 fewer calories.

Sensible Supplements

You've got car insurance, homeowner's insurance, life insurance, and perhaps even pet insurance. Isn't it time for affordable, proven, and sensible *nutrition* insurance?

Maybe you think you don't need it. Or you're already taking a bunch of pricy, super-duper, high-end supplements. Or you have a single dusty bottle of something hidden somewhere in the medicine cabinet. In all these cases, it's time for a sensible new approach. Experts say that after age 50, your best "nutrition insurance" is taking an inexpensive multivitamin plus a calcium supplement every day, with a few fish-oil capsules thrown in if you don't eat fish at least twice a week. "A multivitamin and a calcium supplement are all most people will ever need to cover any shortfalls," says O'Rourke. "You don't need high doses or fancy supplements or overpriced pills. Just the basics."

We'll say it again: You don't need high-dose supplements for everyday good health (unless, of course, your doctor has a good reason to prescribe one). In recent years, study after study has shown that big doses of vitamins like A, E, and even C don't provide any health advantages—and could be dangerous. In the largest-ever analysis of antioxidants—a look at 68 studies involving 232,606 people conducted by researchers at Copenhagen University Hospital in Denmark—people who regularly took beta-carotene, vitamin A, and vitamin E supplements had a 4 to 16 percent *increased* risk of death. Some experts have criticized the study's design, but everyone agrees that getting disease-fighting antioxidants from fruit, veggies, and whole grains is a smarter move.

Even if you're among the 2 percent of us who never, ever indulges in fast food or junk-food, your diet may no longer completely cover all the special vitamin and mineral needs that crop up in your fifties, sixties, and beyond.

Convinced? Here's how to buy—and use—your new "nutrition insurance" policy!

Multivitamin Magic

Our definition of supplement magic? Not crazy, pie-in-the-sky claims or extra ingredients—such as added minerals, herbs, or antioxidant extracts—that sound promising but that, research shows, probably don't deliver any discernible health benefits. To us, multivitamin magic means finding the right multivitamin at the right price—and not letting the vast array of nutritional supplements crammed on drugstore shelves confuse you or tempt you to spend extra money for stuff you simply don't need.

Here's how to find, store, and take the perfect multivitamin.

Spend like a cheapskate. A multi that provides sufficient levels of important vitamins and minerals shouldn't cost you more than $30 a year. You can keep costs lower by buying on sale; just check the expiration dates to be sure you'll take them all before then. Multivitamins will keep for about a year in a cool, dry place. "You don't need a fancy, expensive pill," Moores says. "A moderately priced name brand or store brand is usually just fine."

Find out what a "serving size" is. Some vitamin labels provide nutrient info for a serving that's actually two pills, not one. Don't make the mistake of thinking that one is all you need!

Trouble swallowing? Ask your pharmacist about alternatives. Find out which brands are easy to cut in half, then invest in an inexpensive pill splitter (they cost as little as $1) to get the job done easily and correctly. Liquid and chewable multis are another option, but they may be more expensive and may not contain the levels of nutrients that you need.

Look for 100 percent of the Daily Value (DV) for the "big nine" nutrients. Make sure your multi has 100 percent of the DV (the amount a typical, healthy person needs in a day) for thiamin (B_1); riboflavin (B_2); niacin (B_3); vitamins B_6, B_{12}, C, D, and E; and folic acid. Avoid megadoses, Moores says. "Just getting recommended daily levels is enough to fill in gaps, which is all you're trying to do with a multi. The goal is to get what you'd normally get from food, not to flood your body with extras that will usually just be excreted in your urine (for water-soluble vitamins) or stored in fat tissue (for fat-soluble vitamins)."

Limit intake of retinol-based vitamin A. More than 5,000 IU per day of vitamin A from retinol may increase osteoporosis risk. Look for supplements containing no more than 2,500 IU of retinol-based vitamin A (it may be listed on the label or in the ingredients as vitamin A acetate or palmitate). Less risky: vitamin A that comes from beta-carotene, which your body converts to A as needed. A big caution: If you smoke, keep levels of even supplemental beta-carotene low since studies suggest high levels may raise lung cancer risk.

Go easy on iron. You don't need it. "Increased iron is associated with a higher risk of heart disease," notes Dr. Blumberg. "Once women stop menstruating, they stop losing iron, and men have been storing it all along." Most older people get plenty of iron from their diets and a low-dose supplement. Aim for 8 milligrams or less. If your current multi contains more, toss it and switch. Getting too much can lead to gastrointestinal discomfort and, for 1 in 250 people, may trigger a potentially fatal iron-overload condition called hemochromatosis.

Take three daily supplements.

Don't exceed 100 percent of other minerals. You just don't need more than the Daily Value for chromium, copper, iodine, manganese, molybdenum, and zinc. And most of us take in sufficient quantities of chloride, magnesium, phosphorus, and potassium from a healthy diet. Don't worry about sci-fi-sounding trace elements like boron, nickel, silicon, tin, and vanadium. Experts aren't sure we need them at all.

Consider getting more vitamin D from a separate supplement. Researchers have warned that not getting enough vitamin D—from food, supplements, or sunlight—could raise the risk of a wide variety of cancers, including breast, ovarian, colon, and prostate. More recently, an intriguing study suggested that getting more vitamin D could cut your risk. In a Creighton University study that followed 1,179 healthy postmenopausal women for five years, those who got 1,400 to 1,500 milligrams of calcium plus 1,100 IU of vitamin D from supplements every day had a 60 to 77 percent lower risk of cancer than those who didn't get those amounts. The connection? Lab studies suggest that vitamin D helps stop cancer from proliferating, promotes the death of tumor cells, and helps stop tumors from developing blood vessels that allow them to grow larger.

Food sources alone can't raise the amount of vitamin D in your bloodstream to protective levels. A 3.5-ounce serving of salmon, a top source, packs just 360 IU; a glass of fat-free milk, 98 IU; and fortified breakfast cereal has about 40 IU per serving. And while ultraviolet B (UVB) light in sunshine synthesizes vitamin D in your body, rays are too weak from November to May in northerly climes—and not everyone can or should sunbathe in shorts or a bathing suit for 15 to 30 minutes a day anyway. (Plus, after age 50, your body simply makes less D!)

Your best bet? Look for D supplements. The safe upper limit for adults is 1,000 IU per day, experts say.

Read the label before buying a "silver" or "senior" formula—or any formula designed specifically for women, men, or a particular ethnic group. Judge these trendy "customized vitamins" against our standards. Some may offer slightly more or less of certain nutrients, but in most cases, experts say, a low-cost multivitamin is just as good.

Skip types with added herbs and antioxidants. A rising tide of studies shows that antioxidants in pill form simply don't work—or may even be dangerous. And added herbs for memory or your prostate may be present in tiny, ineffective doses or create unwanted side effects and interactions with prescription drugs you may be taking.

Don't be swayed by marketing ploys. Your body doesn't care if the vitamin C comes from rose hips or was produced in a big vat somewhere. And unless you've got an allergy or sensitivity to ingredients such as wheat, lactose, or rice, you shouldn't pay extra for allergen-free types.

Calcium Supplements

No multivitamin could possibly contain a day's worth of calcium, simply because this bone-building mineral is made of big molecules that couldn't be packed into a single pill small enough for a human being to swallow. Unless you faithfully get three to four servings of dairy products every day, plan to keep a calcium supplement on your shelf—and to take it. Research proves that it can cut your risk of developing brittle bones and of the debilitating fractures that change the lives of millions of people each year. Here's how to buy and take this important supplement.

For best absorption, buy a brand name or look for the USP symbol. Calcium won't do your bones any good if the supplement doesn't break down in your digestive system so your body can absorb it. Usually, name brands, types labeled "purified," and those with the United States Pharmacopeia (USP) symbol will be tops for absorbability, the National Osteoporosis Foundation says. Or go with a chewable or liquid supplement.

Test it yourself. Wondering about your pill's absorbability? Place one in a small glass of warm water for a half hour and stir occasionally. If it hasn't dissolved in 30 minutes, it probably won't break down in your stomach either.

Check for "elemental calcium." That's the amount that's available for absorption in your gastrointestinal system. The less elemental calcium per pill, the more pills you'll need to reach your goal. How much is there? Check the Daily Value column on the nutrition facts label. The DV is based on 1,000 milligrams per day, but remember that we are recommending 1,200 milligrams. If the label says a serving provides 50 percent of the DV, you're actually getting 500 milligrams of calcium. If it says 10 percent, you're getting 100 milligrams.

Carbonate or citrate? It depends on your personality and your schedule. Both types work equally well. If you eat most meals at home and are already in the habit of taking supplements or other pills regularly, choose carbonate. It's the least expensive, provides the most elemental calcium per pill (40 percent versus 21 percent for citrate) so you need fewer pills per day, and is best absorbed when stomach acid levels are high—about an hour or so after a meal.

If you're busy, eat away from home frequently, or are forgetful, choose calcium citrate. It's a little pricier, but it's better absorbed on an empty stomach than calcium carbonate.

What about other types of calcium? You could choose calcium gluconate, calcium lactate, or calcium phosphate, but they contain only about 9 percent elemental calcium, so you'd need lots of pills to reach your goal of 1,200 milligrams. And we suggest avoiding brands made with bonemeal, dolomite, or oyster shells because they may contain lead or other heavy metals.

New to calcium supplements? Start with a comfortable 500 milligrams a day. Take this amount for one week and see how you feel. Some types may cause gas and constipation. If this happens, switch to a different type.

Never take more than 500 milligrams at a time. Your body can't absorb more than that. If you take two 500-milligram calcium supplements a day, space them at least three hours apart for maximum absorbability.

Balance pills and food. If you have a glass of milk and a slice of cheese with lunch, you've just gotten at least 500 milligrams of high-quality calcium and don't need a supplement right now. If you have just a smidge of calcium at dinnertime (say, a serving of broccoli sprinkled with almond slivers), and you haven't had much other calcium during the day, adding a supplement could bring you up to your daily goal of 1,200 milligrams. Don't forget—calcium-fortified foods count, too.

Love cereal and milk in the morning? Do some math before adding a breakfast calcium supplement. A cup of fat-free milk plus a cup of fortified breakfast cereal could provide nearly a day's worth of calcium. If your morning calcium quota's being met in your bowl, don't bother adding a supplement—save it for lunch, dinner, or snacks so you'll get the most benefit, Moores suggests.

Think 500-500-200. Plan to get most of your calcium in before dinner. That way, you'll have time to catch up in the evening if you've missed a supplement or somehow had a day without many high-calcium foods.

Stash calcium everywhere. Keep a bottle at your desk, in the kitchen, in the car. Put chocolate-flavored calcium chews or flavored antacids made with calcium carbonate in your purse or briefcase, too. Why? Calcium protects bone only when you take it faithfully—several times a day, every single day of every single month of every single year. When Tufts University researchers followed women and men in their late sixties and early seventies for three years, those who took calcium increased bone mineral density and slashed their fracture risk. But all those bone-guarding benefits disappeared when the volunteers stopped taking their supplements for the subsequent two years.

Don't mix calcium with meds that must be taken on an empty stomach. It can interfere with absorption of antibiotics like tetracycline, thyroid hormones, corticosteroids, and even iron supplements.

Fish Oil

Fish-oil capsules are among the best way to get the benefits of omega-3 fatty acids quickly and easily. And as we've said, those benefits are substantial. Omega-3 fatty acids can cut heart attack risk by a whopping 73 percent when consumed daily as part of a healthy diet. Omega-3s can also cut triglyceride levels up to 40 percent. There's also some evidence that omega-3s from fish can reduce the stiffness and joint pain of rheumatoid arthritis and may also cut stroke risk as well.

If you don't have heart disease, the American Heart Association recommends getting 1,000 milligrams of the two most powerful omega-3s—

eicosapentaenoic acid (EPA) and docosahexaenoic acid (DHA). Higher levels may work better for cutting triglycerides and easing rheumatoid arthritis symptoms, but keep your intake below 3,000 milligrams a day unless you talk with your doctor, since more could cause bleeding. Fish oil's anticlotting powers could be dangerous for people with bleeding disorders and those taking anticoagulant medications such as warfarin (Coumadin). Here's how to buy and take these golden orbs of good fats,

Don't worry about pharmaceutical-grade capsules. It's reassuring to know that two major tests of fish-oil supplements found no significant amounts of mercury in top-selling brands. That means you don't have to pay extra for pharmaceutical-grade fish oil: The stuff in the drugstore is fine. The one good reason to pay for pricier pharmaceutical capsules is that you can get all you need from fewer capsules (they're more concentrated).

Decide on your dose, then find it on the label. Most of us could use 500 to 1,000 milligrams of supplemental EPA and DHA per day, though some experts say a great way to up your omega-3 intake every day is to go for 2,000 to 3,000 milligrams. (Check with your doctor first if you take an anticoagulant.) A single 1,000-milligram capsule contains about the amount of these two fats found in a 4-ounce serving of salmon. Since capsules vary in strength, read the label to figure out how many you'll need to reach your desired dose.

Don't confuse fish oil with cod-liver oil. Fish oil is actually made from the bodies of fish, unlike cod-liver oil, which is made exclusively from—you guessed it—fish livers. The danger: Cod-liver oil contains high concentrations of vitamin A; taking it in the same quantities recommended for fish oil can harm your kidneys.

Long Life Pantry *and* Refrigerator makeover

HEALTH PROJECT

When your cupboards and fridge are packed with delicious, convenient, healthy foods, eating the Long Life way is a snap. To get there, do this pantry makeover project. Here's how to get started.

Supplies to have on hand:

A sturdy stepstool so you can access high cupboards and hard-to-reach spots at the backs of shelves safely. Trash bags. Zipper-seal bags to contain messy items you're keeping—or tossing. Cleaning supplies for pantry and refrigerator shelves. A pencil and notepad to make notes about things you need to buy.

Best time for a pantry makeover:

The day before trash pickup, so discarded food won't sit around to attract pests or go bad.

How much time to set aside:

Two to 10 hours, depending on the size of your kitchen. You can break the job into small, manageable chunks if it seems too big to tackle all at once. Do one or two pantry shelves each day or each week, for example. Or tackle just the refrigerator today and save the freezer for next week. If you'd rather do the whole pantry or fridge in one day, start with the highest shelf and work your way down to the lowest.

What to do just before you begin:

Clear off your kitchen table and countertops so you have room to place things. Designate one area for foods you'll keep and one for items you'll discard. (If you can't bear to toss food that's still edible, take unopened treats to a social event or donate it to a local food pantry. Or designate one shelf for items you'll use up and not buy again.)

Step 1 CLEAR OUT YOUR PANTRY

As you remove foods from your pantry shelves, put these in the discard pile.

Out-of-date foods, as well as anything that's dried out, spoiled, or rancid. Exposure to oxygen can make cooking oils and whole-grain products go bad even before the expiration date; give yours the sniff test and throw away any that smell stale or bad.

Processed foods containing trans fats and/or saturated fats. Get rid of shortening made with hydrogenated or partially hydrogenated oils as well as cookies, crackers, baking mixes, and store-bought cakes and other processed foods that list these oils or saturated fats as one of the top four ingredients.

High-sugar and/or refined-grain cereals, breads, baked goods, and pastas. You'll replace these with whole-grain, low-sugar versions.

Empty-calorie snack foods. Toss 'em in the trash bag. When you snack for long life, you'll be eating crunchy, juicy fruits, veggies, nuts, and whole-grain crackers instead of high-sodium, high-fat, low-fiber chips, pretzels, and crackers.

High-sodium condiments and processed foods. Toss or give away items that pack more than 20 percent of the recommended daily amount of sodium per serving (roughly 300 milligrams).

"Best intentions" foods that you haven't used for six months to a year. That canned octopus and those ingredients for Thai cooking seemed like such good ideas at the time, but if you're never going to serve exotic seafood snacks or concoct an elaborate meal with coconut milk, curry paste, and fish sauce, it's time to find them a new home.

Step 2 RESTOCK YOUR PANTRY

Keep these items—or put them on your next shopping list.

Canned beans: Pinto, black, red kidney, and navy beans and chickpeas

Canned diced tomatoes, tomato paste, and tomato sauce (lower-sodium versions are best)

Canned fruit in juice or light syrup

Canned vegetables

Dried fruits, including single-serving boxes of raisins

Nuts: unsalted, unflavored almonds, walnuts, pecans, etc.
(store extras in the freezer to keep them fresh longer)

Brown rice: regular and quick-cooking varieties

Other whole grains, such as pearled barley, bulgur, and quinoa
(store in the freezer to retain freshness)

Old-fashioned oats

Whole-grain breakfast cereals that list a whole grain as the
first ingredient and have at least 4 grams of fiber per cup and
not too much fat or sugar

Low-sodium, low-fat canned soups

Whole-wheat pastry flour (store in the freezer for longer shelf
life)

Salt-free seasoning blends and individual herbs and spices

Whole-grain pastas and noodles

Water-packed canned light tuna

Canned salmon

Canola and extra-virgin olive oil

Balsamic vinegar for flavorful dressings and cooking

Low-sodium vegetable juice

Seltzer or sparkling water (delicious mixed with a little fruit
juice)

Popcorn if you have an air popper or no-salt, low-fat
microwavable popcorn if you don't

Fresh garlic

Small onions

Sweet potatoes

Step 3 PURGE YOUR REFRIGERATOR

These refrigerator and freezer items belong in the discard
pile—or can be used up and replaced with healthier choices.

Soda, fruit punch, sweetened commercial tea, and other
sugar-laden drinks

Full-fat milk, cream, half-and-half, cheese, cream cheese,
cottage cheese, and/or yogurt

High-sodium processed cheese spreads and slices and
processed meats

Margarine with trans fats

Full-fat mayo

High-sodium condiments

Fatty ground beef, cuts of beef with visible streaks or
margins of fat, pork (even "lean" pork has more fat than
chicken), bacon, and sausage

Full-fat and premium ice cream as well as high-sugar
sorbet and fruit pops

Frozen dinners and side dishes that contain trans fats or
more than 25 percent of the recommended daily intake of
saturated fat and/or sodium.

Step 4 RESTOCK YOUR REFRIGERATOR

Organize your shelving to best hold the following items.

Low-fat or fat-free milk, half-and-half, cheese, yogurt,
cream cheese, and cottage cheese

Low-fat canola-oil mayo

Boneless, skinless chicken breasts and thighs, turkey
breast, ground skinless chicken, or lean beef

Eggs high in omega-3 fatty acids

Jars of chopped garlic

100% orange juice, Concord grape juice, or pomegranate
juice

Seasonal fruits such as berries, cherries, oranges, tangerines, peaches, grapefruit, grapes, kiwifruit, plums, peaches,
and watermelon or other melons

Seasonal vegetables such as spinach, broccoli, cauliflower,
eggplant, cucumbers, romaine lettuce, mushrooms, radishes, snow peas, sugar snap peas, cabbage, carrots, green
beans, asparagus, or tomatoes

"Convenience" fruits and veggies: Presliced carrots,
pineapple, or salad bar fruit; shredded cabbage; prechopped broccoli and/or cauliflower florets; red and green
bell pepper slices from the salad bar; boxes of cherry
tomatoes; single-serving bags of baby carrots; prewashed
salad greens; precut green beans

Single-meal portions of boneless, skinless chicken or
turkey; lean beef; ground skinless chicken or turkey; frozen
fish (plain—not breaded or in sauce), shrimp, or lobster

Bags of frozen unsweetened fruits such as blueberries,
cherries, peaches, raspberries, or strawberries

Bags of plain frozen vegetables such as spinach,
edamame (green soybeans), corn, green beans, peas, or
mixed vegetables

Healthy frozen dinners for occasional quick meals—look
for brands with less than 400 calories, no trans fats, and
less than 25 percent of the recommended daily intake of
saturated fat and/or sodium.

Low-sugar fruit sorbets and pops—look for brands with
just 4 to 8 grams of sugar per serving

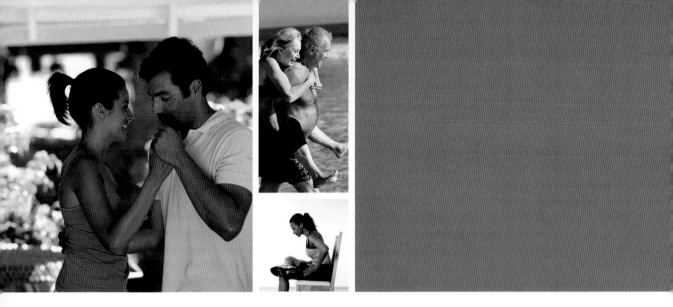

Move to Feel Good

In the summer of 1966, five healthy 20-year-old men went to bed for three weeks. They weren't tired; they were participating in what would become known as the Dallas Bed Rest and Training Study, a landmark study on the effects of exercise (and the lack thereof) on our bodies.

After three weeks of complete inactivity—the men even used wheelchairs to get to the bathroom—their muscle function deteriorated to the point where they could barely stand. As researchers later noted, "Those three weeks of bed rest had a greater effect on their aerobic fitness than 30 years of aging."

After the bed rest part of the study, the men completed eight weeks of intensive exercise training that included treadmill workouts and long-distance running. The results? They completely reversed the damage from the bed rest, proving conclusively the amazing power of physical activity.

move to fee

Fitness at All Ages

Fast-forward 30 years. Researchers contacted the original five men, now age 50, to participate in a follow-up study. All had become sedentary, gaining an average of 50 pounds and doubling their overall body fat (ah, the joys of aging!). They had also lost significant cardiovascular fitness. Not all of that loss was related to the natural effects of aging; about 40 percent was due to inactivity.

But here's the thing: After walking, jogging, or cycling five hours a week for six months, the men *again* completely reversed their age-related drop in cardiovascular fitness. Their resting heart rates, blood pressure levels, and hearts' maximum pumping ability, or aerobic power, returned to the levels of 30 years earlier!

The message? It's never too late to begin exercising.

Don't believe us? How about this one, then. When 50 men and women with an average age of 87 worked out with weights for 10 weeks, they more than doubled their muscle strength and improved their walking speed—even though they weren't doing any walking exercises.

The bottom line: Your physical strength, heart health, and breathing ability aren't bottoming out because you're getting older. If they've declined, it's most likely because you've been sitting around instead of working your muscles regularly.

"Muscle mass seems to be very important to longevity," says Mark Davis, a research associate at the Centre for Sport, Exercise, and Health at the University of Bristol in England.

That's because the amount of muscle you have affects nearly every function in your body. Maintain good muscle tone, and you'll probably gain less weight, have a lower percentage of body fat, and prevent insulin resistance. Your LDL cholesterol and blood sugar levels will be lower, and your HDL cholesterol levels will be higher. You'll also avoid constipation, keep your blood thin and moving smoothly through veins and arteries, improve your sleep, and reduce your risk of depression and memory lapses.

It doesn't take much to reap these benefits. Just a few weeks of regular, moderate- to high-intensity physical activity each day, and almost every health measure is likely to improve—no matter *what* your age. Sure, the benefits are greater if you've maintained an exercise program throughout your life. One study, for instance, found that people who took long swims three to five times a week delayed their natural physical decline by decades. In other words, while the swimmers might be 60 years old, they had the medical measurements of 40-year-olds.

But even if the Beatles were still touring the last time you laced on a pair of sneakers, it's not too late to see dramatic changes in your health and quality of life if you start exercising *today*. Consider this: A study from researchers at Ohio University in Athens found that men between the ages of 60 and 75 could increase their strength at the same rate as men in their twenties by performing basic weight-training exercises twice a week for 16 weeks. By the end of the study, these older men were raising about 600 pounds on a leg-press machine, compared with the 375 pounds they pressed when they began. They also had lower LDL and higher HDL cholesterol levels. All in just four months.

> *Just as the human body needs food for life, so must we all have exercise to survive.*

good

Meanwhile, a study of 1,020 healthy people ranging in age from 54 to 100 (average age, 80) found that for every extra hour a week spent being active, their risk of becoming disabled dropped by 7 percent. By "disabled," we mean having joint pain, being depressed and/or overweight, and even being unable to walk—the kinds of problems that lead to the type of old age you're trying to avoid.

Plus, the more time the older participants spent being active, the lower their risk of dying. Those who spent 2 1/4 hours a week being physically active were nearly one-fourth less likely to die during the 2 1/2-year study than their couch-potato peers. When the physical activity was upped to 7 hours a week, their risk of dying during the study plummeted 57 percent. And remember—these were all healthy people to begin with!

It's not that exercise significantly extends your life. "If you start exercising four times a week at the age of 20, by the end of your life, you've gained three extra years, but those extra years were spent doing the exercise," notes Jere Mitchell, MD, professor of internal medicine and physiology at the University of Texas Southwestern Medical Center in Dallas and one of the original investigators for the Dallas Bed Rest Study. What exercise does, however, is add *life* to your years. "There's a big difference in the quality of life if you drop dead playing tennis at 90 or if you've been in a nursing home since age 60," says Dr. Mitchell.

Yet despite our lip service to an active life, working adults spend little to none of their time exerting their bodies. The problem is particularly bad in the United States: 65 percent of US adults ages 45 to 64 and 78 percent of US adults ages 65 to 74 don't even get *10 minutes a week* of vigorous leisure-time physical activity, i.e., brisk walking, bike riding, or swimming. That's one reason that middle-aged adults are shaping up to be the first generation in modern history that will be *less* healthy in their older years than the generation before.

Don't let yourself be lumped into this generational deficiency. Push yourself out of that easy chair and vow that today begins the rest of your life, the day on which you will pull on a comfortable pair of shorts and a T-shirt, a thick pair of white socks, and a good pair of walking shoes and hit the sidewalk.

You won't go it alone, we promise. In the pages ahead, you'll learn not only more about the health-related benefits of exercise but also *why* something as simple as a walk can have the same effect on your heart as squirting some WD-40 on a squeaky door, what type of physical activity works best for your personality and your goals, and how to get started and motivate yourself. As a bonus, we've included three workout routines of varying difficulty that you can pick up in no time at all.

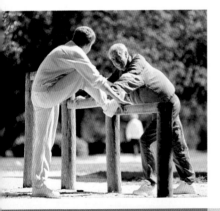

The more energy you expend today, the more energized you will be tomorrow.

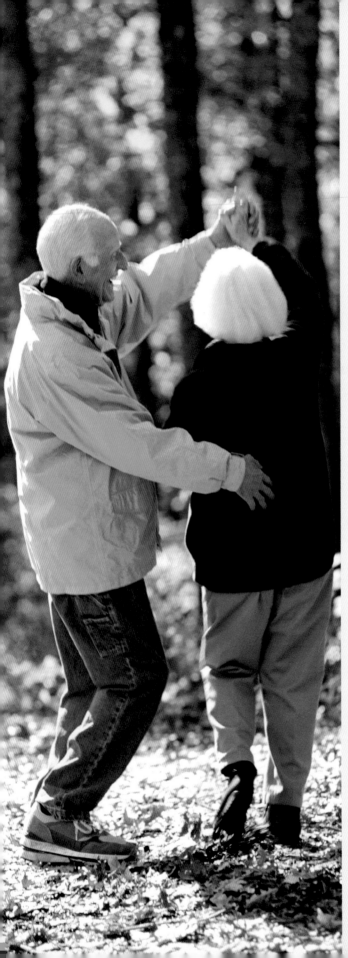

The Benefits of Exercise

Here are several ways that moderate physical activity (the equivalent of walking at a 3-mile-per-hour pace) can help your health.

CARDIOVASCULAR HEALTH

- Improves cholesterol levels
- Improves endurance
- Improves blood pressure
- Improves the ability of the heart to contract and expand

BODY COMPOSITION

- Reduces abdominal fat
- Increases muscle mass

METABOLISM

- Increases the number of calories you burn, even at rest
- Reduces LDL cholesterol
- Reduces very low density cholesterol (vLDL), the type most likely to stick to artery walls
- Reduces triglycerides
- Increases glucose tolerance and decreases insulin resistance

BONE HEALTH

- Slows decline in bone mineral density
- Increases total levels of bone-building calcium and nitrogen

PSYCHOLOGICAL WELL-BEING

- Improves perceived well-being and happiness
- Reduces levels of stress-related hormones
- Improves attention span
- Improves sleep

MUSCLE STRENGTH AND FUNCTION

- Reduces risk of muscle- or bone-related disability
- Improves strength and flexibility
- Reduces risk of falls
- Improves balance

move 175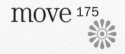

10 Reasons to Move

Ask nonexercisers why they don't get up and move, and you're likely to hear many similar stories. They don't have time. They're not in shape. They have too many aches and pains. And most tellingly, it's just too darn late to bother.

We hope we've convinced you that it's *never* too late to start exercising. But if your brain needs more evidence, here are 10 major health improvements you're likely to see in as little as six months if you begin exercising regularly.

1. Improved memory and cognition

When you work out, whether it's walking through a forest or lifting weights in a gym, you're doing more than just strengthening muscle. You're also stimulating numerous areas in your brain and central nervous system, each of which controls one tiny portion of the movement. Plus, you're stimulating the release of a variety of chemicals, including human growth hormone (HGH). Yes, this is the same hormone given to kids who don't grow; the same one that certain "anti-aging" doctors give to patients at their clinics, even though it's usually illegal to use it for that reason.

Among its youth-promoting benefits, HGH triggers a hormonal and biochemical cascade that releases brain-derived neurotrophic factor (BDNF), a hormone that helps your brain sprout new synapses, or connections between neurons. One study of 59 healthy but sedentary people ages 60 to 79 found that working out aerobically for six months (and we're not talking about marathon training!) increased their brain volume, an improvement missing in a control group that didn't work out. It's probably why several studies find that regular physical activity significantly slows mental decline in people who already have Alzheimer's or other forms of dementia.

It's also why the more BDNF you have circulating in your brain, the greater your ability to learn and remember stuff. The less BDNF, the less learning sticks. Another benefit: High levels of BDNF control appetite and reduce the risk of obesity. They also stimulate the release of neurotransmitters in the brain, such as serotonin and dopamine, that control mood and play a role in depression. Scientists suspect that these exercise-induced BDNF boosts may partially explain the benefits of exercise on people with depression.

Upping your BDNF levels doesn't take much; for rats, a week of running on a wheel is enough. In humans, a single high-intensity workout triggers results. Of course, the increase is short term, which is why regular physical activity is so important.

In fact, some researchers suggest that what we think of as "age-related" mental decline—memory loss, some slowing of our thinking, etc.—is actually "revenge of the sit." We've fallen away from our genetic tendency to be physically active nearly 100 percent of the day, and the resulting loss of BDNF and the neurotransmitters it affects, including serotonin, contributes to our current high rates of obesity, forgetfulness, dementia, and depression.

Now, we're not suggesting that you buy yourself a human-size hamster wheel or begin testing your blood levels of BDNF after every 2-mile jog. Focus on the visible benefits. Simply walking briskly for 45 minutes three days a week for six months can make a huge difference in the kind of mental acuity that allows you to be more attuned to the world around you. It can even reduce the effects of a traumatic brain injury if begun two weeks after a serious concussion.

It's never too late to exercise.

So stick with an exercise program for just three months and see what kind of memory, learning, and decision-making benefits *you* get from it!

2. Lower risk of Alzheimer's disease

Exercise has other brain benefits beyond improved memory and reasoning. A long-term study that followed nearly 1,500 people for an average of 21 years found that just two rounds of leisure-time physical activity each week cut their risk of Alzheimer's in half. You can get benefits in an even shorter amount of time; exercising just three or more times a week during a six-year period, one study found, reduced the risk of dementia by a third in older people compared to those who exercised less.

Some of this risk reduction is thought to be related to changes in the hippocampus, the part of the brain that controls higher thought and the part first affected by the physical changes that lead to Alzheimer's. The bottom line is that physically active people have healthier hippocampuses. So do rats. When rats specially bred to develop Alzheimer's get steady exercise over several months, they show a remarkable reduction in the plaques and other brain changes that signal the development of the disease.

3. Fewer hot flashes

If you're on the younger end of the aging spectrum and still haven't gone through menopause, you have yet another reason to lace up your Nikes: A Spanish study at the University of Granada found that three hours of exercise a week could significantly reduce severe hot flashes and other menopausal symptoms, increasing a woman's overall quality of life. While half of the exercising group had severe symptoms when they began working out, after a year, just 37 percent did (and no, they hadn't

The Real-Life Fitness Test

There are many scientific ways to measure fitness. But for most of us, the signs of being fit are measured daily in what we can or can't do. For a person over the age of 45, you are probably in pretty good physical shape if you can:

- Dance to a fast beat for more than 10 minutes without feeling winded.
- Walk for 30 minutes straight without getting tired.
- Feel energized 14 hours after you woke up (so if you got up at 7 a.m., you should still be awake and active at 9 p.m.).
- Carry large containers of milk or water in each hand without feeling strain.
- Load your luggage into the storage bin above your airplane or train seat without strain.
- Jump up and down 10 times without causing your heart to race.
- Carry a large basket of clothing up or down two staircases without struggle or strain.
- Trim your toenails without any discomfort from the bending.
- Easily sit down on the floor and then stand up.
- Raise your foot as high as your hip when kicking.
- Twist and look behind you without moving your feet.

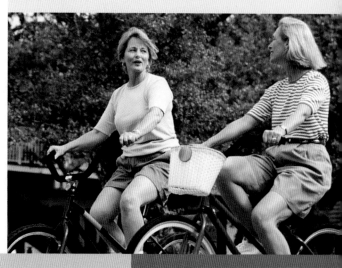

reached menopause yet). Meanwhile, the percentage of women with severe menopausal symptoms in a control group that *didn't* exercise rose from 58 to 67 percent.

4. Improved self-esteem

We talk a lot about self-esteem in our children, but what about our own? Self-esteem, or put another way, simply how you feel about yourself, can play a major role in your health and quality of life. If you feel good about yourself, you're more likely to live a healthier lifestyle, to remain active, to interact socially, and to participate in community activities. All this works in a kind of circular way to keep you healthier. And now we know that exercise helps maintain or improve self-esteem in older people.

For instance, one study measured changes in self-esteem in overweight women ages 60 to 75 who participated in either a stretching and toning exercise program or a brisk walking exercise program for six months. Both programs enhanced their self-esteem, although the stretching-toning group showed greater improvement. All the women, however, felt better about their body images and strength. The message? You don't have to up your heart rate to achieve a better feeling via exercise!

The New Exercise Classes

For more than two decades, most fitness centers have offered classes that provide a limited range of aerobics options. Some add a step, some integrate martial arts moves, and others use stationary bicycles, but the basic class—loud music, a high-intensity instructor, and even higher-intensity workouts—hasn't changed much. Until recently.

Happily, most recreation and fitness centers today offer a plethora of programs that hark back to ancient Chinese traditions, borrow from professional ballerinas, and even pull from the boxing ring. Many are far less intense as well, making them perfectly suitable for an older or out-of-shape exerciser. Here are some to look for and what they're best for.

Tai chi chuan. The name of this ancient Chinese martial art form (called tai chi for short) loosely translates to "the supreme ultimate boxing system." It involves slow, steady movements that incorporate both the physicality of the body through the motions and the mental strength of the mind through meditation. Most of the movements are performed in a standing position, with inner calm a key component.

Numerous studies attest to tai chi's benefits in improving balance, flexibility, and cardiovascular health in people of all ages, but particularly in older people with and without chronic conditions. It can reduce pain and disability from arthritis, significantly reduce the risk of falls, lower blood pressure, relieve stress, and improve aerobic capacity.

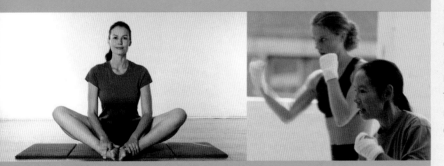

5. Better stress management

There's a reason we counsel people to take a walk when they need to "let off steam." All that steam—or stress—triggers a chemical cascade designed to ready you to run. Your heart beats faster and harder, your lungs take in more oxygen, your liver releases glucose to provide energy for muscles, and your immune system revs up in preparation for injury.

If all you do is sit there, however, all that physiological energy has nowhere to go. Given the kind of chronic stress most of us experience, this constant ready-for-flight-with-nowhere-to-go response damages key body systems over time.

It suppresses the immune system; contributes to bone loss, muscle weakness, and atherosclerosis; and increases insulin levels (you need more insulin to get all that glucose into cells), leading to higher levels of dangerous abdominal fat.

Enter exercise. Just a 20-minute jog or stair-climbing stint does more to soothe stress-induced anxiety than simply sitting still in a quiet room for 20 minutes. Not only does physical activity reduce anxiety, but being physically fit acts as a buffer against the damaging effects of stress, such as high blood pressure. We're not talking a lifetime of physical activity, either; just six months. In fact, such activities can do more to

Pilates. Pilates was created by German fitness instructor Joseph Pilates in the early 1900s both as a way to rehabilitate from injury and to strengthen the body to reduce future injuries. It utilizes a series of low-impact, controlled, precise movements that are designed to improve balance, flexibility, and core strength, accompanied by slow, steady breathing. Programs sometimes involve certain machines Joseph Pilates invented.

Unlike with tai chi, which has been the subject of hundreds of research studies, researchers are just beginning to uncover the health benefits of Pilates. So far, they've found it can relieve lower-back pain better than standard medical treatments and improve flexibility as well. Best of all, the risk of injury is very low with a trained instructor. Look for an instructor certified by the United States

Pilates Association who has had months, not a couple of weekends, of training.

Ball classes. You've probably seen those oversized rubber balls at the store or fitness center. They're wonderful tools for strengthening your abdomen and back and improving your balance. What do you do with them? Try lying across a ball on your back to do situps. The combination of the abdominal exercise and the added effort required to balance on the ball supercharges the motion. Or simply sit on the ball with your feet hip-width apart and lift one foot at a time. Can you keep your balance? Classes that integrate balls offer a low-impact option for improving muscle strength and flexibility.

Kickboxing. You might call kickboxing the high-impact aerobics of the 21st century. This is the class for you if you're look-

ing for a great endurance exercise with a dollop of strength training thrown in. You'll even get a bit of stretching for that flexibility flavor. In kickboxing, you incorporate movements from the boxing world, including kicks, punches, and squats, for a full-body workout. Come to class prepared to work hard.

Kettlebells. Coming soon to a gym near you, kettlebells is a Russian fitness routine that incorporates solid cast-iron weights that look like bowling balls with handles. Like Pilates and yoga, kettlebell routines focus on strengthening core muscles; unlike those two programs, however, you also get an aerobic workout because you move quickly. The program is designed to work several muscles at a time in a dynamic fashion rather than a static "lift-lower-lift-lower" approach.

reduce stress-related high blood pressure than changing your diet.

6. Stronger immunity

Ever notice that people who work out a lot tend to get fewer colds and bouts of flu than those who avoid the gym like a burning building? There's a reason for that. Every time you exercise, it puts stress on your entire body, stimulating the release of certain immune system hormones and chemicals. If you exercise too much, this has a negative effect, increasing inflammation and eventually *suppressing* the immune system. But if you exercise moderately on a regular basis, you're able to maintain a higher level of immune activity without triggering that suppression response.

Again, this is not a lifetime-of-exercise-needed kind of response. The response of your immune system to a single physical workout is intense enough to supercharge the effects of a pneumonia or influenza vaccine, particularly in the elderly, who tend to have weaker immune systems to begin with. Exercise regularly, and those vaccines are more likely to work in you. (It's a little-known fact that flu vaccines simply don't work in many people, particularly the elderly.) With or without a vaccine, physical activity significantly reduces your risk of developing an infection, studies find. When researchers examined the risk of hospitalization for infectious disease in 1,365 women ages 55 to 80, they found that those who were inactive were more than three times as likely to be hospitalized for infections. Other studies find a much lower risk of upper respiratory tract infections like colds and bronchitis, as well as pneumonia, among older adults who remain physically active. Again, we're not talking about training for a marathon. Something as gentle as the ancient Chinese martial art of tai chi can boost your immune system enough that it can better fight off the virus that causes shingles, a painful nerve disease more common in those over 50.

7. A better sex life

Just 30 minutes a day of vigorous exercise is enough to slash a man's risk of erectile dysfunction by between 37 and 58 percent, depending on the intensity of the physical activity. Sexual frequency, enjoyment, and satisfaction in older people is also directly linked to their fitness levels; the fitter you are, the more often you're having sex!

8. Less abdominal fat

Here's another good reason to get outdoors and be active: Exercise is a critical factor in reducing the size of fat cells around your abdomen, the so-called visceral fat. This is the fat that gives men their beer bellies and women an apple shape. It's also the type of fat that accumulates within your abdominal organs and liver, contributing to inflammation, insulin resistance, and diabetes. Plus, it's associated with metabolic syndrome, a cluster of health markers that significantly increases your risk of heart disease as well as diabetes.

We now know that the *size* of these fat cells, as well as the number, is directly related to your risk of developing diabetes, regardless of your weight. Simply cutting calories won't shrink those cells; you *must* add exercise to the equation. That's what researchers from Wake Forest University Baptist Medical Center in Winston-Salem, North Carolina, found when they studied three groups of women. All cut 2,800 calories a week, either through dieting alone or through a combination of dieting and exercise.

Both exercise groups burned 400 calories a week through walking and shrank their visceral fat cell size by 18 percent; the dieters, who reduced their body fat, weight, and waist and hip measurements exactly as much as the diet-

Don't think exercise . . . think ha

and-exercisers, saw no change in the size of those fat cells. A similar study found that while diet alone and diet plus exercise reduced total and abdominal fat in overweight women to the same degree, *only* exercise reduced blood levels of chronic inflammation markers like C-reactive protein (CRP) and interleukin-6.

9. Relief of depression

Researchers took 156 people between ages 50 and 77 who had been diagnosed with major depression and randomly assigned them to one of three groups: either exercise (30 minutes of bike riding, walking, or jogging three times a week), medication (the prescription drug sertra-line, better known as Zoloft), or a combination of the two. After 16 weeks, all three groups showed similar improvements in depression, but only the exercise groups also improved in their cognitive abilities. Plus, when researchers checked on the participants six months after the study ended, they found much lower relapse rates in the exercisers than in the medication group.

10. More muscle strength

Sometimes it's easy to overlook the obvious—in this case, that exercise makes you stronger! Exercise your arms, and carrying groceries becomes easy. Exercise your legs, and stairs become a nonissue. You may not be able to see it when you put on a bathing suit, but as little as two to four weeks of weight training can create the kind of microscopic molecular changes in your body's production of hormones—including growth hormone and other chemicals, as well as proteins related to muscle growth—that con-tribute to muscle repair and strengthening. Researchers have even seen significant improvements in as few as four workouts.

This is critical, says Dr. Mitchell, because the more muscle you have, the better your cells use insulin and take in glucose. Those two factors

Slow or Fast?

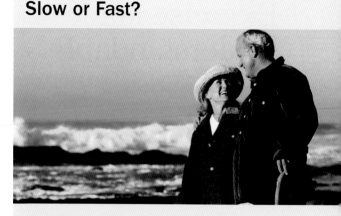

Is it better to walk slow or fast? Researchers at the University of Michigan in Ann Arbor won-dered the same thing, so they tracked nine overweight, sedentary women ages 50 to 65. The women walked 3 miles a day for a total of 15 miles a week for eight months. At the end of the study, those keeping a modest pace—cover-ing a mile in roughly 20 minutes—increased their insulin sensitivity and thus reduced their risk of diabetes, although the improvement tapered off as their speed increased. The slow-er walkers also lost more body fat than the faster walkers.

On the other hand, faster walkers (who aver-aged a 15-minute-per-mile pace) secreted more growth hormone, while growth hormone levels in the slower walkers actually declined.

The message: Just get out there and walk. Whether you walk fast or slow, you still gain important health benefits.

play a major role in inflammation, obesity, heart disease, and diabetes, and are behind many of the health-related benefits of exercise and its ability to keep you feeling young as you age.

Yet, he notes, "There's no magic pill you can take to train your muscles." He's not just touting the company line; Dr. Mitchell, 79, walks an hour a day most days and works out with weights two or three times a week.

Exercise Made Understandable

Put simply, exercise is any activity that exerts your body beyond the point reached in normal daily activities. Sometimes we forget the simplicity of the definition. We get so caught up with shoes, gyms, programs, stopwatches, science, clothing, and fads with funny names like "yogilates" and "super power sets" that we give up on the whole idea of exercise.

Throw all those complicated notions aside. Exercise is nothing more than moving your body for good health. Of course, some exercise is better than others, and different types of movement do affect your body in different ways. But understanding the different types is easy—and so is doing it!—if you don't let marketers or trainers or overwrought health magazines complicate things.

Here's what we suggest: Throw out all you think you know about exercise and start over, beginning right now. In the following pages, we'll give a concise explanation of the four essential types of fitness—**endurance**, **strength**, **flexibility**, and **balance**. Then we'll tell you precisely which ones *you* need to focus on for optimal health today and tomorrow. Finally, we'll provide specific exercise sequences for you to consider doing most mornings or evenings that deliver the best results for the minimum investment of time and effort.

Fitness Type 1
endurance

Endurance activities are those that challenge large groups of muscles, such as those in your legs or arms and shoulders, for at least 10 consecutive minutes. The most obvious examples are walking, biking, and swimming, but endurance activities also include lifestyle movements such as washing windows, vacuuming, sweeping, mopping, gardening, mowing the lawn, raking, and pruning. A round of golf—without a cart—also counts!

These activities provide the biggest bang for the buck when it comes to protecting against the effects of chronic diseases associated with aging, such as heart disease, diabetes, and osteoporosis. One major reason: Endurance exercises strengthen not only the muscle groups being used but also your heart, lungs, and circulatory system. That's why endurance exercise is also called aerobic exercise: the word *aerobic* basically means it involves oxygen, which is what your heart, lungs, and circulatory system are all about.

Endurance exercise is also the most straightforward. To build endurance, you just do your preferred activity at a high rate of intensity for as long as you are comfortable. Come back to it in the next day or two, and you'll be able to do it a little longer. And so it goes.

So what is a high enough rate of intensity? It's simple: Work hard enough to make yourself breathe harder than usual. Want us to be more

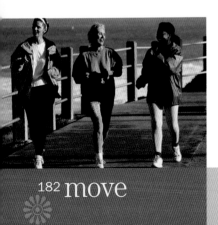

Endurance exercise provides the best defense against most chronic diseases.

10 Ways to Exercise Naturally

Here are ways to get a moderate level of activity without setting foot in a formal exercise environment. Each burns up to 7 calories a minute; your goal is to get at least 10 minutes of sustained activity at a time.

1 Take a daily fitness walk. This is in addition to any other walking you would do as part of your day. Commit to a pace slightly faster than your normal gait. Don't let weather stop you—light snow or misty rain is no excuse to stay home! If the weather is too challenging for an outdoor walk, then hit the shopping mall—only no window-shopping. Hoof it from one end to the other with no stops at the food court. You'll find that your daily walk not only strengthens your body but is also a great way to relax, think, and socialize.

2 Sign up for dance classes. Ballroom dancing, line dancing, folk dancing, ballet, and even disco or other forms of modern dance are fabulous endurance exercises.

3 Take up table tennis. Who knew? But an intense game of table tennis gets your heart rate up, increases the amount of oxygen going to your lungs and brain, and provides all the other amazing benefits of aerobic physical activity.

4 Coach a kids' sport. Got some extra time on your hands? How about volunteering to coach a youth soccer or baseball team? In addition to the fun you'll have and the appreciation you'll garner, you'll also get an unexpected workout at least twice a week (more if you call more practices!).

5 Play with the kids or grandkids. Try throwing a Frisbee or teaching them how to play badminton. Heck, dance around the living with them for 10 minutes.

6 Go canoeing. Many parks offer canoes or rowboats for rent, and rowing at a moderate pace of less than 4 miles per hour provides the moderate workout you need.

7 Ride a horse. We're not talking at a gallop, although that's certainly something to build up to. But even a gentle trot or canter helps; you get an extra boost of physicality if you learn how to groom and saddle the horse.

8 Audition for a musical. Most communities have local theater groups that rely on volunteers for their talent. Singing while moving, as in walking across the stage, provides a moderate level of activity.

9 Clean the old-fashioned way. For a cleaner house and a healthier you, get down on your hands and knees to scrub the floor, hang laundry out on a clothesline, and wash the windows yourself instead of calling someone to do it. All will provide a good, moderate workout with a bonus at the end: a sparkling house.

10 Join a sports team. Maybe you're beyond the over-40 soccer team, but what about the local softball team? Or a doubles tennis team? Even joining a bowling team will provide a decent-enough workout once or twice a week.

specific than that? There are measurements you can take to more objectively gauge your ongoing exertion, but they often involve purchased gear such as a heart rate monitor. Instead, just measure your own rate of perceived exertion (RPE). This simply means your innate sense of how hard you're working.

In determining your RPE, 10 is the highest level of intensity; it essentially means you can't catch your breath and are about to fall over from exertion. Zero is the lowest level of intensity; it means you've probably been lying comfortably on your sofa for the past hour. When you're engaged in endurance activities, aim for somewhere between 5, which is moderate, and 7, which is strong.

Another way to know that you're working hard enough is that you'll be sweating and slightly out of breath but still able to talk. Increase the intensity, and you may find yourself only able to gasp out "yes" or "no." Any higher, and you need to bring it down a level.

Next question: How long do you exercise? Answer: Ideally, for up to 30 minutes of consecutive exertion. For now, though, start with 10 minutes. That's the minimum length of time in which you can get the respiratory and cardiovascular benefits you seek.

Ten minutes doesn't sound like much, but if you've been inactive for several years—or even a few months—start slowly. This is not

the time to head out for a 30-minute hill climb. Instead, start with a 10-minute walk. Every day, add another five minutes and increase your speed until you're doing 30 minutes at the "breathing-hard-but-can-still-talk" level. As you get into shape, you'll find your workout gets easier. And as it gets easier, you can either choose to up the intensity or settle in at a healthy fitness plateau.

Even better, start to diversify your endurance activities. If walking comes easily, then perhaps it's time to take up swimming or tennis or to get out your bicycle and take to the road. One great thing about endurance activities is that they tend to be done outdoors, making them much more natural and fun than being in a gym.

Fitness Type 2
strength

Strength exercises increase the power of a specific muscle by challenging it with some form of resistance. That could be weights, exercise bands, or even your own body weight. The usual method is careful, slow lifting and lowering of a weight to target a specific muscle or muscle group.

If you think this form of exercise is best left to the young'uns, think again. This is probably the most important form of exercise you need when it comes to preventing the frailty and disability associated with aging.

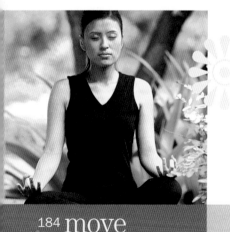

Forget measurements at first: You know when you are exerting yourself, and when you've had enough.

Why? Without muscle strength, your ability to walk, sit, stand, and bend gradually fades. Welcome then to sarcopenia-land, the land of wasted muscles. When you observe seniors who struggle to stand or walk, it's for one reason only—their muscle strength has gone. Yes, injury or disease may have curtailed their capacity for exercise or activity, but at the end of the day, it's still weak muscles that limit their mobility. And only healthier muscles—achieved through strengthening exercises—can return that mobility.

Strength training has other important benefits. It reduces the risk and symptoms of osteoporosis, heart disease, arthritis, and type 2 diabetes. It helps improve your sleep and reduces your risk of depression. At least one study also found that it improves balance—even in middle-age people you wouldn't think would have balance problems. And don't worry about injuries; the risk is low with strength activities, particularly in older adults.

Think strength training is too hard or too awkward for you? Think again. The fact is, strength training is often *less* tiring than endurance workouts. It can be done in limited space and limited time. You need minimal gear—often just a few dumbbells. Best of all, you'll see the results in as little as a few weeks. Plus, strengthening exercises can boost metabolism as much as 15 percent, which is a bonus when it comes to losing weight. Maybe that's why more than ever, people 65 and older are taking up strength training.

But let's get rid of one exercise myth right now: Muscle does *not* weigh more than fat. How could it? A pound is a pound is a pound, whether it's muscle or fat. However, a pound of muscle takes up less space in your body than a pound of fat, just as a pound of lean beef takes up less space than a pound of shortening. Muscle is *denser* than fat, not heavier. That's why

Time to Move Up?

How do you know if you need to move to a lighter or heavier weight? Here's what the experts say.

REDUCE THE WEIGHT IF:

- You can't complete 2 sets of 10 repetitions in good form.

KEEP THE WEIGHT THE SAME IF:

- You need to rest after 10 reps because the weight is too heavy to complete more reps in good form.

INCREASE THE WEIGHT IF:

- You could have done a few more reps in good form without a break. At your next workout, do the first set of reps with your current weight and the second with the next highest weight. For example, if you're currently using 1-pound dumbbells, use 2- or 3-pound dumbbells for your second set.

- You could do all 20 repetitions at once without a break. At your next session, use heavier dumbbells for both sets.

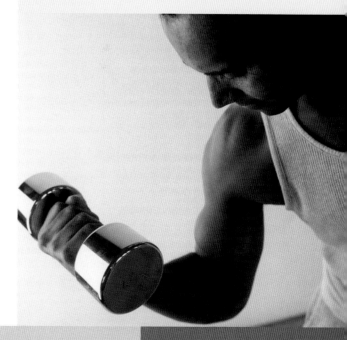

Ask the expert ?

I am a 58-year-old former athlete. I used to play soccer pretty seriously and was in good shape until I hit 40. But everyday life today is busy, and in my free time, I just want to sit and relax. How can I reclaim my body and strength?

answer: Congratulations on your decision to reclaim your body. It is never too late! Listed below are eight steps to getting you back on the "active, healthy, and fit" track.

1 Arrange to get a complete physical with your doctor, including blood work, especially blood lipids and glucose. If possible, undergo a graded exercise test on a treadmill to assess your cardiovascular response to physical stress.

2 Once cleared for training, address any musculoskeletal issues that can present real problems when training. Ex-soccer or football players typically have chronic knee pain. Any chronic muscle or joint pain should be addressed before you start training by getting to the root of the problem. Don't cover it up with medication! If you have chronic pain or lingering injuries that might affect exercise, I recommend a physical therapist who can evaluate you and recommend corrective exercises.

3 If your eating and drinking patterns are an absolute disaster, book a few sessions with a registered dietitian or enroll in a weight management program. Steer clear of programs that promise a quick fix.

4 Buy some decent workout gear, especially footwear. You don't need any plastic suits, heavy sweats, or other athletic paraphernalia.

5 Bury your old training methods and avoid the "weekend warrior" approach. Plans, patterns and progressions (the three Ps) are the keys to permanent lifestyle changes.

6 Establish short- and long-term goals. Be realistic and specific as to what you would like to achieve through regular training and lifestyle modifications. These might include:

• I don't want to end up like my father, sitting in a chair all day long. I want to be a healthy and fit 80-year-old.

• I want to be able to carry my golf bag for 18 holes and not have to take a cart.

• On my next vacation to the mountains, I would like to be able to hike _____ Peak.

• I need to slim down so I can move quicker on the tennis court.

• I just want more energy, and by getting fitter, leaner, and stronger, I know I will have it.

7 Cardio, strength, and mobility training are all integral components of a well-rounded training program, regardless of your goals. The frequency, intensity, mode, and rate of progression should be based on whether you're training for health, fitness, sport performance, and/or fat loss.

8 To get started ...

• Gradually build up to 30 to 60 minutes of brisk walking five or six times a week.

• Stretch after you walk.

• For basic strength, complete 2 sets of 10 to 12 chair squats and desk pushups every other day.

• When you're ready for more, work with a certified personal trainer or join a reputable facility with qualified staff. Educate yourself through a variety of reputable resources from reputable publishers.

Remember, changing your lifestyle is a process, not a program, not a diet, not a six-week course. It takes effort, hard work, and persistence to form new habits. Oh, and don't forget to have some fun along the way!

Expert: Patricia A. VanGalen, MS, a certified personal trainer who specializes in working with older adults.

you can be working out and seeing your measurements change, but your weight remains the same. The same weight is simply taking up less space. In fact, some experts estimate that the space used by a pound of muscle is 22 percent less than the space used by a pound of fat.

Okay, back to the strength workouts. In general, there's just a handful of exercises you'll ever need to know. We'll show them to you in our routines beginning on page 201. Strength training has a very simple process and lexicon.

A repetition, or "rep" is lifting and then returning a weight to its starting position once (or if you are using rubber bands, stretching and then releasing the band). In general, you want to lift carefully and steadily, completing the lift in a slow count of 2. Pause for a second at the peak of the lift, then return at half the speed of the lift (that is, to a count of 4) until you are at the starting position. A rep should take 8 to 10 seconds. Typically, you exhale during the most difficult part of the movement—in most exercises, that's the lift—and inhale during the easier part. Whatever you do, *don't* hold your breath. That could increase blood pressure to dangerous levels. One rep done!

A set is 8 to 12 reps in a row. A set should take anywhere from one to two minutes. When you complete a full set, pause for a minute or two to rest, then repeat the same exercise for a second set. If you really want to push yourself hard, pause again, then do one final set. Doing 2 sets of the same exercise takes between four and eight minutes and is the perfect amount for everyday strength training. Weightlifters and athletes may add a third set because they need particular muscles to be strong and have extra endurance, but that's probably not necessary for you.

If you pick a workout that includes six exercises, it would take about 30 minutes total to do the routine properly and safely. Think about it: You can complete a full strengthening workout in the span of a typical TV comedy show—and you can watch the show while doing it!

As to how much weight to use, that's simple: The amount you can just handle for 2 full sets. Those last few reps should be challenging but not painful or exhausting.

Over time, strengthening exercises get easier. When you get to the point where 2 sets of an exercise don't provide much challenge, move up to the next weight level. Simple!

New to all this? Consider not even using weights at first and just going through the motions with your hands closed in fists. You'll find that 2 sets of 12 movements without a weight can be strenuous enough. Soon, however, you'll be ready for that first dumbbell. And from there, who knows?

Here are some other important considerations when it comes to strengthening exercises.

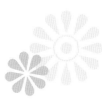

Strength exercise takes little time or space and doesn't tire you out.

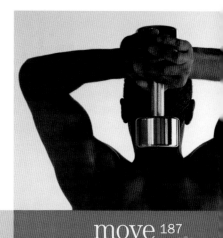

Nordic Walking

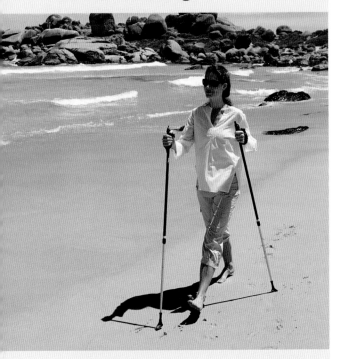

If you're interested in getting a full-body workout while taking a walk, consider Nordic walking, which uses poles similar to ski poles. A relatively new sport, it was born in the late 1990s as a way to train Finnish cross-country skiers in the summer. Using the poles is simple: You plant one pole in the ground and "push off" against it with the foot on the same side. So if you're about to step with your left leg, you plant the pole on the right and use your right foot to push off.

Studies find that pole walking can burn up to 50 percent more calories than regular brisk walking, as well as work out up to 90 percent of your body's muscles, thanks to the abdominal and upper-body strength required to plant the poles and push off. A bonus for people with achy knees or hips is that some of the force of walking is transferred to the poles instead of your joints.

You can buy a pair of walking poles at most sporting goods stores or online for about $70.

Build in recovery time. Always give yourself a day off between strength activities to give your muscles time to rebuild and recover. It's this recovery period that leads to stronger muscles.

Emphasize legs over arms. When you think of weight training, you tend to think of lifts involving your arms and shoulders. That's not quite appropriate. Although you should incorporate both upper- and lower-body strength-training exercises into your routine, strengthening lower-body muscles around your hips, knees, and ankles is particularly important for healthy aging and mobility. Be sure that at least half of your exercises target your legs, hips, and lower back.

Posture matters. Whether you're lifting a small dumbbell over your head or doing a leg lift, how you hold your body determines whether you get the most out of that movement. Stand or sit erect with your back straight, your hips aligned, your shoulders pulled down, and your neck stretched high. Most important, as you exercise, try to move just the target muscles. Don't swing your whole body to help lift a dumbbell. If the exercise is for your arms, for instance, only your arms should move.

Don't rush. You'll get twice as much benefit if you take your time returning the weight to its starting position. For instance, once you lift that weight over your head, count to 4 as you slooowly bring your arm down.

Keep your joints loose. Locking your knee and elbow joints can result in pain and injury since you put all the stress of the weight on the joint instead of the muscle, where it belongs.

Good technique matters a *lot.*

Fitness Type 3
flexibility

The first two fitness types—endurance and strength—focus mostly on the capabilities of your major muscle groups. Flexibility, however, is in large part about your joints.

The definition of flexibility is simple: It's the range of motion your body can go through. With age, range of motion naturally decreases. The goal of stretching and other flexibility exercises is to keep your range of motion as wide as possible. "You have to maintain a certain range of flexibility and mobility," says Mark Davis of the University of Bristol in England, because without that, you start restricting your activities. That creates a vicious cycle in which you engage in less activity, further reducing not only your flexibility and mobility but also your strength and endurance. Before you know it, you're grunting just trying to get out of a chair and saying no to invitations to walk, shop, or visit because it's just too challenging to bother. Unacceptable!

Flexibility exercises strive to do a few things. They wash the key parts of your joints—the bones, tendons, ligaments, and cushionlike substances between—with nutrients and blood. They also keep the tendons and ligaments strong and stretchable. And, just as important, they keep the muscles attached to your joints loose and flexible. After all, that's the key function of a muscle:

To move your body through constant stretching and compressing.

Stretching, in other words, does a lot of important things. However, it's also one of the easiest and most pleasurable types of exercise there is. And it requires no gear whatsoever.

To properly stretch a muscle and its related tendons and ligaments, you want to slowly get into the extended position, then hold it for 20 to 30 seconds. This is much different from what many people do, however. Too often, people jerk and pull their muscles, holding the stretch for just a few seconds, if at all. Be patient! By slowly stretching a muscle and then holding the stretch for the suggested time, you are maximizing the benefits and minimizing the chances of injury.

Aim to do flexibility exercises at least twice a week. These include basic stretching, reaching, and bending. Activities like yoga, tai chi, and Pilates provide excellent opportunities for improving your flexibility. The beauty of these is that you can do them anywhere—even sitting on a plane. But many of your daily activities also provide good opportunities for stretching, including:

Waking. Stand up and slowly reach for the ceiling. Hold for the requisite 20 to 30 seconds. First thing in the morning, when you're in your pajamas, is a perfect time to do a little stretching. In fact, it's perfectly natural. Think of how many animals naturally stretch themselves out after a nap or night's rest.

Stretching is one of the easiest and most pleasurable exercises you can do.

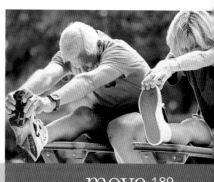

Exercise Gear

buying worth

A high-quality pedometer. This little gizmo tracks the steps and miles you walk throughout the day (10,000 steps equals 5 miles). Numerous studies find that wearing one is a great motivation to increase your steps. It becomes almost like a game: "Can I get more steps today than I got yesterday?" Take it to the next level by forming a pedometer club (a fitness-oriented version of a book club) in which all members compete to see who can rack up the most steps on a monthly basis. Once a month, meet for a group walk and a healthy lunch to compare notes. Don't buy the cheapest pedometer, however; research shows they're not very accurate. You should be able to find a good one for about $20.

A heart rate monitor. The key to aerobic or endurance activities is to get your heart rate up to a certain level and keep it there for 10 minutes or more. Using the breathing-heavy-but-can-still-talk approach generally gets you to the right pace. But if you want a more precise measurement, first determine your maximum heart rate by subtracting your age from 220. Your target heart rate is between 50 and 75 percent of that. So if you're 50, your target heart rate is between 85 and 130 beats per minute. To monitor their heart rates continuously, athletes and serious exercisers use a heart rate monitor. The typical unit includes a band you wrap around your chest and a wristband or armband that picks up the signals from the chest monitor. It's an easy way to see if you need to pick up the intensity—something that will become more important as you get fitter.

Dumbbells. Exercise experts have a saying: "Dumbbells are smart." That's because they make it difficult to push yourself too hard, thus avoiding injury. They're also flexible. You can use them anytime, nearly anywhere. Increasing the weight as you get stronger is as simple as picking up another set of dumbbells. You can even buy some that allow you to change the weight by turning a knob, but for durability, choose fixed-weight dumbbells. A popular type is hex dumbbells. The ends resemble hexagons so they don't roll when you set them down. If you want to take your weights with you when traveling, look for hollow weights that you fill with water when you're ready to work out.

An inflatable exercise ball. As described on page 179, these exercise balls are terrific when it comes to strengthening core muscles and improving balance. Even just sitting on one when you're at the computer can provide some benefits. Size is important when it comes to balls. Buy one large enough so your feet are flat on the floor when you sit on it. If you're under 5 feet 5 inches, try a 55-centimeter ball; if you're over 5 feet 11 inches, aim for a 75-centimeter ball. Everyone else should do fine with a 65-centimeter ball. And don't inflate it completely; a little give in the ball helps with stability.

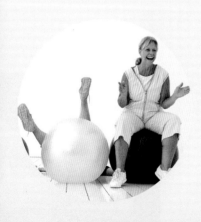

Vacuuming. As you vacuum, you reach forward, then back. You bend to move things and stretch to reach the corner or under the sofa. You think you're cleaning, but you're really stretching! Have a house full of hard-surfaced floors? You can get the same benefits from mopping.

Washing windows. The up-and-down motion of washing the windows and the stretching as you stand on your tiptoes to reach the higher parts provide a good flexibility workout.

Bowling. Every time you bend and stretch to throw the ball, you're extending muscles beyond their typical range. Take advantage of that by completing a few extra stretches while you wait to see how many pins you've hit.

Golf. Reaching down to pick up your ball, swinging your arms, and twisting your body as you move the club head to meet the ball are movements that can help keep you flexible.

For best health, however, you should do a stretching routine as well. You can stretch all the major joints with just a few simple stretches. If you hold each stretch for the appropriate 30 seconds, that means in five minutes, you can do a complete body stretching sequence with enormous positive benefits. As part of the Long-Life Fitness Routines that start on page 198, you'll see that we call for you to do four stretches each day, focused on a single body area.

Fitness Type 4
balance

Balance activities are particularly important for people as they age because good balance prevents falls. "But I have no intention of falling," you say. Right. None of us does. Yet one out of three people 65 and older falls every year. These are not people living in nursing homes but rather those typically living in their own homes.

Falls are the most common reason for injuries treated in emergency rooms among those 65 and older, and 5 to 10 percent of those falls cause serious injuries, including major head trauma. Most important: Falls are one of the most common reasons people find themselves in nursing homes.

There are two types of balance, static and dynamic. Static balance involves the ability to maintain your balance without moving, such as while standing on one foot. Dynamic balance refers to the ability to maintain your balance while moving.

The good news is that many other forms of exercise already challenge and improve your sense of balance. Examples include tai chi, yoga, dance, and even strength training. If you're an avid exerciser, it's unlikely that you need to do additional balancing exercises—but try some anyway. This is one area of fitness in which there isn't a lot of science or precision. Just do

Start every morning with a stretch.

move 191

things that force you to stay up on your feet in awkward situations. Here are some ideas.

Do basic balance challenges each day at home. For instance, stand on one leg and lift the other, or walk in a straight line heel to toe. If you're just starting, hold on to something when you try these. Eventually, the goal is to be able to perform these exercises for longer times without holding on to anything.

Dance. Balance is about being light on your feet and having a good sense of your body and its movements. What teaches you that more than dancing? For the most benefits, sign up for ballroom dancing classes, You'll get the physical benefits of the dancing and the emotional and life-enhancing benefits of the social interaction.

Get off the beaten path. Taking walks on an unpaved nature trail forces you to step over or around roots, boulders, and other obstructions. It's the perfect activity to improve your balance.

Do more side-to-side activities. Sports like badminton, basketball, and soccer all force players to constantly move frontward, backward, and sideways, making these sports terrific for helping players develop balance and a sense of assuredness on their feet. If you are relatively fit and have a willingness to play and laugh about it, consider a gentle round of these sports with kids or your spouse. You'll get a wonderful aerobic and balance workout.

Take up tai chi. One study of 256 physically inactive people ages 70 to 92 found that participating in this ancient Chinese martial art form for six months reduced falls by half compared to a similar group who did stretching exercises for six months. Plus, those in the tai chi group who did fall had much less serious falls, with just 7 percent resulting in injuries versus 18 percent in the stretching group.

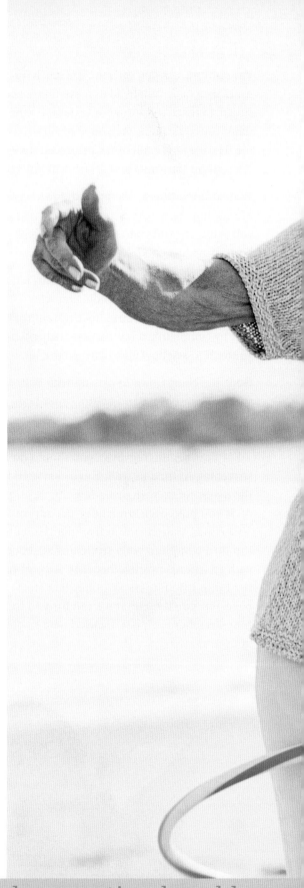

Balance can be practiced and learne

When *Not* to Exercise

You want to do some form of physical activity every day, if possible. However, if you have any of the following conditions or symptoms, either take a day off or check with your doctor first.

- A cold, the flu, or an infection with a fever
- More fatigue than usual
- A swollen or painful muscle or joint
- A new or undiagnosed symptom
- Chest pain or an irregular, rapid, or fluttery heartbeat
- Shortness of breath
- A hernia with symptoms

If you do only one thing ...
garden

Gardening is one of those rare multiple-benefit activities, providing endurance, strength, and flexibility activities all in one. How? Picture an early spring day when you're preparing your vegetable garden for the first planting. Digging in the dirt builds muscle strength as well as endurance. So does loading shovels of compost and topsoil into the wheelbarrow, wheeling it over to the garden, dumping it, and turning the earth over as you work it in. When the time comes to plant the tomato and squash seedlings, you bend and stretch to get them in the ground.

Other benefits of gardening?

- Cutting the grass with a walking mower (preferably manual) provides a great endurance workout.
- Raking leaves provides flexibility and endurance benefits.
- Hauling compost, dirt, and weeds is a good strength-building workout.
- Pulling weeds is a wonderful way to stretch muscles stiff from too much sitting.

The Best Fitness of All: *Daily Living*

If you follow what trainers and experts tell you, a well-rounded fitness regimen would have you actively engaged in some type of formal exercise for an hour a day six or seven days a week. A lot of effort, a lot of time, but not unreasonable if you want to be truly fit for a long life. But what of the other 15 hours a day that you're awake?

When you think about it, it's thoroughly illogical to believe that the optimal fitness schedule is "1 hour on, 15 hours off." Sure, thinking that way helps sell gym memberships and lots of fancy fitness gear. But the truth is, fitness is best thought of as a lifestyle, not as a task.

Every moment of your day, every task you do, is an opportunity to move in ways that help your health. When you think of fitness as a lifestyle, it means you walk a little faster, stand a little taller, stay outside a little longer, do tasks a little more intensely. It means you bypass the easy or lazy options and instead take the steps, fetch the item from the garage yourself, and take care of that fallen branch or broken step right now, by yourself.

When fitness becomes a lifestyle, it means that you are naturally walking more each day, so you don't have to formally schedule it, get dressed for it, and recover from it. It means that you are naturally stretching your muscles, using your strength, and challenging your sense of balance. It means that not a half hour goes by when you haven't done some small thing with a little more exertion as a matter of habit.

And does this kind of living pay off! More energized living burns calories, strengthens muscles, builds endurance, improves your mood, and makes you sleep more deeply. Science proves it, and living it quickly reveals it.

So how do you start living a fitter lifestyle? Again, it's all in the choices. Here are some simple life rules to start.

- Always take the steps if you are going up or down two or fewer flights of stairs.
- Always walk a little faster.
- Always stand when talking on the phone.
- Always get up and move when TV commercials come on.
- Always get the mail, take out the garbage, walk the dog, and pick up the newspaper yourself.
- Always strive to be outdoors more (it's virtually impossible not to be more active outside than inside).
- Always get up and move after 30 minutes of sitting.

Can you add to the list? These are all easy to do, and the benefits will be enormous!

Does living the fit lifestyle mean you can stop thinking about exercise? No. Active living will do a great job of keeping you slim and maintaining your body's current physical condition. But remember the definition of exercise—using your body in ways that go *beyond* normal exertion levels. Only by mixing in a some formal exercise can you improve strength, endurance, flexibility, and balance.

To help put all this in perspective, we've created the Long-Life Fitness Pyramid. Whereas the well-known food pyramid tells you how much of each type of food you should eat in a day, our fitness pyramid is meant to be a general guide to the range of exercise you should strive for in a week and in what amounts. Make a copy and post it by your desk or on your refrigerator! With it, you'll have a terrific understanding of your fitness needs.

Yes, you can do it!

The Long-Life
FITNESS PYRAMID

The comprehensive approach to a strong, healthy body

Balance Exercise

FREQUENCY: A FEW MINUTES PER DAY

Examples: agility games and challenges, tai chi

Flexibility Exercise

FREQUENCY: AT LEAST TWICE A WEEK

Examples: stretching, yoga, pilates

Strength Exercise

FREQUENCY: EACH MAIN MUSCLE GROUP EXERCISED
TWICE A WEEK

Examples: weight training, exercise bands, calisthenics

Endurance/Aerobic Exercise

FREQUENCY: 30-MINUTE SESSIONS AT LEAST THREE TIMES A WEEK

Example: fast walking, biking, aerobics, rowing

Hobbies and Passions

FREQUENCY: SEEK A DAILY DOSE

Examples: sports, fishing, knitting, gardening, bird-watching

Active Daily Living

FREQUENCY: ALL WAKING HOURS

Examples: taking the stairs, getting outdoors, living energetically

Finding Your Inner Motivation

So you've decided that all you've read makes sense: You're going to get out there and become more physically active. A week from now, however, you're slumped back on the sofa watching television. Don't feel bad. Half of all people who begin exercise programs drop out within the first six months. So how do you motivate yourself day in and day out? It's a question researchers have been struggling with for decades. While they don't have any one answer, they do have some suggestions.

Reread this chapter. It turns out that women who believe in the health benefits of exercise tend to work out more often and more intensely or for longer periods than those with negative thoughts about working out (i.e., "I'll be sore in the morning." "It's too cold to walk." "I'm too old to lift weights.").

Don't watch yourself exercise. Stop looking at the mirror and don't think about the movements, just *do* them. One study found that women who concentrated on their body movements during exercise tended to exercise less often, less intensely, and/or for less time than women who didn't.

Switch from negative to positive thinking. For instance, if you hate sweating during exercise, turn it into a positive such as, "Sweating clears toxins from my body and makes my skin look better," or "The more I sweat, the more my muscles are working." If you get out of breath when you exercise and perceive it as harmful, you'll stop, but what if you viewed it as an indication that you're building endurance? You'd be more likely to continue exercising.

Track your progress. Use our fitness test (page 177) to track your workouts and benefits. Research finds that you're more likely to stick with a physical activity if you can see or quantify the progress.

Join a class. The socialization that occurs in an exercise class serves as a powerful motivator for anyone of any age. As one woman told researchers trying to learn what motivates older people to exercise, "Most of us live alone, so it's better to come and exercise in a group. I do not do too well at home, as I cheat a little. When I am in the class, I've got to keep up. You do not want to cheat with the instructor."

Set rewards for yourself. Maybe tell yourself that every week in which you complete at least four 30-minute exercise sessions, you'll treat yourself to a massage or, if you have a certain hobby, like woodworking, you'll buy a new tool.

The toughest exercise is convincing yourself to stick with it. Don't just rely on willpower!

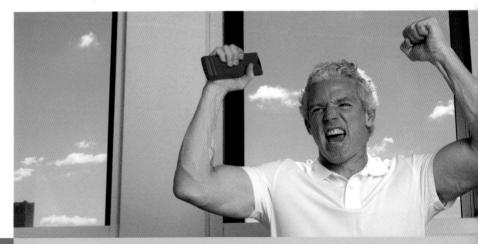

Active living—

Find a caring instructor or personal trainer. Having someone who knows you and cares about your progress provides a powerful incentive. "We need supervision!" one woman explained when addressing issues of motivation with researchers. "We need the instructor to help us keep it up, or else we do not do it. At least once a week, we need that external boost. It's not easy to do the exercise on your own!"

Sign a health contract with your doctor. This is a written agreement to accomplish a health goal. In your case, that health goal is to walk 30 minutes a day five days a week. Or to spend 45 minutes two days a week doing resistance training. Or to sign up for a tai chi class or a Spinning class. The contract should include a calendar for you to track your progress and to reinforce your commitment.

Tell everyone you know. It turns out that social support for your exercise program keeps you motivated—so call your kids and e-mail the grandkids. Let your next-door neighbor and the nosy lady at church know that you're starting a new physical fitness program. They'll keep asking how you're doing, and to avoid the embarrassment of telling them you quit, you'll keep at it.

Sign up for a 5K walk or run two months in the future. Having a goal you're working toward is one of the best motivators. You can get help training for the event from the Internet, books, or your local gym.

Have we convinced you of the age-defying benefits of physical activity yet? Are you ready to take up a sport, lift a weight, try to touch your toes? We hope so. Because the simple truth is this: There is no more effective prescription for living a long, healthy life than exercise. To borrow from one of the leaders in the area: Just do it!

Matching Goals to Exercises

If you want to ...

LOSE WEIGHT:

■ Walk slowly but for longer distances. A study at Colorado University in Boulder found that obese people who walk a mile at a leisurely pace burn more calories than if they walk a mile at their normal pace. And there's a bonus: The slower pace puts less stress on your knee joints. Another approach is to tackle your cardio workout before breakfast, forcing your body to break into fat reserves for fuel.

PREVENT DIABETES:

■ Add strength training into your life. By building muscle, you increase the ability of your cells to take in glucose, reducing insulin resistance and your risk of diabetes.

PREVENT FALLS:

■ Do 10 minutes of balance training four or five days a week.

PREVENT HEART DISEASE:

■ Participate in some kind of endurance activity several times a week for at least 30 minutes.

PREVENT OSTEOPOROSIS:

■ Get some form of weight-bearing exercise that forces you to work against gravity. This could be endurance or resistance. It includes activities such as walking, running, dancing, climbing stairs, weight lifting, and calisthenics. And don't forget gardening! One study found that gardening was second only to weight training when it came to reducing the risk of osteoporosis in 3,310 women age 50 and older.

RID YOURSELF OF BACK PAIN:

■ Try a program that focuses on your core, like Pilates, yoga, or tai chi. These programs stretch and strengthen all the muscles in your trunk, including the abdomen, back, and shoulders, which can relieve an aching lower back.

the best exercise of all.

The Long Life Fitness Routines

Can you spare a half hour to rejuvenate your health, spark your energy, and improve your mood? We've come up with three fitness routines that combine simple moves into an anytime, anywhere 30- to 45-minute session. They are:

routine **1 Easy Does It!**

routine **2 The Antidote-to-Aging Program**

routine **3 The Spread Stopper**

While these routines vary in their intensity and requisite skill and strength levels, they are all structured the same.

- Four strength exercises and four stretches per day.
- Each day focused on one of three body regions—upper (arms, shoulders, and neck), core (chest, back, and abs), or lower (hips, legs, and feet).

Many of the exercises identify which muscles are being targeted. However, for the exercises targeted at your body's core section, we've skipped the list since so many small muscles in the back and abs area are simultaneously challenged by these moves.

The Plan

Each routine is made up of three 30-minute stretching and strengthening sequences, each focused on a different part of your body. Do the three sequences on consecutive days, then take the fourth day off.

The Process

- Do strength exercises first, then stretches.
- Do the indicated number of sets and reps of each strength exercise, as noted.
- Take no more than 2 minutes of rest between sets.
- Take no more than 2 minutes of rest between exercises.
- To improve endurance, shorten rests to under 30 seconds.
- Hold each stretch for the times noted— never more than 30 seconds.
- Concentrate on what you are doing and feeling! Music is good, TV isn't.
- Focus on deep, long breathing throughout the routine.
- No eating during the exercise sequence. Sips of water are okay.

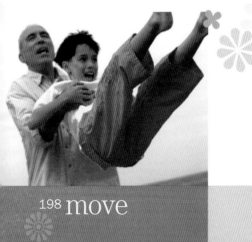

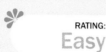

routine **1**

Easy Does It!

A routine for **beginners** or people recovering from illness or injury.

☀ RATING:
Easy

Perfect for people who:

- Have not exercised for two years or more
- Are overweight or have limited movement
- Are recovering from prolonged injury or illness
- Are new to formal fitness plans

WHAT'S NEEDED:

- ☐ Light dumbbells
- ☐ Towel
- ☐ Mat, bed, or daybed
- ☐ Supportive chair
- ☐ Wall space

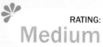

routine **2**

The Antidote-to-Aging Program

A medium-challenge routine for healthy, **active people** who currently lack any formal exercise in their lives.

☀ RATING:
Medium

Perfect for people who:

- Middle-aged people with busy lives
- Sedentary people in good health
- Active, healthy seniors
- People who have noticed a recent decline in energy

WHAT'S NEEDED:

- ☐ Light to medium dumbbells
- ☐ Towel
- ☐ Pillow
- ☐ Supportive chair
- ☐ Wall space

routine **3**

The Spread Stopper

A more difficult fitness routine for **fit people** that delivers a leaner body and stronger muscles.

☀ RATING:
Hard

Perfect for people who:

- Are seeking to tone their abs, back, and legs
- Are active on weekends
- Used to play sports but now lack the time
- Are seeking to lose weight
- Have experience working out

WHAT'S NEEDED:

- ☐ Medium to heavy dumbbells
- ☐ Towel
- ☐ Supportive chair
- ☐ Stairs

The promise: If you live in a higher-energy way, pursue an active hobby, and add one of these routines, you will achieve a level of healthy, comfortable fitness that could have a huge positive impact on all parts of your life. Get started!

day 1	Upper-body sequence
day 2	Lower-body sequence
day 3	Core sequence
day 4	Rest
day 5	Upper-body sequence
day 6	Lower-body sequence
day 7	Core sequence

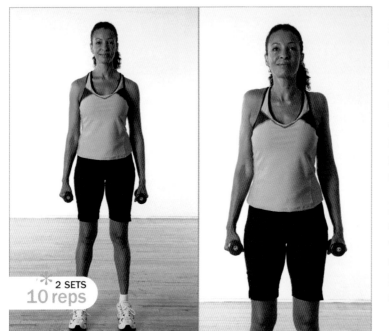

2 SETS
10 reps

Shrug
Tones upper back, midback, and shoulders

1. Stand with your feet hip-width apart. Hold a dumbbell in each hand and let your arms hang straight down so your hands rest by the sides of your thighs, palms facing in.

2. Keeping your arms straight, slowly raise your shoulders toward your ears as if you were shrugging. Roll your shoulders back as far as comfortably possible, then return to start.

Water Pitcher Raise
Tones shoulders

1. Stand with your feet hip- to shoulder-width apart and hold a dumbbell in each hand. Bend your elbows, keeping them close to your body, so your forearms are straight out in front of you and form 90-degree angles, palms facing each other. It should look as though you're holding two water pitchers.

2. Keeping your hands in front of you, raise your upper arms and elbows to the side. The weights should rotate toward each other as if you were pouring water down in front of you. Pause, then return to start.

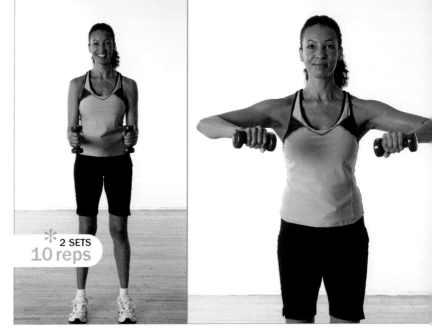

2 SETS
10 reps

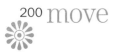

STRENGTH EXERCISES

Reverse Raise
Tones triceps*

1. Stand with your feet about hip-width apart with your knees slightly bent. Hold a dumbbell in each hand, allowing your arms to hang naturally by your sides, palms facing in.

2. Keeping your arms straight, slowly raise them behind you as high as comfortably possible, rotating your palms so they face the ceiling. Pause, then slowly lower back to start.

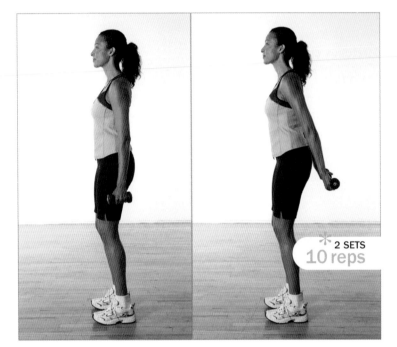

*✻ **2 SETS**
10 reps*

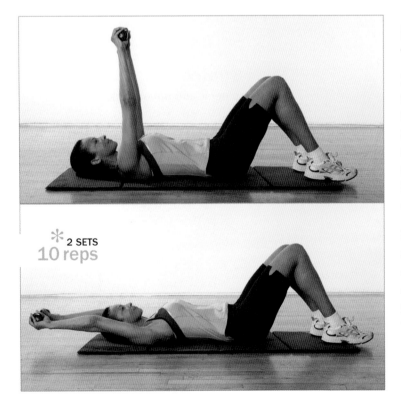

*✻ **2 SETS**
10 reps*

Pullover
Tones chest and back*

1. Lie on a mat on the floor with your knees bent and your feet flat on the mat (if this is uncomfortable, you can do this exercise on a bed). Grasp a dumbbell by the ends with both hands and raise it above your chest.

2. Keeping your elbows straight, lower your arms back and over your head as far as comfortably possible (don't arch your back). Pause, then return to start.

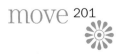

Wall Twist
Stretches chest and shoulders

Stand to the right of a wall, then reach out with your right arm and place your hand against the wall. Gently turn your torso toward the right, away from your arm, as far as comfortably possible. Hold, then switch sides.

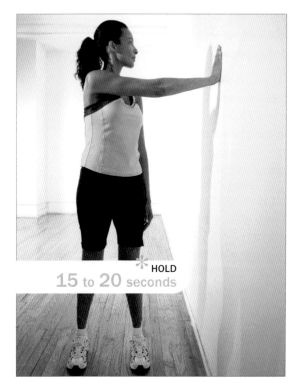

*HOLD
15 to **20** seconds

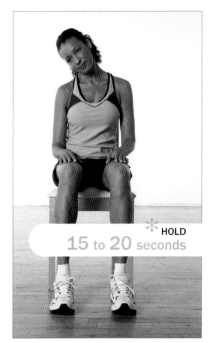

*HOLD
15 to **20** seconds

Neck Stretch
Stretches neck and upper back

Sit up straight in a supportive chair and drop your chin toward your chest. Slowly drop your head toward your right shoulder, trying to touch your ear to your shoulder as you let your shoulders drop. Hold, return to center, then switch sides.

Hand Pull

Stretches hands, wrists, and forearms*

Sit up straight in a chair and extend your right arm with your wrist flexed and your fingers pointed toward the ceiling. Using your left hand, pull your right fingertips back toward your body as far as comfortably possible. Hold, then switch sides.

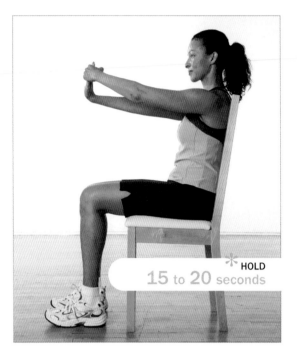

*HOLD
15 to **20** seconds

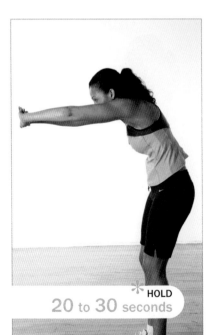

*HOLD
20 to **30** seconds

Back Stretch

Stretches upper back*

Stand with your feet hip- to shoulder-width apart. Extend both arms straight in front of you and lace your fingertips together, turning your hands so your palms face outward. Press your palms away from you, straightening your arms and rounding your back as far as comfortably possible.

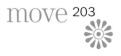

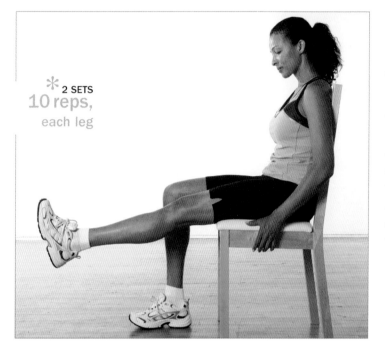

* **2 SETS**
10 reps,
each leg

Seated Leg Extension
Strengthens quadriceps*

Sit on a chair with your feet flat on the floor and hold onto the sides of the seat for support. Slowly lift your left leg until it's straight in front of you. Pause for 1 to 2 seconds, then slowly lower your leg. Repeat with the opposite leg. Alternate 10 times for 1 set.

Standing Leg Curl
Strengthens hamstrings*

Stand facing a wall with your feet about hip-width apart and place your hands against the wall for support. Keeping your back straight, slowly bend your right leg at the knee, raising your heel toward your rear until your shin is parallel to the floor. Pause for 2 seconds, then return to start. Complete a full set with one leg before switching to the other.

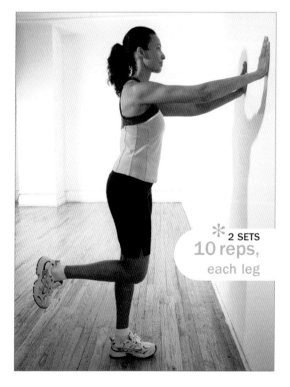

* **2 SETS**
10 reps,
each leg

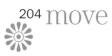

STRENGTH EXERCISES

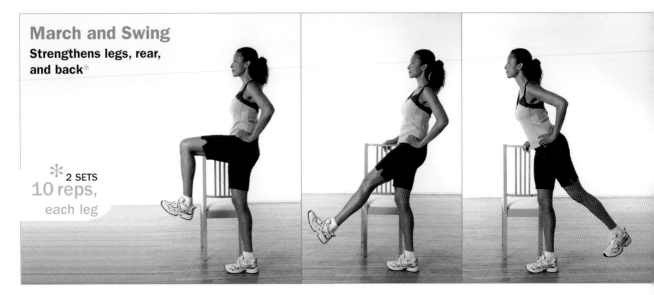

March and Swing
Strengthens legs, rear, and back*

*** 2 SETS
10 reps,
each leg**

1. Stand with your left hand on your hip and the other on a chair back or tabletop for support. Raise your left knee until the thigh is parallel to the floor, with the foot flexed.

2. Straighten your left leg, pressing the heel forward and toward the floor as you lean your torso slightly backward.

3. Return to the knee-lifted position, then straighten your left leg behind you, leaning forward with your torso. Complete a full set with one leg before switching to the other.

Tip-Toes
Strengthens calves*

1. Stand behind a chair with your feet hip-width apart and one hand planted on the chair for support.

2. Using your calf muscles, slowly rise onto your toes as high as comfortably possible. Pause, then slowly lower your heels back to the floor.

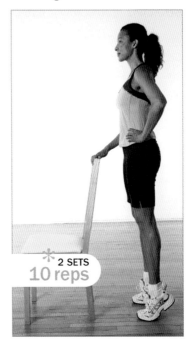

*** 2 SETS
10 reps**

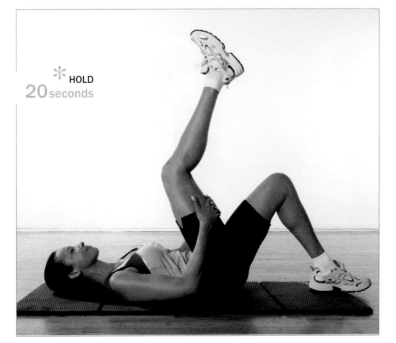

✳ **HOLD**
20seconds

Hamstring Stretch
Stretches hamstrings✳

Lie on your back with your knees bent and both feet flat on the floor. Raise your right leg toward the ceiling, then clasp your hands around the back of your right thigh and gently pull it toward your chest (use a towel if you can't reach). Hold, then switch legs.

Seated Figure 4
Stretches glutes, lower back, and hips✳

Sit on a chair with your feet flat on the floor. Cross your right ankle over your left knee so your calf is parallel to the floor and your right knee is pointing to the right. Keeping your back straight, lean forward from the hips until you feel a stretch deep in your right glute muscle. Hold, then switch legs.

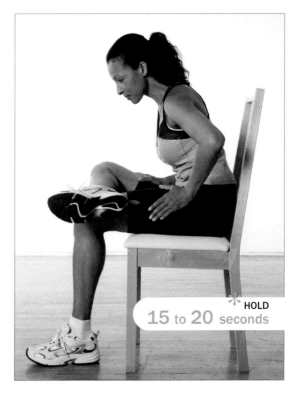

✳ **HOLD**
15 to **20** seconds

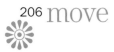

Seated Calf Stretch
Stretches calves✳

Sit on the edge of a chair with your left foot flat on the floor and your right leg extended with the foot flexed. Loop a towel around the ball of your right foot and, keeping your back straight, gently pull your foot toward you as far as comfortably possible. Hold, then switch legs.

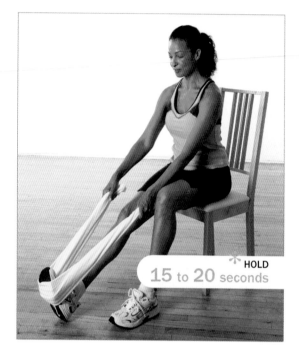

✳ HOLD
15 to **20** seconds

Knee Drop
Stretches groin and inner thigh✳

✳ HOLD
15 seconds

Lie on a mat on the floor (or if more comfortable, on a bed) with your knees bent and your feet flat. Place your hands on the inside of your knees and gently let your knees fall out and down toward the floor or bed. Then gently press down to deepen the stretch as far as comfortably possible. Hold, relax, then repeat.

Pelvic Tilt

1. Lie flat on your back with your knees bent, your hands behind your head, and your elbows extended to the sides.

2. Lift your pelvis up and toward your ribcage, tightening your lower abdominal muscles and gently "pushing" back into the floor. Hold for 2 seconds, then relax and let your pelvis rotate back to its normal position. Repeat the exercise in a slow, controlled manner.

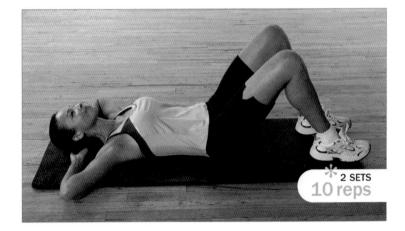

2 SETS
10 reps

Standing Twist

1. Stand straight with your legs hip- to shoulder-width apart. Hold a dumbbell with two hands and extend your arms straight in front of you, keeping your elbows soft.

2. Keeping your arms extended, contract your abdominal muscles and turn your torso to the right as far as comfortably possible. Pause, then return to start. Repeat on the opposite side. Continue alternating for a full set of reps on each side.

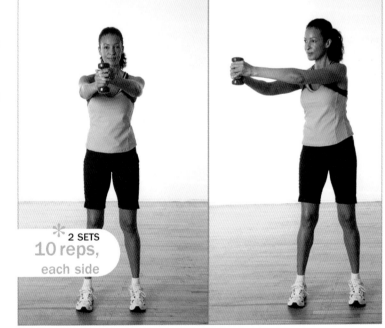

2 SETS
10 reps,
each side

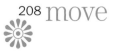

Seated Toe Lift

Sit straight all the way back in a chair and place your hands on the sides of the seat in front of your hips or on the chair arms. Contract your abdominal muscles and slowly lift your feet off the floor as far as comfortably possible. Pause, then lower your feet back to the floor.

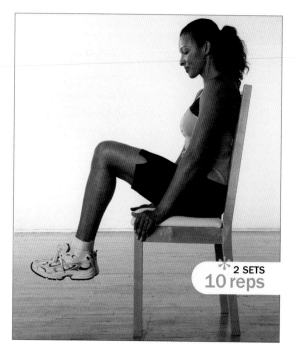

2 SETS
10 reps

Navel Pull

Sit in a chair with your hands on your stomach. Contract your abdominal muscles and pull your navel in toward your spine. Keeping your abs tight, slowly inhale for 4 to 5 seconds and exhale for 8 to 10 seconds. Relax and repeat.

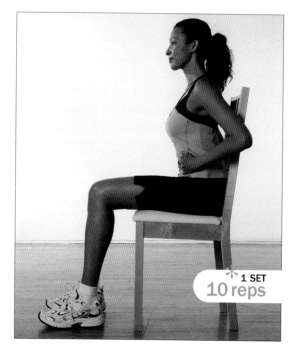

1 SET
10 reps

Morning Stretch

Lie on a mat on the floor (or if more comfortable, on a bed), raise your arms overhead, and extend your legs so your body forms a straight line from your heels to your head. Imagine that strings are pulling your arms and feet in opposite directions and try to extend your limbs as far as you can. Keep your feet flexed. Hold for 10 seconds, then relax.

*REPEAT
3 times

Lying Rotation

Lie on a mat on the floor (or if more comfortable, on a bed) on your right side with your right arm bent and right hand under your head. Bend both legs (you can put a pillow between your knees for added comfort). Extend your left arm straight in front of you. Then slowly rotate it up toward your head and all the way around (your torso will naturally roll back and your palm will flip so it's facing up; but keep your lower body stable) past your head, behind your back, and over your hips until it's back to the starting position. Switch sides.

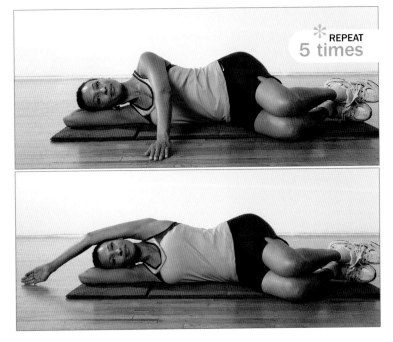

*REPEAT
5 times

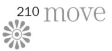

STRETCHES

Side Stretch

Sit in a chair (preferably one without arms) and grasp the back of the seat by your left buttock with your left hand, palm facing your body. Hold on as you gently lean forward and drop your right ear toward your right shoulder. Hold, then repeat on the other side.

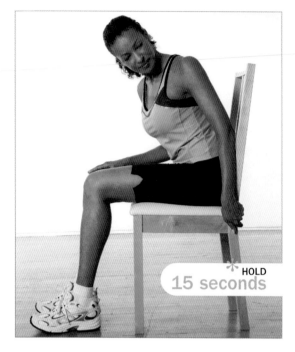

* **HOLD**
15 seconds

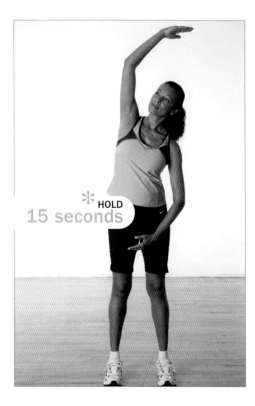

* **HOLD**
15 seconds

Reach and Bend

Stand straight with your feet about shoulder-width apart. Gently lean to the left as you raise your right arm toward the ceiling, curving it slightly overhead, palm facing down. Hold, then repeat on the other side.

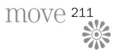

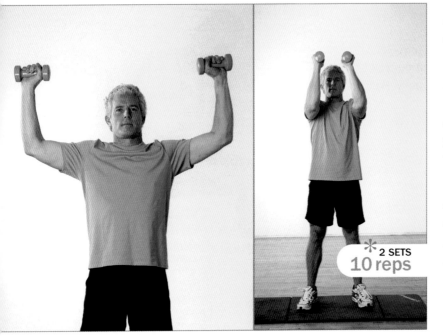

*2 SETS
10 reps

Chest Squeeze
Tones chest and shoulders✳

1. Stand holding a light dumb-bell in each hand. Bend your arms at a 90-degree angle and extend them to the sides so your upper arms are parallel to the floor, palms facing forward.

2. Squeezing your chest mus-cles, bring your elbows toward each other until they are about shoulder-width apart. Return to start.

Back Fly
Tones upper back and shoulders✳

1. Sit in a chair with your feet flat on the floor about hip-width apart. Hold a dumbbell in each hand with the weights at about chest level and about 12 inches from your body, palms facing each other and elbows slightly bent (imagine you're hugging a beach ball).

2. Bend forward from the hips (don't hunch your back) about 3 to 5 inches. Keeping your back straight, squeeze your shoulder blades together and pull your elbows back as far as comfortably possible. Pause, then return to start.

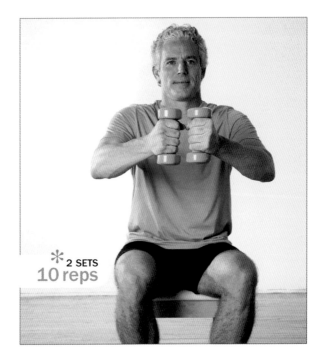

*2 SETS
10 reps

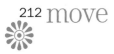

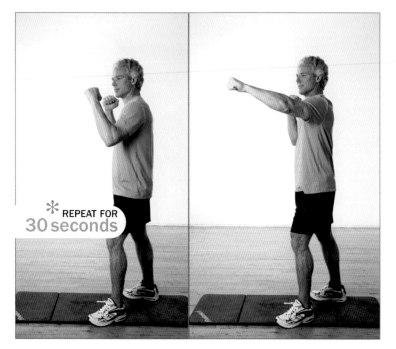

* **REPEAT FOR**
30 seconds

Jab
Tones shoulders and upper and midback*

1. Stand with your feet hip-width apart with your left foot about a stride's length in front of your right foot, keeping your knees slightly bent. Raise your arms in front of you as though sparring. Your elbows should be bent, with your left hand in front of your face and your right hand just below your chin.

2. Punch straight out in front of you with your left arm (don't fully extend or lock the elbow), then bring it back to start. Repeat, then switch sides.

Flutter Curl
Tones biceps*

1. Stand with your knees slightly bent and your feet hip-width apart and hold a pair of dumb-bells down at your sides with your arms rotated so that your palms are facing out as far as comfortably possible.

2. Keeping your back straight and your elbows tucked close to your sides, slowly curl the weights up toward the outsides of your shoulders. Pause, then return to start.

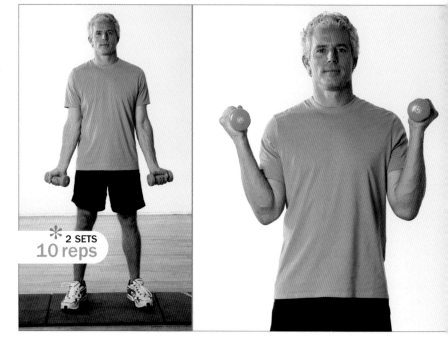

* **2 SETS**
10 reps

Lift and Arch

Stretches chest, shoulders, and abs*

Sit on the floor with your legs crossed and hold a towel overhead with both hands so your arms form a V. Keeping your lower back in the neutral position (don't arch it), lift your chest and arch your upper back slightly as you gently pull on the ends of the towel.

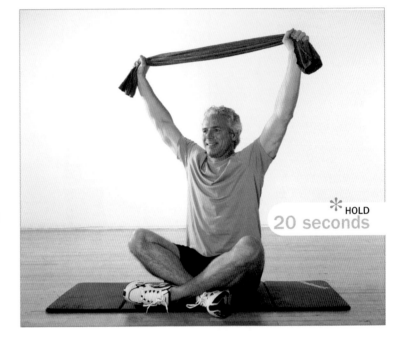

***HOLD**
20 seconds

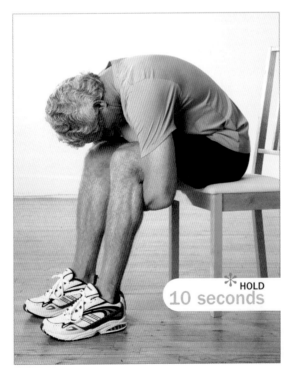

*HOLD
10 seconds

Rag Doll

Stretches back and shoulders*

Sit on the edge of a chair and slump your body forward over your legs so your chest rests on your knees and your arms hang down. Wrap your arms under your knees and press your back up toward the ceiling (your chest will rise off your legs). Hold, repeat 3 times.

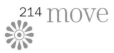

De-Hunch Stretch
Stretches chest, shoulders, and upper back*

Sit on the edge of a chair with your legs open and your pelvis tilted slightly forward. Lift your chest and squeeze your shoulder blades together and down away from your ears. Extend your arms at 45-degree angles from your body and then slightly behind you, palms facing forward. Hold, repeat 3 times.

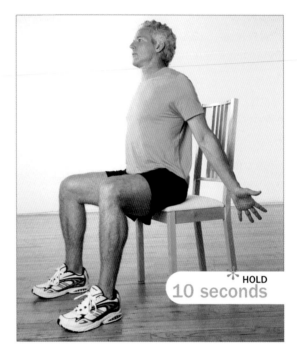

HOLD
10 seconds

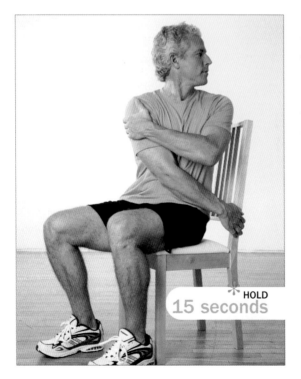

HOLD
15 seconds

Sit and Reach
Stretches back, shoulders, and sides*

Sit straight in a chair with your feet flat on the floor and place your left hand on your right upper arm. Twist to the left and grasp the back of the chair with your right hand, bringing your chin over your left shoulder as you turn. Hold, then switch sides.

move 215

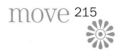

Pillow Squat

Tones inner thighs and glutes∗

1. Stand with your feet hip- or shoulder-width apart. Place a pillow between your legs just above your knees.

2. Keeping the pillow in place, extend your arms straight in front of you and simultaneously lower your rear as if to sit in a chair. Your legs should be bent at about 45 degrees. Pause, then return to start.

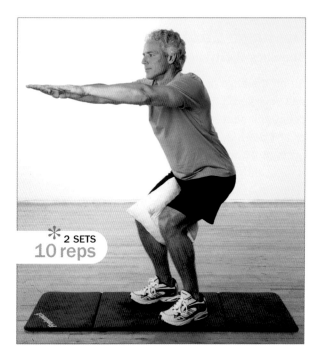

∗ **2 SETS**
10 reps

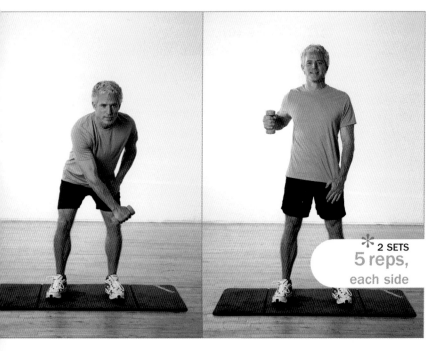

∗ **2 SETS**
5 reps,
each side

Lawnmower Pull

Tones glutes and thighs∗

1. Stand with your feet hip-width apart and hold a light dumbbell in your right hand. Squat slightly until your legs are bent at about 45 degrees and place your left hand on your left thigh for support. Reach across your body with your right arm, placing the hand with the dumbbell right in front of your left knee.

2. In one smooth motion, pull your right arm back across your body (as though pulling a lawnmower cord) and stand up slightly, though not fully. Complete a full set with one side before switching to the other.

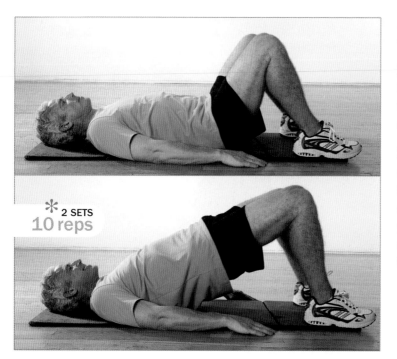

2 SETS
10 reps

Bridge
Tones hips and glutes*

1. Lie on your back with your legs bent and your feet flat on the floor. Rest your arms at your sides, palms facing down.

2. Contract your buttocks and raise your hips toward the ceiling until your body forms a straight line from your knees to your shoulders with your knees aligned with your hips. Pause, then return to start.

Chair Tap
Tones thighs, hips, and glutes*

1. Stand tall facing a chair with your feet about hip-width apart and your hands on your hips. (You can also place one hand on a wall for balance if you need to.)

2. Keeping your abdominal muscles tensed for back support, raise your left foot and tap the seat of the chair with your toes. Return to start. Complete a full set with one leg before switching to the other.

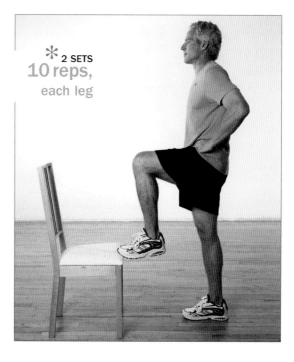

2 SETS
10 reps,
each leg

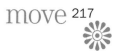

Standing Calf Stretch
Stretches calves*

Stand at arm's length from a wall and place your palms flat against the wall. Extend your left leg 2 to 3 feet behind you and press your left heel to the floor. (Your right knee will bend naturally as you extend your left leg.) Keeping both heels flat on the floor, press against the wall until you feel a nice stretch in your calf. Hold, then repeat with the other leg.

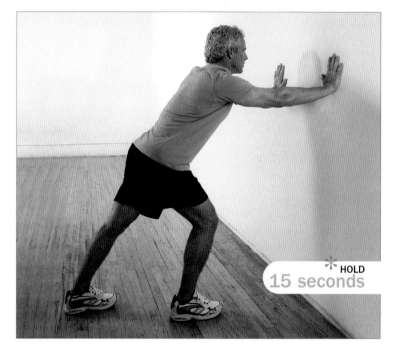

✻ HOLD
15 seconds

✻ HOLD
15 seconds

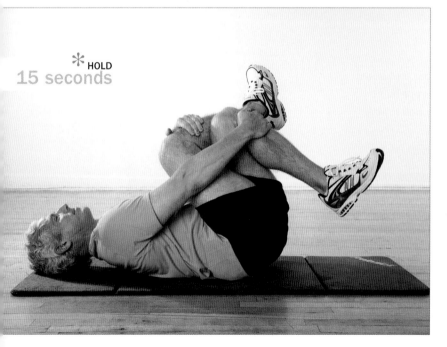

Cross and Pull
Stretches glutes and lower back*

Lie on your back and cross your right leg over the left. Lightly grasp your right knee with your left hand and your left knee with your right hand. Gently pull your knee toward your chest as far as comfortably possible. Hold, then release and repeat on the opposite side.

Downward Dog

Stretches hamstrings, glutes, and calves*

Kneel on all fours with your feet flexed. Press your hands and feet into the floor, raising your hips toward the ceiling (your body should look like an upside-down V). Keep lifting your tailbone toward the ceiling as you lower your heels to the floor as far as comfortably possible.

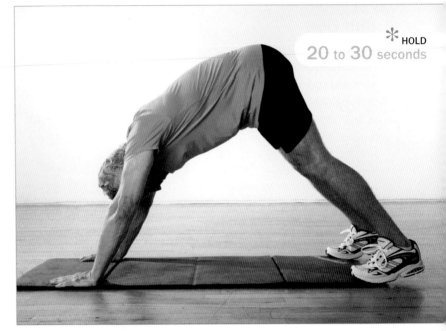

*** HOLD**
20 to 30 seconds

Flamingo

Stretches quadriceps and hips*

Stand (with your right hand resting on a wall for support, if needed) and bend your left leg behind you. Grasp the top of your left foot with your left hand, keeping your back straight. Slowly pull your heel toward your rear, stopping when you feel tension in your quads (the front of your thigh). Keep your hips and knees in alignment and tilt your pelvis slightly forward to deepen the stretch. Hold, then switch sides.

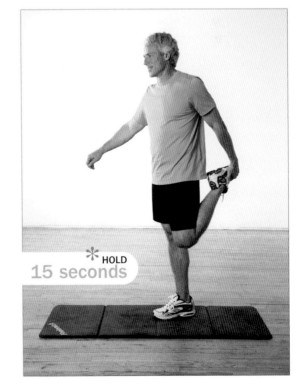

*** HOLD**
15 seconds

 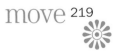

Bird Dog

1. Kneel on all fours with your hands directly below your shoulders and your knees directly below your hips. Keep your head in line with your back (don't tilt it up or down).

2. Slowly extend your right arm and left leg so they're in line with or slightly above your back, pointing the toes of your left foot. Pause, then return to start. Repeat on the opposite side.

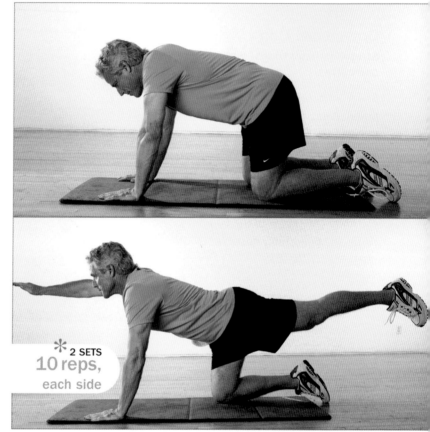

✳ **2 SETS**
10 reps,
each side

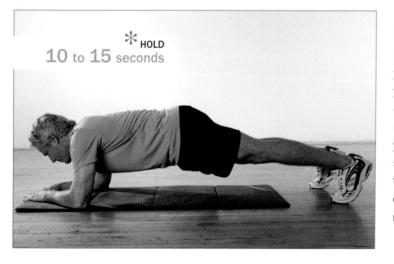

✳ **HOLD**
10 to **15** seconds

Hover

Lie facedown on the floor with your upper body propped on your forearms and your elbows directly beneath your shoulders. Lift your torso off the floor so your body is in a straight line, supported by your forearms and toes. Your back should not arch or droop. Hold, relax, then repeat 3 times.

 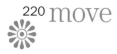

Towel Crisscross

1. Lie on the floor with your knees bent and aligned over your hips, then raise your calves so they're parallel to the floor. Hold a small towel outstretched in both hands with your arms extended so the towel is by your knees.

2. Roll your head and shoulder blades off the floor. Extend your left leg and simultaneously move the outstretched towel to the outside of your right knee. Next, extend your right leg and bend your left knee, moving the towel to the outside of your left knee, keeping your shoulders off the floor. Your neck should stay in a neutral position. Alternate 10 times for 1 set.

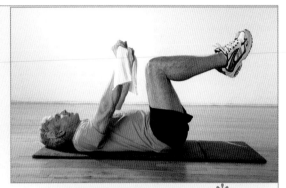

✳ 2 SETS
10 reps

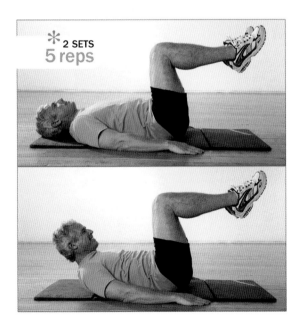

✳ 2 SETS
5 reps

Modified 100

1. Lie on your back with your knees bent at a 90-degree angle and your calves parallel to the floor. Keep your arms straight at your sides.

2. Contract your stomach muscles, pulling your navel toward your spine, and press your lower back into the floor. Roll your head and shoulder blades off the floor, sliding your fingertips forward along the floor as you do so. Hold for 5 breaths, inhaling and exhaling forcefully, then roll back down to the floor.

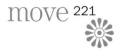

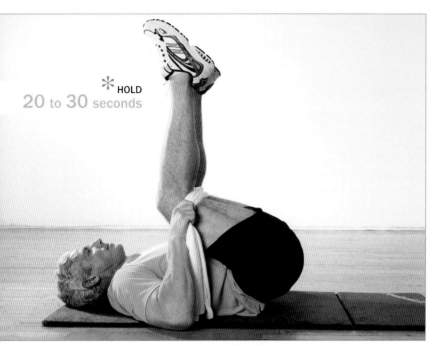

HOLD
20 to 30 seconds

Back Curl

Lie on your back with your feet off the floor and your knees bent toward your chest. Wrap a towel around the backs of your legs just below your knees, then grasp one end of the towel with each hand and pull your knees toward your chest until your lower back rolls off the floor slightly (or as far as comfortably possible).

Shirt Pull

Stand straight with your feet hip-width apart and your arms crossed at your wrists in front of your body, as though preparing to pull off a shirt. Tilt your chin upward and pull your crossed arms up, raising them and uncrossing them until they are fully extended overhead. Stretch your fingertips toward the ceiling as high as possible. Hold, then relax and return to start. Repeat 5 times.

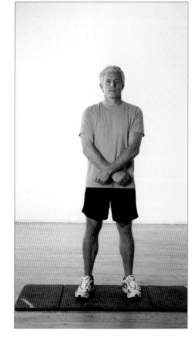

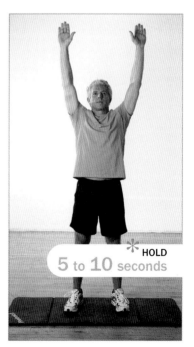

HOLD
5 to 10 seconds

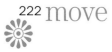

Triangle

Stand with your feet wide apart in a straddle stance with your left toes pointed forward and right toes pointed to the side; extend your arms straight to the sides. Keeping your arms outstretched, bend your torso to the right and run your right hand down the shin of your right leg as far as comfortably possible. Reach toward the ceiling with your left fingertips and look up toward your left hand. Hold, then release and switch sides.

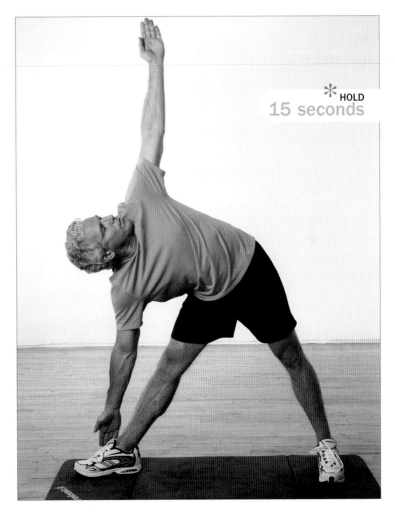

✳ HOLD
15 seconds

Child's Pose

Kneel with the tops of your feet on the floor and your toes pointed behind you. Sit back on your heels and lower your chest to your thighs. Extend your arms and rest your palms and forehead on the floor (or as close as comfortably possible).

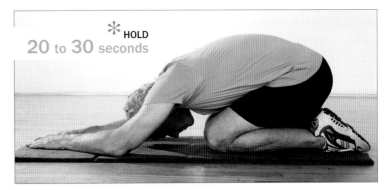

✳ HOLD
20 to 30 seconds

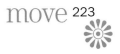

Pec Pull
Tones back and shoulders*

1. Holding a dumbbell in your left hand, stand with your right leg 1 wide step in front of your left with your left heel lifted off the floor. Rest your right hand on your right thigh for support and lean forward slightly.

2. Bend your left arm at a 90-degree angle in front of you, palm facing in. Pull your left arm up until your elbow is even with your shoulder. Pause, then return to start. Complete a full set with one arm before switching to the other.

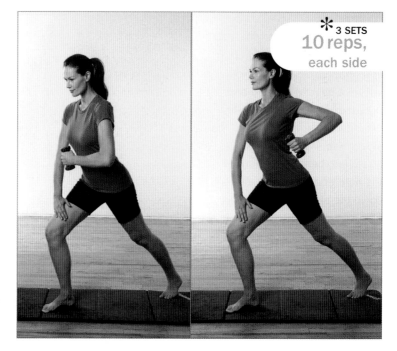

* 3 SETS
10 reps,
each side

Curl and Press
Tones biceps and shoulders*

1. Sit on a chair (preferably one without arms) with your feet flat on the floor. Hold a dumbbell in each hand with your arms down by your sides, palms facing out.

2. Keeping your upper body stable, bend your elbows and curl the weights up to your shoulders. Rotate your wrists so your palms are facing away from you and press the weights overhead. Pause, then reverse the move, lowering your arms to return to the starting position.

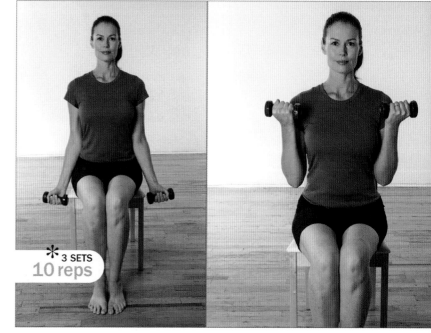

* 3 SETS
10 reps

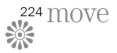

Chair Dip
Tones triceps, shoulders, and upper back＊

1. Sit on the edge of a chair with your hands grasping the chair seat on either side of your rear, and your feet flat on the floor. Slide your rear off the chair and walk your feet forward slightly, keeping your legs at a 90-degree angle.

2. Keeping your shoulders down, slowly bend your elbows, lowering your hips toward the floor until your upper arms are nearly parallel to the floor. Pause, then push up to return to start.

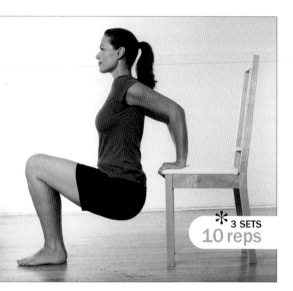

＊ **3 SETS**
10 reps

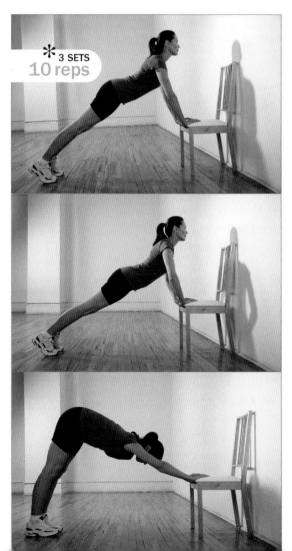

＊ **3 SETS**
10 reps

Chair Press-Up
Tones chest, triceps, and shoulders＊

1. Place a chair against the wall and assume a pushup position with your hands on the third step of a flight of stairs (using the seat will work, too). Your arms should be extended with your hands directly below your shoulders, and your body should form a straight diagonal line from your head to your heels.

2. Bend your elbows, keeping your arms close to your body as you lower toward the chair (or step).

3. Straighten your arms and press your hips back and up toward the ceiling so you're in an inverted V position, dropping your heels toward the floor. Return to start.

Overhead Grasp and Bend
Stretches triceps and sides*

Stand with your feet about shoulder-width apart. Extend your left arm overhead, bend the elbow, and reach down the middle of your back with your left hand, pointing your elbow toward the ceiling. Keep your shoulders down as you gently grasp your left elbow with your right hand and push it as far as comfortably possible into a deeper stretch. Hold, then switch sides.

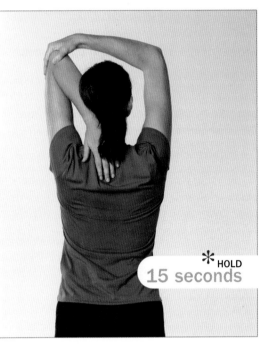

*HOLD
15 seconds

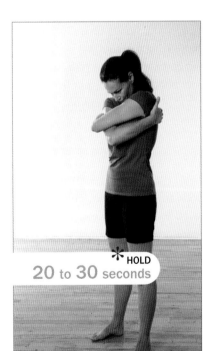

*HOLD
20 to 30 seconds

Self-Hug
Stretches upper back*

Stand with your feet hip-width apart and your knees slightly bent. Wrap your arms around the front of your body as if you were giving yourself a hug, grasping the backs of your shoulders with your hands. Keeping your torso steady, relax your upper back and shoulders and let your head hang forward as far as comfortably possible.

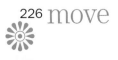

Wall Stretch

Stretches chest and shoulders*

Stand next to a wall and raise your left arm, pressing your hand and forearm against it. Slowly rotate your body toward the opposite shoulder until you feel a stretch across your chest and in your shoulder. Hold, then repeat on the other side.

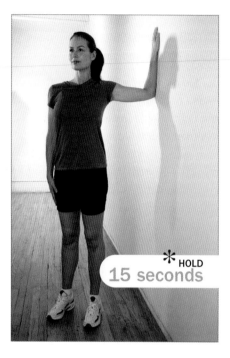

✳ HOLD
15 seconds

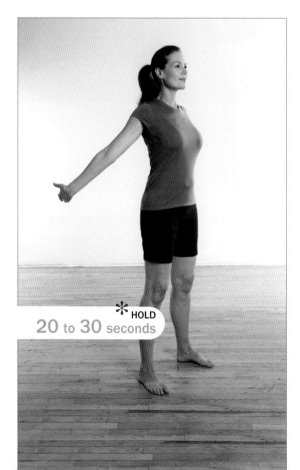

✳ HOLD
20 to 30 seconds

Open Arms

Stretches biceps, forearms, and chest*

Stand with your feet hip-width apart and your knees slightly bent. Slowly raise your arms out to the sides until they reach shoulder level. Then, with your palms facing forward, gently stretch your arms behind you, keeping them just slightly below shoulder level. When you've pulled back as far as comfortably possible, bend your wrists back until you feel a stretch in the fronts of your arms.

Single Bridge
Tones glutes and thighs*

1. Lie on your back with your knees bent and your feet flat on the floor about hip-width apart. Contract your buttocks and lift your rear up so your body forms a straight line from your knees to your shoulders. Support your hips with your hands, keeping your elbows and upper arms planted on the floor.

2. If you can, straighten your left leg toward the ceiling, pointing the toe, then flex your foot.

3. Lower your leg until your knees line up, then raise the leg again. Repeat 3 times, then switch sides. (If this is too difficult, skip step 2 and just raise your leg so your knees are in line with one another.)

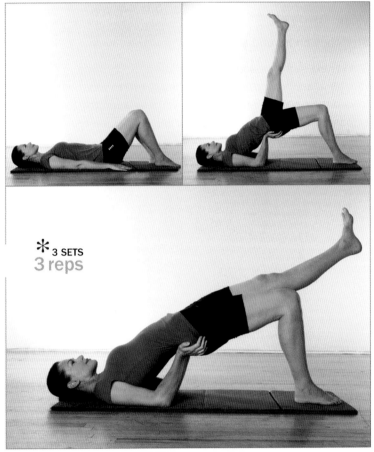

* 3 SETS
3 reps

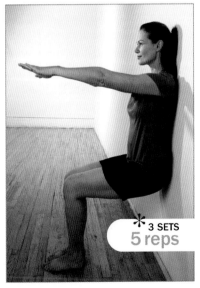

* 3 SETS
5 reps

Wall Squat
Tones glutes and thighs*

1. Stand against a wall with your legs straight and your feet about 2 feet from the wall and slightly apart. Raise your arms straight in front of you and slide down the wall until your thighs are nearly parallel to the floor. Hold for 3 to 5 counts, then slide back up to the starting position, lowering your arms as you stand.

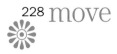

Step-Up
Tones thighs and glutes*

1. Stand facing a step and hold dumbbells at your sides, palms facing in.

2. Place your left foot on the step, then press up so your right foot is also on the step. Next, step down with your left foot, followed by the right. Repeat, starting with your right leg. Alternate 10 times for 1 set.

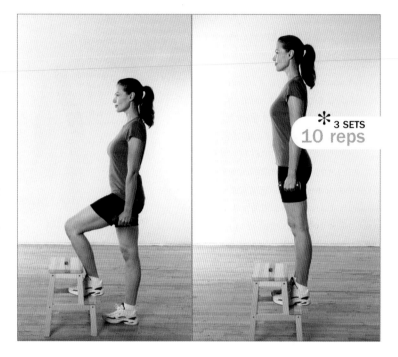

* **3 SETS**
10 reps

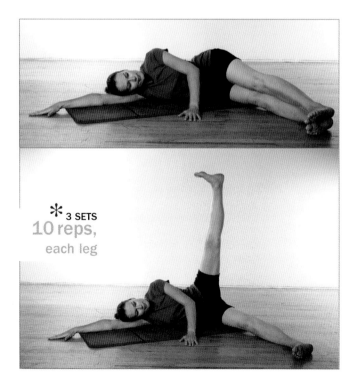

* **3 SETS**
10 reps,
each leg

L-Lift
Tones hips and glutes*

1. Lie on your right side with both legs extended straight in front of you so your body forms an L shape. (If your hamstrings or back is tight, angle your legs at 45 degrees). Extend your right arm overhead, resting your head on your upper arm, and place your left hand on the floor in front of you for support.

2. Keeping your feet flexed and your abdominal muscles tensed for back support, lift your left leg toward the ceiling as high as comfortably possible. Pause, then return to start. Complete a full set with one leg before switching to the other.

move 229

Lying Rope Stretch

Stretches hamstrings*

Lie on your back with a towel or tie looped around the arch of your left foot. Contract your left quadriceps (front of thigh) and pull the towel back, lifting your left leg as far as comfortably possible. Keep your right leg straight, or bend it slightly if your back or hamstring is very tight. Hold, then switch legs.

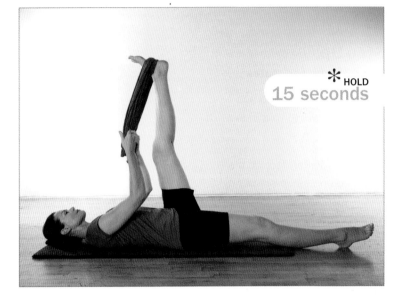

* HOLD
15 seconds

Cross-Body Leg Stretch

Stretches glutes and outer leg*

Lie on your back with a towel or tie looped around the arch of your right foot. Pull the leg off the floor as high as comfortably possible (you can bend your knee slightly if you need to). Then place your right arm on the floor and, using your left hand, pull the leg slowly across your body as far as comfortably possible, keeping your hips on the floor. Hold, then switch sides.

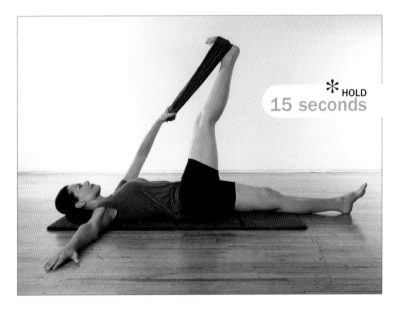

* HOLD
15 seconds

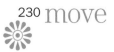

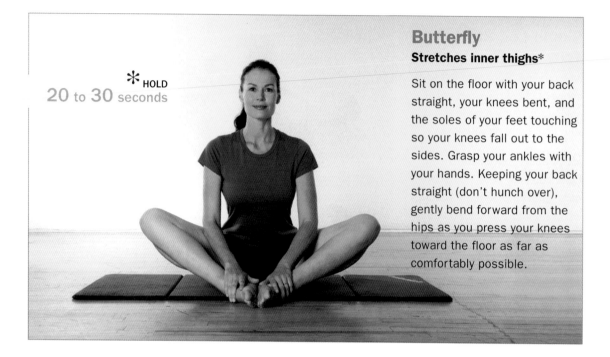

* HOLD
20 to **30** seconds

Butterfly
Stretches inner thighs*

Sit on the floor with your back straight, your knees bent, and the soles of your feet touching so your knees fall out to the sides. Grasp your ankles with your hands. Keeping your back straight (don't hunch over), gently bend forward from the hips as you press your knees toward the floor as far as comfortably possible.

Lunge Stretch
Stretches fronts of hips and thighs*

Stand with your feet together and place your left hand on a wall for support, if needed. Take a giant step back with your right leg, placing the top of your right foot on the floor. Gently bend your left leg and drop your hips toward the floor, pressing your pelvis forward until you feel a gentle stretch down the front of your right hip and leg. Hold, then switch sides.

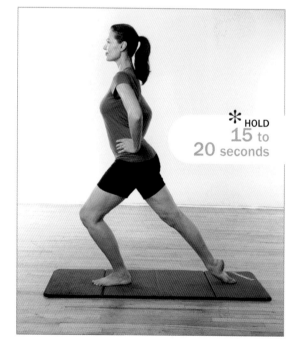

* HOLD
15 to
20 seconds

Single Leg Stretch

1. Lie on your back with your legs straight. Bring your left knee into your chest. Grasp your left ankle with your left hand and put your right hand on your knee.

2. Keeping your abdominals tight, curl your head and shoulders up off the floor, pull your left knee into your chest, and lift and stretch your right leg straight out, with your heel a few inches off the floor. Pause, then return to start. Alternate 10 times for 1 set.

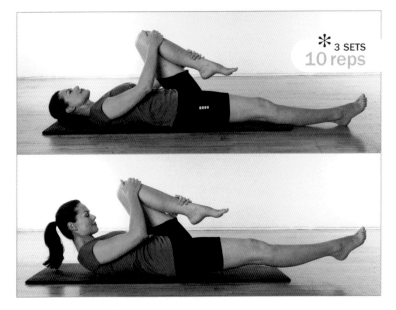

✳ 3 SETS
10 reps

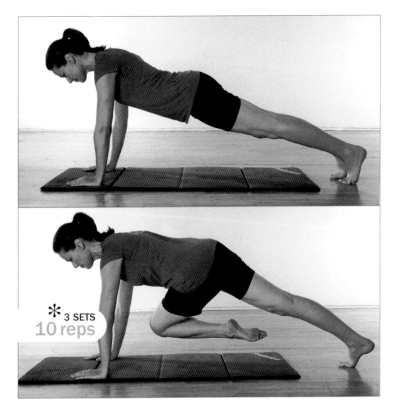

✳ 3 SETS
10 reps

Plank Torso Twist

1. Assume a pushup position with your arms extended, your hands directly below your shoulders, and your legs extended and supported on the balls of your feet. Your body should form a straight line from your head to your heels.

2. Keeping your upper body stable, bend your left knee toward your right shoulder, twisting your hips slightly to the right. Pause, then return to start. Repeat with your right leg. Alternate 10 times for 1 set.

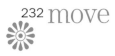

Boat

1. Sit on the floor with your back straight, your knees bent, and your feet flat on the floor.

2. Keeping your back straight, contract your abdominal muscles, lean back, and extend your legs so your body forms a right angle. Extend your arms straight out on either side of your knees. Hold for 3 to 5 seconds, then return to start.

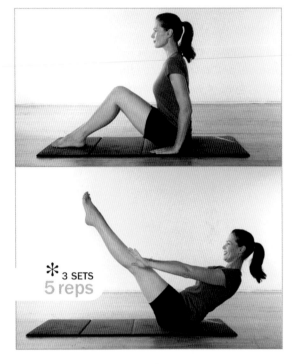

✳ 3 SETS
5 reps

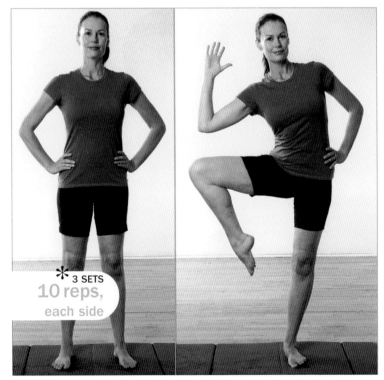

✳ 3 SETS
10 reps,
each side

Standing Side Crunch

1. Stand with your feet hip-width apart. Slightly point your right toes out to the side. Place your left hand on your hip and extend your right arm straight overhead.

2. Raise your right knee out to the side, raising it to waist height as you bring your right elbow down to meet your knee. Complete a full set with one side before switching to the other.

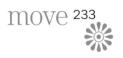

Cobra

Lie facedown with your feet together, your toes pointed, and your hands on the floor, palms down, just in front of your shoulders. Lift your chin and gently extend your arms, raising your upper body off the floor as far as comfortably possible. (If you feel any strain in your back, keep your elbows bent and your forearms on the floor.)

✳ HOLD
20 to 30 seconds

Cat Stretch

1. Kneel on all fours with your hands directly below your shoulders and your knees directly below your hips. Pull your abdominal muscles in, drop your head, and press your back up, rounding it up toward the ceiling. Hold.

2. Then raise your head and drop your belly toward the floor, arching your back in the opposite direction. Hold.

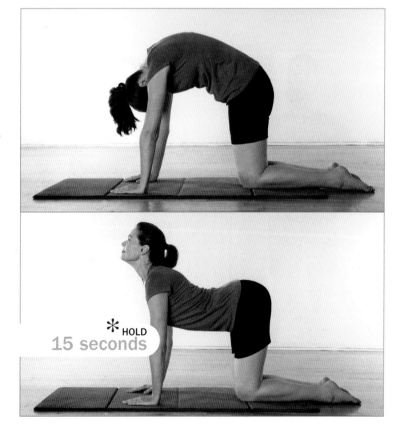

✳ HOLD
15 seconds

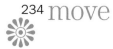

Spinal Twist

Kneel on all fours with your hands directly below your shoulders and your knees directly below your hips. Extend your right arm underneath and across your body (your left arm will bend slightly) until your right shoulder is near or on the floor. Hold, then switch sides.

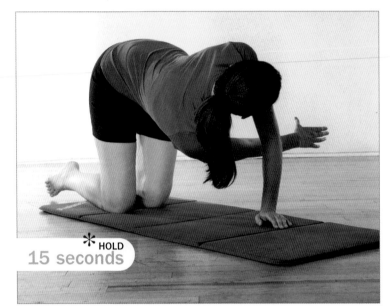

*HOLD
15 seconds

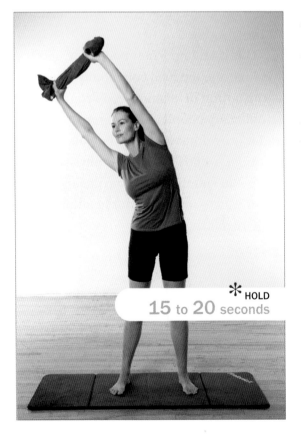

*HOLD
15 to 20 seconds

Towel Stretch

Stand with your feet shoulder-width apart and hold a towel overhead with both hands so your arms form a narrow V shape. Gently bend your upper body to the right, twisting ever so slightly in that direction so your left arm and shoulder move toward the floor, until you feel a stretch down your left side. Hold, then switch sides.

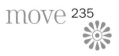

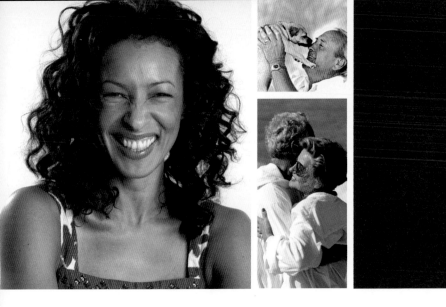

Live to Feel Good

What does it take to age successfully? It's a question researchers only began exploring in earnest in the past 20 years, when it became clear that our understanding of aging no longer sufficed in a world increasingly filled with active adults in their eighties, nineties, and beyond.

What they found is thoroughly fascinating. Yes, nutrition and exercise are key elements of a healthy, disease-resistant body. But what matters as much as, if not more than, the daily details of food and fitness are the attitudes and mind-sets that guide our lives. As it turns out, good health may or may not make us happy, but happiness without question contributes mightily to good health.

This is an important point. For too long, the medical community scoffed at the notion of a "mind-body connection," as did many people. But the research is in, and it is irrefutable: Your thoughts and emotions greatly affect your physical well-being. Put simply, there is no cheaper, easier way to improve your health than to smile regularly.

live to feel g

Happiness
What is it, anyway?

On any given day, we all tend to be a bundle of emotions and moods, from angry to ecstatic and bored to bubbly. It's naive to think that we should all exist in a steady state of smiles. Concepts like joy, purpose, and self-worth are far too complicated to reduce to a yes-or-no question of "Are you happy?" If only there were some type of measuring machine, like a blood pressure kit, that could tell us our happiness levels on a numbered scale. Now that would be useful!

Surprise. Researchers haven't created such a machine, but they have come up with the next best thing: They've identified the specific attitudes, lifestyle choices, and personal traits that best contribute to both long life and long health. We call them the Fabulous Five.

Optimism, resilience, social activities, and faith make today better— and add years to your life.

1. **Resilience** in response to life's changes and challenges

2. A healthy, active **social life**

3. The ability to prevent or manage **depression**

4. Embracing some form of **spirituality** or higher purpose

5. The skill to **defuse** the stresses of daily life

Research definitively shows that people who exercise these five traits are far less susceptible to the diseases and breakdowns of aging. Better yet, they actually do seem more joyous, more purposeful, and more active.

It's no surprise that these positive psychological traits are deeply enmeshed in the cultures of long-lived people. On the Japanese island of Okinawa, home to the world's largest concentration of healthy, happy people over the age of

100, people embrace a "don't worry, be happy" philosophy of life called *taygay* that minimizes stress and protects people's emotions from life's slings and arrows.

Okinawans also practice a deep, meditative spirituality that links them with their ancestors, their gods, and the universe. They stay connected with friends, family, and neighbors. Okinawan village life is based on the value of *yuimaru*, or mutual assistance. Friends, coworkers, or neighbors meet regularly in groups called *moais*, where everyone puts a little money into a pot, and whoever needs it most takes it home.

Elder Okinawans are proud of their status and revered by their communities—something Western cultures would do well to imitate. Here, there's no word for "retirement," and most older people do not feel lonely.

The benefits of positive attitudes and practices like these don't manifest themselves in the distant future. Optimism, resilience, social activities, and faith make *today* better. And, as revealed in Okinawa, they also make you more likely to enjoy life many years from now.

The bottom line: If you think that living a healthy lifestyle is just about food and exercise, you are badly mistaken. Everyday attitudes are as important to your health, short *and* long term, as anything else you can do.

So read on! We'll explore each of the Fabulous Five attributes in detail and show you specific, easy ways to embrace them. Remember: Making change is easier than you think, if you go about it one small step at a time. You can improve your mind-set, your social life, and your direction. The first step is merely gathering enough courage and conviction to take a first step. The second one will follow much more easily.

Trait 1 | Resilience

When Dutch researchers asked 600 people 85 and older to identify the key components of successful aging, they came up with one that surprised even the experts: psychological health. But rather than defining psychological health as the lack of depression or other mental health conditions, they told researchers it meant being able to adjust to circumstances, focus on gains rather than losses, and appreciate your blessings. We have another word for it: *resilience.*

Resilience is why certain kids who grow up surrounded by poverty or cruelty still manage to get into top universities and become successful. It's why some people rebuild after hurricanes, despite the challenges and hardships. It's why you say of someone who's just been diagnosed with cancer or who has just lost a husband or whose business has just failed: "I can't believe how well she's handling this." We like to think of a resilient person as a human rubber band—able to be stretched to the breaking point and still snap back.

What resilience is *not*, says John Stuart Hall, PhD, professor of public affairs at Arizona State University in Phoenix and a pioneer in the area of resilience in older adults, is "positive psychology," or always "looking on the bright side." Instead, he explains, resilience is "having a balanced perspective and understanding that there are going to be daily challenges." It's being able to focus on your assets instead of your weaknesses. Resilient people, he says, "learn to value themselves and to look for measures of their successes, not failures."

Everyone has some measure of resilience, says aging expert Adam Davey, PhD, associate professor at Temple University in Philadelphia. But older adults should be most resilient because of the wisdom they've gained from decades of coping with challenging situations. "This enables them to draw on their wealth of experience to come up with solutions to the current situation," Dr. Davey explains. Thus, if you're faced with financial trouble, for instance, you can think back to another time this happened and draw strength from the fact that you managed the situation then, so you can manage it now.

Resilience really comes into play when you're confronted with stress. If you're resilient, studies find, you recover from stress faster, reducing the damaging impact it can have on your body and readying yourself more quickly for the next challenge.

Researchers have identified certain common traits of resilient people. How many apply to you? Resilient people:

- Adapt to change easily
- Feel in control of their lives
- Are able to bounce back after difficult times
- Have close, dependable relationships
- Remain optimistic even in the face of challenges
- Can function well under pressure
- Have a sense of humor, even under stress
- Have a sense of confidence and strength in themselves as individuals
- Believe things happen for a reason
- Can handle uncertainty or unpleasant feelings
- Know where to turn for help
- Like challenges
- Enjoy taking the lead
- Have hobbies and other activities

No worries. Even if you're on the low end of the resilience scale, you can take steps today to

Have you laughed enough today?

build your inner resilience. While the following tips provide a start, every other tip throughout this chapter will also add to your resilience.

Laugh at least five times a day. Humor and resilience are actually quite similar. After all, what is humor but the ability to make light of real life? Laughter keeps you optimistic, helps you cope, reduces stress, and reminds you of what's important in life. If you don't have a sense of humor, now is the time to work on one. Start with the professionals: Watch comedies on TV, rent funny movies, read funny books. Be less stern and more playful with your family. Have animated conversations about unimportant things with friends. Learn the art of the gentle tease—and be open to teasing in return. Come bedtime, look back on your day and think about whether you laughed enough. Then vow to laugh more tomorrow. Just one warning: Avoid sarcasm, mockery, and any other forms of humor that degrade or hurt others. Humor, when twisted improperly, can be more bitter than sweet.

Choose laughter over anger. Let's be honest: There's no shortage of people and things that can make us angry, be it the government, the clerk at the store, your spouse's insensitive comment, the living room mess, the crazy driver in front of you, your boss, and so on. In every case, you have a choice: Get angry, or don't. We recommend choosing the latter. Getting angry *solves* nothing. But it does accomplish something: It ruins your mood, hurts your health, and gets in the way of constructive responses. Resilient people avoid anger. Rather, if they can control the situation, they work to improve it—and if they can't control it directly, they find ways to cope with it. The next time anger starts to sweep over you, shut it down, smile at the absurdity and frustrations of life, and get busy fixing things.

Have empathy. This is closely related to the tip on controlling anger. Most people do what they do by choice. People who take the time to ponder the other side's perspective almost always sidestep anger and respond constructively. Rather than just getting angry at your boss, for example, take a moment to think through why he said what he said or did what he did (more often than not, he's acting in response to someone else's unreasonable demands!). The ability to see situations from multiple viewpoints is extremely handy for building a more resilient personality.

List your strengths. This could be everything from your ability to interact with anyone at any time to your talent for baking. Don't do this on your own; ask people who know you well to contribute to the list. Knowing your strengths, becoming *aware* of your strengths, is like putting money into the resilience bank. When it's time for a withdrawal, you'll know just how much you have to use.

Write down your blessings. It sounds hokey, but recognizing the many things you have to be thankful for is a sign of resilience. Don't leave

With every challenge comes a choice: Get angry, or get moving to solve it.

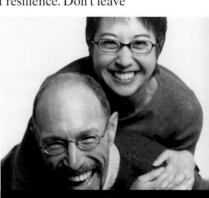

anything out. If you're blessed because you moved into a house with the master bedroom on the first floor and you don't have to climb stairs, add it to the list. Make copies of the list and put one in your bedroom, the kitchen, and the glove compartment of your car. Whenever you're tempted to bemoan your fate, pull out the list and remind yourself how lucky you really are.

Don't panic. When adversity hits, take a deep breath, think about the situation, and then list five things you can do without falling apart. Say to yourself, "In the near future, this will already be worked out, and things will be getting better."

Ask the right questions. People often let situations control them instead of *them* controlling the situation. Many times, this occurs because they haven't bothered to get the information they need. When problems occur, ask questions. Lots of questions. This provides you with enough information to develop alternative responses, at least one of which will enable you to bounce back from the situation.

Identify one positive thing in every situation. We're not recommending that you become a "lemonade-out-of-lemons" kind of person, but no matter how bleak a situation is, there's always something positive to be found. There is a couple whose house burned down on Christmas Eve, just two days after they'd moved in, when the husband tried to light a fire in the fireplace. They lost everything they had accumulated over their 40-year marriage. But they still had each other. And, they said, starting over was kind of fun!

Manage your expectations. If you expect everything to go perfectly when you travel by airplane these days, you're setting yourself up for disappointment. Instead, anticipate long delays and lost luggage by taking extra reading material

or playing cards and not putting anything you can't live without in your checked bags. Then, when disaster *doesn't* strike, you're three steps ahead! This kind of thinking works particularly well for family reunions, house renovations, and medical treatments.

Set daily goals. You need a sense of accomplishment every day to strengthen your own belief in yourself. These goals could be small, such as calling the housebound elderly woman down the block every afternoon, or designed to add up to a larger achievement, such as getting another degree or building a gazebo.

Compare yourself only to yourself. Just because Mary lost her job and had to declare bankruptcy doesn't mean you will. Just because your neighbor Al had lots more good fortune this past year than you did doesn't mean you're a failure. Mary and Al are very different people from you. Focus on your situation in the context of your life, not that of anyone else around you.

Recognize what you can and cannot control. If you have diabetes, for instance, and you're following a healthy diet, taking your medication, and exercising regularly, but you still have fluctuating blood sugar, recognize that you're doing all you can to control the situation, and you may need to put the rest of the problem in your doctor's hands.

Change one thing every day. "With age, we move in tinier and tinier circles," says Dr. Davey, becoming so entrenched in our routines that we don't even notice them any longer. Then, when something happens to change that routine, we lack the flexibility to cope with it. To prevent this from happening to him, he changes one thing about his routine every day. He might brush his teeth with his left hand, take a different route while riding his bike to work, or sleep in a different bedroom in his house.

No matter what our age, there's a child inside each of us, just waiting to play.

If you think aging means pain, disability, or poor health, you're living in the past. A landmark study published in 2002 found that people who perceive aging negatively live an average of 7 1/2 years *less* than people who view aging in a positive light.

Since then, other studies have found numerous connections between the perception of aging and overall health and well-being. For instance, one found that people who viewed aging positively were more likely to remain physically active, a key component of aging well. Those who thought negatively about aging, however, were less likely to remain physically active and more likely to age "unsuccessfully." Other studies found that views about aging affect memory, well-being, the will to live, and overall satisfaction with life.

Your expectations about aging also affect how your body reacts to stress, particularly when it comes to the effect of stress on your heart. View aging as all downhill, and your heart flips out when you're under stress; view aging as a well-deserved benefit of a well-lived life, and your heart reacts to stress as a minor blip in the scheme of things.

Your perceptions about aging also affect how you live your life. For instance, if you believe that brain function inevitably declines with age—a total falsehood—you might refuse to learn to use a computer, cutting yourself off from a valuable tool for learning, staying in touch with people, and finding new activities and interests—all of which, as you now know, are keys to aging well.

All this creates a vicious circle: If you think aging means infirmity, and your health or memory deteriorates because of your belief, it only reinforces that mistaken belief and results in greater problems.

the bottom line:

Your attitudes have the power to program your body to perform as you think it should perform.

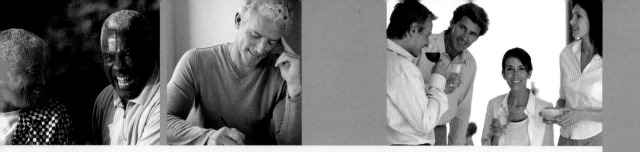

To readjust your perceptions of aging:

Pick up your walking pace.

One study of 47 healthy men and women with an average age of 70 found that those who received subliminally negative messages about aging (senility, dependency, and disease) and then took a walk traveled at the same speed as before they received the messages. Those who received positive messages about aging (wisdom, astuteness, and accomplishment) walked 9 percent faster. It may seem a small change, but other studies found that walking speed is a good way to measure your overall fitness and physical function. Studies also link walking speed to the risk of nursing home admission and death in older people. Generally, your walking speed drops 9 to 30 percent as you age, so any increase is a good thing.

Focus on other successful seniors.

Many of today's greatest authors, orchestra conductors, actors, commentators, teachers, and visionaries are people over the age of 70. Role models abound for people seeking an active path for their later years.

Watch your language.

Instead of chalking up forgetfulness to a "senior moment," call it what it is: a brain blip, a sign you're under too much stress, an indication that you didn't pay close enough attention the first time. When you were 20 and you forgot someone's name, you didn't refer to it as a senior moment, did you? This really works; one major study of 230 60-year-olds found that those who chalked up their difficulty in completing certain tasks like cutting their toenails or walking a half-mile to "old age" were much more likely to have arthritis, heart disease, and hearing loss than those who attributed their difficulties to other reasons.

Learn the ages of the key political figures in your country.

Chances are, most are over 65. If they're healthy and energized enough to run a country, you're certainly able to achieve the health and energy you need to lead a productive and active life.

Get the TV out of the bedroom and living room.

In fact, turn it off altogether. It turns out that the more television older people watch, the worse their perceptions of aging are. That's because older people are depicted so negatively on TV. In one study, participants between 60 and 90 who watched an average of 21 hours of TV a week found that older people were often the brunt of jokes or were left out altogether. As one 68-year-old participant wrote in her viewing diary: "I feel like we've been ignored. I feel like we are nonexistent." Overall, the study found, less than 2 percent of primetime television characters are 65 or older.

Watch the Senior Olympics.

If observing a 75-year-old do the pole vault doesn't change your ideas about aging, probably nothing will.

Trait 2 | Social Connection

Are you lonely? Not "alone," but lonely. There *is* a difference. For instance, you can be married with kids still at home and still feel lonely. Loneliness occurs not only when your social life is less active than you'd like but also when you don't get the level of intimacy you need from the relationships you *do* have.

Loneliness is not just a state of mind. Studies find that feeling lonely significantly increases your risk of heart disease and depression and that lonely people are more than twice as likely to develop Alzheimer's disease as those with stronger social connections. In fact, loneliness is just as threatening to your overall health as obesity!

Researchers from Harvard Medical School discovered one reason: Men who had strong social lives and close relationships with others had lower levels of C-reactive protein, a marker for inflammation that's related to heart disease and depression, and lower levels of fibrinogen, a protein involved in blood clotting. The more fibrinogen, the greater the risk of heart attack or stroke.

The health benefits of social connection are significant whether you are a natural loner or a natural socialite. The only thing that may be different is the quantity of interactions that are beneficial to you. "If you're a loner, it may mean you don't have a lot of intimate relations, but it does mean the social relations you *do* maintain are more important than ever," says Gary Kennedy, MD, chief of geriatric psychiatry at New York's Montefiore Medical Center. "Older people may lose family, friends, and work, but most compensate by optimizing the relationships they make." That means taking that weekly golf game a step further and having lunch or drinks afterward to enhance the relationship and learn more about your golf partners, sharing personal stories and issues with friends so they become more than just acquaintances, and working at friendships rather than putting them on autopilot.

How you perceive your social connections is also important, says Dr. Kennedy. "Some people say, 'No one cares; I'm alone.' But when you ask them about their lives in detail, it turns out their daughter calls every day, they get invited to holidays with family but always find a reason not to go, etc. It's their *perception* that they lack social support when the reality is that they have a frequent and sincere social network." That means you have to learn to think differently about your social connections. For instance, just because your daughter isn't free for lunch every week doesn't mean she isn't an important part of your life.

Now, we will admit that as you get older, it can become more difficult to make friends, especially if you're retired or work at home. It wasn't

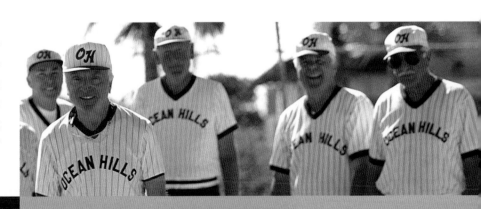

To have friends first takes the willingness to *be* a friend. Are you ready to give what it takes?

always this way. Remember when your kids were little? You made friends at the park and the day-care center and through mother's groups, soccer teams, and Boy Scout troops. Everywhere you turned, someone else was dealing with the same issues you were and was happy to get together for coffee to hash out solutions.

Fast-forward to today. The kids are gone or nearly gone, and chances are your life is more solitary, with fewer external activities than 20 years ago. Even stranger is when you discover you're in a neighborhood filled with families living life on a different plane. All this can be overcome, and in a moment, we'll give you lots of ideas to add social connections to your life.

One thing is crucial to each of these ideas: the willingness to reach out. For some people, making that first phone call, inquiry, or appearance is as tough a task as running a marathon. We understand, but there's no denying it: Making new social connections requires reaching out. It takes courage, but when you acknowledge all your strengths, all your successes, and all that you have to offer, it gets much easier. Do what it takes to confirm your sense of self-worth, and venture forth!

When you reach out to people, you will be astounded at the results. Yes, a minority will be too fearful to accept, and you will occasionally be rebuffed. But most people will be thrilled at your offer. A social invitation is a wonderful thing, whether you are a 6-year-old being invited to a birthday party or a 68-year-old being asked to join a bridge game. For a sense of personal satisfaction, there's little that can match bringing people together.

Here's how to get started.

Revive the dinner party ritual. When was the last time you invited four people over for dinner? Once, dinner parties were a natural part of life. But over time, they've become less com-

Adding Dog Years to Your Life

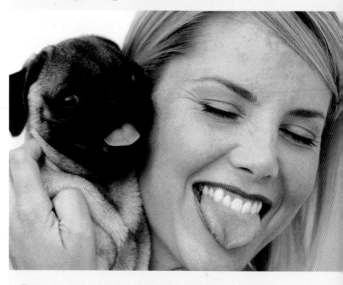

Talk about great companionship! Dogs worship the very ground you walk on. They don't care if you snap at them when you're in a bad mood or if you sit for hours saying nothing. But they do require that you get out of bed and walk them, at the very least. And that, studies find, is a very good thing for older people. When researchers looked at dog owners between 71 and 82 years old, they found that those who walked their dogs were more likely to get 150 minutes of walking a week and have faster walking speeds than those who didn't have dogs.

Other studies find significant health benefits in owning a dog (more so than owning a cat), including faster recovery from heart attacks, a greater ability to live independently, and better overall well-being. If your living situation allows it, seriously consider adding a dog to your immediate family!

Finding Friends on the Internet

Once, letter writing was common. Then it went away. Now it's back better than ever in the form of e-mails and bulletin boards on the Internet.

With the rise of the Internet over the past decade, all the modern rules of communication have changed. On any given day, billions of e-mail messages are flying among friends, families, business associates, and hobbyists around the world. Whether you live on a rural farm in Kansas or in a remote village in England, there are people out there who share your passions. You just have to find them.

Surprisingly, many adults over 50 either don't bother with the Internet or have never been exposed to it. It's worth the effort, though: The more time you spend using the Internet, studies find, the greater your social network. Many seniors find that their lives have been transformed by a few hours a day researching, communicating, and sharing online.

"Portal" Web sites are sites that resemble major airports, with lots of people congregating and then moving on to their specific areas of interest. In the United States, Yahoo.com is among the biggest. A portal site is a perfect place to start your search for information and like-minded communities. Often, there's a "groups" heading on the site's first page. Click there and enter your area of interest. It could be scrapbooking, gardening, bird-watching—whatever intrigues you. Within minutes, you'll be off on an amazing journey through new communities and other similar Web sites.

Just as when you're at an airport or visiting a new major city, however, you want to protect yourself when roaming online. Make sure your computer has all the protective software necessary to prevent intruders. And never, *ever* publicly reveal personal information on the Internet. Be constantly cautious and smart, and your Internet explorations will be safe and fun.

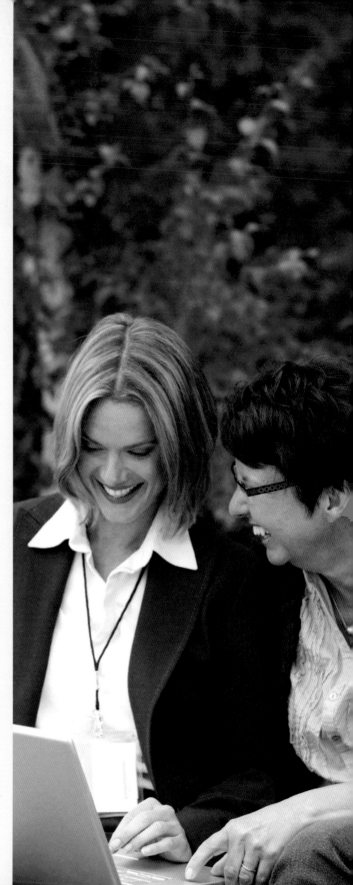

Fill your life with routines that

mon. Change that. The fanciness of your cooking is not important. What's important is the opportunity to sit at a table together, not rushed by a waiter or intimidated by crowds or noise, and to talk freely over a glass of wine and a plate of food. Make a vow: Two Sundays from now, you're having guests!

Be bold and take up a sport. It may sound like a cliché, but try golf. With three to six hours spent on the course, you've got plenty of time for conversation and companionship. Plus, there are the required post-play munchies at the 19th hole. If golf just isn't your thing, other good "companion" sports include tennis, bocce ball, and bowling.

Or take up a game. Chess, poker, bridge, mahjong, billiards, and darts are all great choices. Sitting around a table with friends and jovially playing a game for a few hours is one of the best things you can do for your health. (Be careful, though, of all the snacks and alcohol!) Make it a twice-a-week ritual.

Or join a club. Like to drink wine? Check with your local wine store. They'll have information on wine groups in your community. If not, put a flyer up in the store offering to start one. The store will probably even host the first meeting! The key here is to take something you already enjoy—tasting wine, solving puzzles, scrapbooking, knitting, swimming, fishing, woodworking, gardening—and turn it from a solitary activity into a social one. The wine club formula works for nearly any hobby.

Meet your neighbors. You probably know the FedEx guy better than you know the cat lady you've lived next door to for six years. Bake a plate of cookies and ring her doorbell, throw a barbecue for a few neighboring households, organize a block party, or start a neighborhood newsletter, in print or online, to get to know the people surrounding you.

Become a foster grandparent. Many communities offer programs that let you hang out with kids who either don't have grandparents or whose grandparents live too far away. You'll learn the appropriate time to use the moniker "Dude," how to text on a cell phone, and how to design your own Web page. Most important, however, you'll have a new friend, meet like-minded adults, and find yourself more engaged in life overall.

Get a job. Sure, you've looked forward to retirement for 40 years. But studies find that unemployed people are more likely to be lonely than those who work. You don't have to work full–time; some kind of part-time job that requires you to interact with your co-workers and the public is just the ticket! In other words, no solitary desk jobs!

Register for some college courses. If you never went to college or never had a chance to finish, now is the time. The more education you have, studies find, the more social connections you have as you age. Conversely, the less education you have, the more likely you are to become a loner because you don't trust others enough. A higher educational level means you're more likely to volunteer, and as the next tip shows, that's also a key quality in successful aging.

Volunteer. Nothing makes a person feel more wanted and appreciated than volunteering. We know this instinctively, but researchers around the world have reams of data proving it. When you help others, your own sense of control increases. With a stronger sense of control, you're less likely to become depressed. It also makes you more likely to accept help from others, another key component of successful aging.

Join Elder Hostel. With more than 8,000 opportunities for in-depth, behind-the-scenes learning in more than 90 countries, nothing can keep your brain activated and your social life filled better than this organization.

Hit Starbucks every morning. Instead of drinking your coffee at home alone, have it in the company of the "regulars" at your local coffeeshop (chain or independent). Not only will you get a boost from the caffeine (which studies find reduces the risk of depression by more than 50 percent), but you'll also get another boost from the social scene, and once you become one of the regulars, you'll have new friends.

Commit to connections. Instead of a vague, "we must get together sometime," whip out your datebook and ask what day is best. That which we put off for tomorrow ... well, you know what happens.

Weed out your connections. If you want to get the most from your relationships, quality is better than quantity. To find the time to focus on the best relationships, weed out the people who suck energy and joy from your life (like your friend Carol, who never stops whining about her sore back, her credit card bill, and her 35-year-old son still living at home). Next time she calls, gently extricate yourself from the call. After a couple of times, she'll get the message. If not, be kind but honest: "Carol, I just don't think our relationship is working. I need to pull back for a while. I hope you understand." The short-term pain will be worth the long-term gain.

Develop rituals with others. We know one couple who always hosts an Academy Awards dinner. Another celebrates the first sighting of the spring daffodils with an open house, and a third has an autumn leaf-raking, spiked-cider cookout that's a must on every calendar in the neighborhood. These activities keep you connected with people in your life, provide pleasurable activities to plan for, and ensure that you'll have regular opportunities for meeting new people (tell your old friends to bring a friend).

Visit a nursing home. It may sound depressing, but it's one of the best things you can do for yourself and the residents of the home. Ask the staff to recommend someone who doesn't get many, if any, visitors. Introduce yourself and start talking. Most important: Listen. Ask the person about his family, his former job, and so on. If you don't click with one person, try another. You'll make a friend, and you'll be helping someone else even more than you're helping yourself. It also provides a powerful motivation to keep up with all the other advice in this book to ensure that you maintain your own independence and physical strength.

Sometimes, an exchange of smiles is the best medicine in the world.

A nice walk, soothing massage, a good conversation: Life's simple pleasures can help cure depression.

Trait 3 | The Ability to Manage Depression

When it comes to preventing the frailty and disability of aging, nothing beats preventing or treating depression, says Rene J. McGovern, PhD, professor at Kirksville College of Osteopathic Medicine in Missouri. She's right. While we've known for years that depression significantly increases your risk of death from heart disease, a major Norwegian study found it also increases the risk of death from stroke, pneumonia, influenza, Parkinson's disease, and multiple sclerosis. The only major disease on which depression did not have an influence in the study was cancer.

Another study found that even after taking into account age, education, and chronic health conditions such as diabetes, heart attack, stroke, and high blood pressure, the greater the symptoms of depression in older people, the more likely they were to develop memory and learning problems over a seven-year period.

The link between depression, disease, and death? Amazingly, it's chronic inflammation—that state of heightened immune system activity that doctors now believe is the underlying cause of so many diseases. It turns out that when you're depressed, you're also stressed, and your body releases great waves of inflammatory chemicals in response. This triggers your immune system to switch on—and remain on.

Depression is a complicated disease, a mix of the physical and mental that is often hard to sort out. "Dysthymia (or low-grade depression), just creeps up on you. It's the 'common cold' of mood," Dr. McGovern says, often due to external factors and their affect on your psyche. However, more serious depression is largely about chemical imbalances, caused both by psychology and physical factors.

The good news? When you successfully treat your depression, you erase its impact on your overall life expectancy.

When depression strikes, you need professional help. But there are many things you can do on your own to prevent depression from hitting you and to minimize its effects if it does.

Pick a walkable neighborhood to live in. Instead of settling down in some cookie-cutter closed community, choose a home in a safe urban area in which you can walk to restaurants, theaters, and shops. A study of 740 older adults living in a major city found that living in "walkable" neighborhoods protected older men from depression better than less walker-friendly areas. It wasn't just the exercise that played a role, researchers found, but something within the neighborhood itself, possibly the sense of connection it provided.

Take up yoga. Depression is in large part about the shortage of certain natural feel-good chemicals and hormones in your brain. Interestingly, brain scans of people who practice yoga show a nearly 30 percent increase in levels of an important mood-related chemical called gamma-aminobutyric acid (GABA) after just one hour-long yoga session.

Sign up for a marital satisfaction workshop. It turns out that marriage is a great treatment for depression, with one major five-year study finding that depressed people who got married scored much lower on a depression test than those who stayed single. The improvement occurred regardless of how happy people were in their marriages or how much they fought with their spouses.

Keep a container of flaxseed in the fridge. Sprinkle it over yogurt and salads, mix a tablespoon into pasta sauce, and blend it into smoothies. The seed of the flax plant is one of the richest sources of omega-3 fatty acids available in our diets, and many studies find that this valuable fat significantly reduces the risk of depression.

But consume less vegetable oil. Just as important as adding omega-3s to your diet is cutting back on omega-6 fatty acids, found in vegetable oils used to make everything from margarine to doughnuts to potato chips. One study found that people diagnosed with major depression had nearly 18 times as many omega-6s as omega-3s in their blood, compared with about 13 times as many for subjects who weren't depressed. The depressed patients also had much higher levels of inflammatory chemicals.

Take a B vitamin supplement. A major Finnish study found that taking B supplements boosts the benefits of depression treatment. Other studies found low blood levels of vitamin B_{12} and folate (another B vitamin) in depressed people, with older women with vitamin B_{12} deficiencies having twice the risk of depression compared to women with normal blood levels of the vitamin. The benefit is probably related to the importance of B vitamins in brain health and their ability to reduce levels of homocysteine, a marker of inflammation that has also been linked to depression.

Touch your loved ones. The bottom line—particularly for women—is that the more loved you feel, the less likely you are to become depressed. Here are some simple ways to "feel the love."

Set a standing lunch date with your closest friend. If she happens to live 200 miles away, have your "date" on the phone.

Work on your relationship with your children. Sure, they can be annoying, they don't take your advice when they should, and you're tired of bailing them out of one fix after another. But if their love helps you stay healthy, it's worth it.

Tell your partner "I love you" every day. He or she should feel compelled to tell you the same, and the constant sweet talk will spread a veil of love and comfort over your day.

Light candles. And get out the massage oil. The kids are gone, and this is *your* time to bring grownup sex back into your life. What better way to feel loved than to make love?

Get a full physical. As mentioned, your depression may not be related to anything emotional but rather to something physical. Researchers from the Institute for the Health of the Elderly at the University of Newcastle upon Tyne in England examined the brains of 40 people who had died, half of whom had had at least one major episode of depression. They found significant hardening of the arteries, or atherosclerosis, in the brains of those who had been depressed. If your doctor spots this early, medication and lifestyle changes can make a big difference.

Take a brisk 15-minute walk a day. You probably know that exercise can help prevent or treat mild depression. For years, though,

Depression is not a prolonged bad mood. It is a serious disease that is connected to many major causes of death.

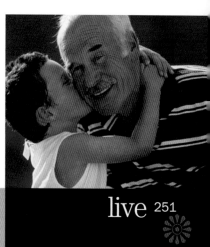

researchers thought you needed a pretty high level for it to have any effect. Now a study from researchers at the University of Iowa has found that just 15 minutes at a brisk pace could help, bringing greater energy, less tiredness, more pleasurable feelings, and a greater feeling of calmness.

Volunteer at the animal shelter. You'll get countless benefits: the altruistic benefit of "giving back"; the social benefit of interacting with others; the physical benefit of moving around (walking dogs or cleaning cages). And, if you play with the dogs and cats, their joy provides a virtual vaccine against depression. Just playing with Fido for a few minutes a day boosts levels of feel-good brain chemicals like serotonin and oxytocin.

Hit the day spa. Just 12 minutes of a massage (sign on for the 30-minute back rub) provides a natural mood boost, significantly reducing the risk of depression according to numerous studies. The reason? There are big boosts in serotonin levels and big drops in levels of the stress hormone cortisol in those being stroked. Ask for lavender or rosemary massage oil; six weeks of aromatherapy massage may also reduce anxiety.

Mix up a bowl of guacamole. Filled with healthy monounsaturated fat, the avocados in this tasty snack are also great sources of folate. A Finnish study found that people with the highest amounts of folate in their diets had the lowest risk of depression. Other good sources include fortified breakfast cereals, beans, leafy green vegetables (try dicing an avocado into a spinach salad), and sunflower seeds (also good on that spinach salad).

Walk outside in the sun, particularly during the winter. You need a daily dose of sunlight to keep seasonal affective disorder, or SAD, at bay. This form of depression is related to a lack of ultraviolet light. If the weather is too awful for walking, read the newspaper sitting under a full-spectrum light, which you can buy at most large discount and department stores.

Visit your public gardens once a week. Walk around the gardens in all seasons and note what's new and how the winter landscape differs from that of spring and summer. The peacefulness of the place will help reduce stress hormones and improve mild depression.

Catch the beat. Drumming—whether on real drums or banging on the bottom of a pot with a wooden spoon—helped 112 retirement community employees in Pennsylvania feel more energetic and less depressed and angry. Why? Drumming helps connect your physical body with your feelings, creating synergy between the external beat of the music and the internal beats of your heart, breathing, and hormone cycles. You can drum alone, but you'll get a better boost from a drumming circle. Look online or in your local newspaper—you'll be surprised how easy it is to find one!

Stress is a bad reaction to external stimuli. You can train yourself to react differently.

Are you depressed?

To determine if you might be depressed—or close to it—choose the best answer for the following questions, focusing on your emotions and thoughts of just the past week.

yes/no

1 Are you basically satisfied with your life? ☐ ○

2 Have you dropped many of your activities and interests? ○ ☐

3 Do you feel that your life is empty? ○ ☐

4 Do you often get bored? ○ ☐

5 Are you in good spirits most of the time? ☐ ○

6 Are you afraid that something bad is going to happen to you? ○ ☐

7 Do you feel happy most of the time? ☐ ○

8 Do you often feel helpless? ○ ☐

9 Do you prefer to stay at home rather than going out and doing new things? ○ ☐

10 Do you feel you have more problems with memory than most? ○ ☐

11 Do you think it is wonderful to be alive now? ☐ ○

12 Do you feel pretty worthless the way you are now? ○ ☐

13 Do you feel full of energy? ☐ ○

14 Do you feel that your situation is hopeless? ○ ☐

15 Do you think that most people are better off than you are? ○ ☐

uiz

NOW COUNT THE NUMBER OF circles YOU CHECKED AND FIND YOUR SCORE

0–4: Relax; you're doing great and have nothing to worry about in terms of depression. But retake this test every six months just to be sure.

5–8: You may have some mild depression. Now is the time to talk to a friend, spiritual adviser, or therapist to make sure it doesn't become any worse and to identify steps you can take to improve it.

9–11: You may have moderate depression. You should make an appointment with your health–care professional for a full physical. Be sure you tell the doctor how you scored on this test. You may need therapy, medication, or both.

12–15: You are at risk for severe depression. Call your doctor immediately and tell the reception-ist it's an emergency. If the diag-nosis is confirmed, you will proba-bly need medication and therapy, but you should feel better in just a couple of months.

Trait 4 | Spiritual Engagement

Are you a spiritual person? Spirituality occurs when you recognize a "why" in your life or perceive things with your inner heart. It's a sense of the mystery of life, a belief that there is more to life than what you can see or fully understand. As one researcher in the field noted, "Spirituality is the ability to stand outside of ourselves and consider the meaning of our actions, the complexity of our motives, and the impact we have on the world itself." That could be religion—or not.

Spirituality is also strongly connected with resilience and successful aging. For instance, a spiritual outlook on life enables you to focus beyond any physical disabilities because the spiritual perception views such functioning as just one aspect of living. It also helps you answer and cope with the question of "Why me?" when bad things happen because it helps you view yourself as part of something bigger, not the center of the world.

A spiritual perspective also helps you cope with situations you can't control, a key component of stress. If you view the world as bigger than yourself and admit to the existence of some "greater power," whether it's God or something else, it becomes easier to relinquish control.

Spirituality also focuses your mind on the present, emphasizing mindfulness over the rushing and focus on the future that are so much a part of modern life. Finally, a spiritual perspective recognizes the importance of social support, in terms of both giving and receiving. All have been found to improve overall health and well-being and to help people age better, regardless of any physical or mental disabilities.

For instance, one study of 400 elderly Brazilians found that those who perceived their health to be good or very good were 5 times more likely to be "aging successfully" than those who perceived their health as bad. However, those who said their personal beliefs gave meaning to their lives were *10 times* more likely to be classified as aging successfully.

Other studies of older adults find that attending religious services once a week significantly reduces levels of inflammatory markers in the blood and leads to lower death levels over a 12-year period regardless of a person's weight, diseases, social support, depression, or age.

Scottish researchers from the University of Dundee found that people who had strong religious beliefs were less likely to be lonely in older age (and you know how important *that* is!), while Canadian researchers found that older people who participated in church-related activities were much healthier overall over a six-year period than those who didn't take part in such activities. In fact, other researchers found that once-a-week churchgoers had lower blood pressure, less abdominal fat, higher HDL cholesterol (the good kind), and lower levels of inflammatory stress hormones than people who skipped Sunday services.

For many, spirituality and organized religion are one and the same—but they needn't be. A passion for nature; a belief in healing energy; faith in science and the natural laws of existence; or merely a strong sense of good versus evil can all provide purpose and direction in your life. What ultimately matters to your health isn't *what* you believe in but merely that you believe in *something* with your heart and soul.

Even if you aren't religious or spiritual today, you're likely to become more so as you age. Studies find that religion appears to increase with age as spirituality becomes more important.

While we strongly believe in the power of spirituality to help people live longer, healthier lives, we also acknowledge that this is particu-

Pause and give thanks—it enriches

larly personal topic, fraught with emotions, traditions, history, and even politics. That said, here are a few suggestions that you may find useful in growing your personal spirituality.

For health, focus on yourself. As we all know, there is a difference between personal spirituality and organized religion. Spirituality is about one person—you. Organized religion can be a path to personal spirituality, but it also encompasses much more. Whatever path you choose, it's what happens in your *own* heart and soul that matters to your health.

Find a spiritual adviser. This could be a pastor, rabbi, yoga instructor, professor, close friend, or even someone from your church who is grappling with the same questions you are. The two of you should meet weekly for an hour to talk about your week and address larger questions about the meaning of various events. Spiritual growth is achieved more easily through shared experience and discussion than in isolation.

Take up music or art. Both enable you to express yourself beyond the literal, allowing you to reflect that sense of something larger than yourself in your work. Not only that, but these new skills have added benefits in terms of keeping your memory sharp and your mind clear.

Devote time to the spiritual. Whether it's going to a church, meditating, taking a nature walk, reading a spiritual guide, or saying a nightly prayer, spending regular time cultivating your sense of the greater good is rewarding for your mind, heart, and overall health.

Pray. Prayer can happen anywhere, anytime and shouldn't be reserved for times of need. One way to think about prayer if you're not religious is as a quiet conversation with the deepest part of yourself.

Are You Spiritual?

Answer the following true-or-false questions to assess your current level of spirituality. Be honest—no one but you will know your answers. Remember too that there are no right or wrong answers, however, "true" answers reflect a greater level of spirituality than "false" answers. Retake the quiz every six months to see if your spiritual attitudes are evolving.

- I believe in the existence of a higher power.
- I often experience a heartfelt connection to nature.
- During spiritual moments, such as when praying or meditating, I often feel a joy beyond ordinary happiness.
- I believe that things happen that have no rational, scientific explanation.
- My religion or spirituality is the main source of moral guidelines in my life.
- Overall, I'm at peace with the world around me.
- Sometimes I ask for the help of a higher spiritual power.
- I genuinely feel thankful for all that I have.
- It is important to me to help others.
- I accept others even when they do things I think are wrong.
- I take time out at least once a week to focus on my spiritual or religious needs.
- I belong to a spiritual community or organization.

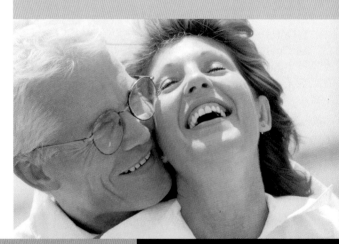

your heart, and protects it, too!

Trait 5 | Resistance to Stress

The word *stress* is so overused today that it has nearly lost its meaning. So, we want to introduce some new words.

First, say hello to norepinephrine, epinephrine, cortisol, vasopressin, and aldosterone. These are all hormones your body releases when a psychological or physical challenge suddenly confronts you. These chemicals play a major role in the inflammation we've talked about frequently in this book. Recall that this inflammation damages cells, leading to a host of health problems. Every time you are scared, pressured, angered, or frustrated, your body releases chemicals that lead to inflammation, and this is one of the major harms caused by acute stress.

But there is new news in the world of stress. To understand it, you first need to know that there's a second type of stress that's much more problematic than the type caused when someone shouts an insult at you. *Chronic* psychological stress is when troubles gnaw at you persistently over time. Think of ongoing financial woes, mean-spirited bosses, out-of-control children, tough daily commutes, an underlying sense of insecurity, and even deep resentments about politics or neighbors. It turns out that chronic stress ages you cell by cell. It does so by literally shortening a part of the cell called a telomere.

Telomeres are caps on the ends of the cell's chromosomes that help keep the chromosomes stable, just as the cap on a pen prevents ink from leaking. Every time a chromosome unzips to make copies of its genetic material so the cell can divide, however, the telomere gets a tiny bit shorter. The shorter the telomere, the worse the cell functions. Studies link shrinking telomeres to numerous age-related conditions, including high blood pressure and cholesterol, insulin resistance, and early death, primarily from infection and cardiovascular disease.

Telomeres get some help in maintaining their length from an enzyme called telomerase, which is released by immune system cells. Telomerase builds up telomeres after replication, keeping the cell alive longer and functioning better. Eventually, however, the telomere gets so short it disappears, and the cell self-destructs and dies.

The new discovery: Chronic psychological stress can shrink telomeres the same way hot water shrinks a wool sweater. It also seems to lower the amount of telomerase that immune cells release. And, in a vicious cycle, the less telomerase you have, the greater your body's response to stress and the more inflammatory chemicals are released.

These findings are important because they show how psychological issues like stress have a harmful physical effect on our cells. The findings also provide crucial good news: It's how you *perceive* stress, rather than the actual cause of the stress, that leads to the harm.

If you can find ways to inoculate your body against overreacting to perceived stressors, you will halt the flow of inflammatory chemicals and stop the unnatural damage to your cells' telomeres. One famous study found that people who practiced transcendental meditation for 16 weeks had significantly improved blood pressure, insulin resistance, and heart rate readings when exposed to stress compared to those who didn't meditate.

This all becomes even more important as you age, since studies find that your body's reaction to stress *increases* with age.

Along those lines, then, here's our advice for inoculating yourself against the aging effects of stress and changing your conscious perception of the stress you encounter. Add these tips to those in the sections above, and you will have every idea you need to live more calmly, happily, and for a longer time.

Conquering clutter

There—in that pile of month-old mail. There—in that stack of newspapers. There—on the fireplace in the collection of sea glass scattered across the mantel, in the overstuffed hall closet, in the maze of junk under your bed. Clutter! The bane of a long-lived life.

Clutter means more than a messy living room. It takes away your sense of control ("I just don't know what to do with all this stuff."). It isolates you ("I can't invite anyone over to the house until I get the clutter under control."). Clutter can even be physically dangerous, leading to tripping accidents, increased allergens, and insects and other vermin.

The key

to controlling clutter is to start with a little at a time and maintain the clear space as you move toward the next cluttered area. Here, then, is our clutter-control prescription.

1 Make a list of cluttered spaces you wish to clear out. It could include drawers, closets, or counters. Do not list an entire room, like "living room."

2 Schedule "clutter-control" mornings or evenings, giving yourself enough time to complete one item on your list.

3 Approach the cluttered area with three boxes labeled "keep," "donate," and "trash."

4 Pull every item out of or off the cluttered area. Don't put anything back without asking yourself the following questions.

"Have I used this in the past six months?"

"Will I need to use this in the coming six months?"

"Does this hold significant sentimental value?"

If the answer is **no** to any of these questions, put the item in the donation or trash box. If the answer is **yes** to any of these questions, ask yourself one more:

"Does this need to be in this location, or is there a better place for it?"

Then put it in the appropriate spot.

5 Once you've completed the decluttering, take a picture. Tape the picture to the bottom of the decluttered drawer, stick it on the inside of the door of the decluttered closet, or tuck it under an item on the decluttered shelf/mantel/desk.

6 Make sure you give away your donations within a week of the cleanup. You may need to do some research about who accepts what and whether they will pick up. Likewise, some trash—like old cans of paint or glue—need special treatment. Whatever you do, don't just transfer the clutter from one space to another. The job isn't done until trash and giveaways are long gone.

Every week, look at a photo you took of your cleaned and organized room. It will motivate you like nothing else to keep it clutter-free.

Just choose no. There's an old expression: "Don't take the bait." It means that when given the opportunity to get angry or stressed, choose not to. Make this your mantra. The next time someone does something that would typically anger you or increase your stress, choose not to react that way. Smile, let the hostile emotions pass right by, and deal with things calmly. Over time, you can teach yourself an amazing amount of healthy self-restraint, even in the face of constant pressure. Not only will you improve your health, but you'll also be in a better mind-set to successfully deal with the underlying issue.

Walk away. Anytime—and we mean *anytime*—you can feel your heart rate rising due to stress or anger, excuse yourself from the situation and do what it takes to recover. Breathe deeply, think positive thoughts, go outside, have some cold water, force yourself to smile, and remind yourself that you are in control. Re–enter the situation only when you know that you can handle it calmly and positively. You'll not only help your health but also prevent challenging situations from deteriorating further.

Practice mindfulness. "The skillful use of attention" is how James Carmody, PhD, director of the Research Center for Mindfulness at the University of Massachusetts, describes mindfulness. "It's noticing the things that come up in our mind or environment that compel our attention or that our attention gets stuck on," he says.

Once you notice where your attention sticks, you can begin to redirect it to an object or thought of your choosing. For instance, you might choose to redirect your musings about the big car repair bill to the day you spent last year fishing with your grandson. "We find that when people do this every day for about 30 minutes, not only do their stress levels fall significantly, but their sense of feeling overwhelmed drops, while their sense of being able to cope increases,"

Dr. Carmody says. And, although he's still conducting the study, he predicts that levels of stress-related hormones also drop significantly.

You can learn this form of mindfulness meditation through classes, tapes, or books.

Turn on Beethoven. People who feel stressed are more likely to listen to music than they are to do anything else, including eating, crying, or sleeping. Who can blame them? Numerous studies find that listening to music during stressful situations, including surgery, reduces stress hormones. Our advice is to skip the rock 'n' roll and stick with the classics. One study comparing Mozart to New Age music found that people listening to classical music relaxed more and reported greater levels of "mental quiet," "awe and wonder," and "mystery," suggesting that the music provided a sense of spirituality as well.

Make yourself laugh. Really. Start by smiling. Then say "ha, ha, ha." Then think about how ridiculous you look and get out a real laugh. Not working? Then try some of the ideas in our laughter advice for building resilience. Laughter helps shut down your body's stress response, cutting off the release of harmful stress hormones. When researchers compared people who received an hour of quiet time to those who had an hour of humor and laughter, they found that the laughter group showed significant drops in blood levels of several key stress hormones, while the group sitting quietly had no change.

Build bonding into your schedule. We talked about social networks and friends earlier. This is so important to successful aging that it's worth addressing again. Particularly for women, having close friends with whom to vent and bond makes more of a difference in chronic stress levels than the most luxuriant bubble bath.

Surround yourself with stress-relieving tools. That would be fresh flowers, peppermint or vanilla candles or diffusers, pictures of people you love, photographs of a particularly wonderful vacation, works of art, and a sign that says, "Breathe." All can reduce stress levels, studies find.

Stop multitasking. All you're doing is increasing stress hormones on a regular basis, even when nothing particularly stressful is happening. Instead, do one thing at a time. When that one thing is particularly stressful, take a break before you move on to the next task. During that break time, practice your mindfulness meditation or deep breathing or simply lie down with a cold cloth over your eyes and drift.

Clean a closet. There is simply nothing that puts more control into your life than cleaning up a mess you encounter frequently.

Take up yoga. Just one class is enough to reduce stress hormone levels, studies find.

Hold hands with your partner. A good relationship is a great stressbuster. In fact, simply holding hands with someone you love reduces brain activity related to stress better than holding a stranger's hands. The better your relationship, the calmer the brain response.

Munch some pistachios. After four weeks of a heart-healthy diet containing 1.5 to 3 ounces of pistachios daily, participants in a Pennsylvania State University study had reduced stress responses, including lower blood pressure and greater artery relaxation.

Spend time in a garden. If you live in a condo or high-rise, try a container garden. The greenery has a tremendous effect when it comes to reducing stress. The best gardens are "healing gardens," which contain some form of water, green vegetation, and flowers, in either an indoor or outdoor environment. Develop it correctly, though. The garden should be easily controlled and tended, offer social opportunities (with a bench or small table and chairs), allow for physical movement (an indoor or patio garden can do this with a variety of potted plants in different spaces and at different levels), and provide natural distractions (plants that attract butterflies are ideal).

Go for the sugar. When stress hits, let an ounce of dark chocolate or some other sweet treat dissolve in your mouth. Just make sure it's made with real sugar, not corn syrup or other sweeteners. Animal studies find that a quick sugary treat can reduce stress hormone levels after a stressful event without increasing weight. Artificially sweetened drinks have much lower effects.

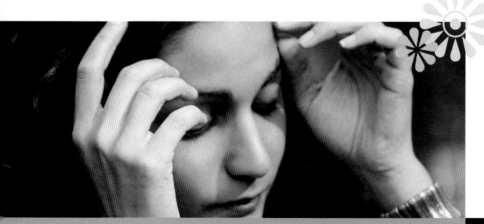

Stress isn't just in your mind. Stress affects your entire body in strong, measurable ways.

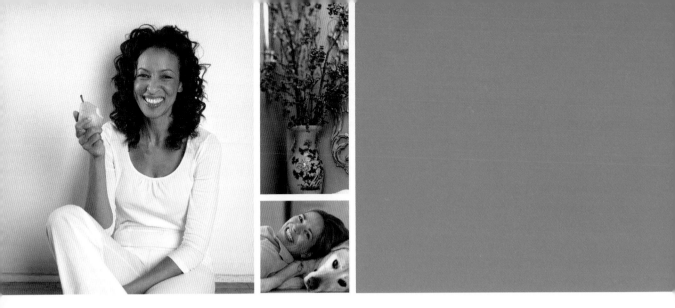

Take Charge of Everyday Health

Your body speaks to you all the time. Do you listen to what it is saying?

Most people don't. Life is much easier ignoring those little pains, that bad week of sleep, the occasional stomachache, these recurrent colds. Most of the time the problem just goes away on its own, you reason. What's different this time?

And the truth is, a lot of people seem to get by just fine ignoring their symptoms and health problems. But that doesn't change the important fact: Your body has told you something is wrong, and you chose to ignore it. Perhaps your stomach pain was merely a reaction to a bad piece of fruit, or maybe it meant that your stomach is beginning to have serious troubles. You just don't know.

Is this how you would treat an automobile that suddenly made odd noises, or if a wet spot started to reveal itself on a ceiling in your home? We hope not.

One of the truisms of life is that a problem ignored is a problem that will soon grow worse. This holds true in relationships, the workplace, the government, your home, and with your own body. Perhaps it's time to turn your ear inward.

Listening and Reacting

It's easy to categorize health into two parts. The first part is healthy everyday living and covers issues like food, exercise, sleep, stress control, and energy. Up until this point, *The Long Life Prescription* has been focused entirely on just this—how to live every moment in a way that will extend and enrich your health and happiness for decades to come.

The second part of health is what you could call "capital-letter" diseases: formally titled health issues like Diabetes, Arthritis, Asthma, Cancer, and hundreds of other diagnosable chronic conditions. These are the age robbers, the killers, the conditions that researchers focus on, all of us fear, and each of us wants to avoid. These conditions are the focus of the next part of this book; there we'll show you all the best ways to prevent these health traps of the future from snagging you.

But there's a third part to health, and that's the focus of the next pages. It's the small health problems, the symptoms, the nagging little health issues that fall between being healthy and having a serious chronic disease.

Starting around the age of 45, most adults start experiencing more nagging symptoms than when they were younger. The main reason is simple—after four decades of life, natural wear-and-tear is beginning to catch up with you.

Suddenly, your joints hurt more, your digestion isn't so reliable, your hearing is not as sharp, and your alertness is in decline come mid-afternoon.

More often than not, these health issues are small. But our message is big: By taking strong action to remedy small health issues now, you are taking strong action to lengthen your life and stay vibrant when older.

Why? Because symptoms are exactly that: the way an emerging problem reveals itself to you. The pain isn't the real problem, for example; it's the cause of the pain that often matters more. Or take a cold. You may be focused on stopping your runny nose, but that's not the important task—it's stopping the underlying virus from spreading. One doesn't have much to do with the other.

Your body constantly alerts you to potential health trouble ahead. Your job is to listen—and respond.

In the pages ahead, you will discover clever ways to remedy several of the most common symptoms and simple health problems of people ages 40 and above. More importantly, you will find these remedies also address the underlying health issues.

We bet you'll recognize most of these problems—from sore gums to aching leg veins, regular colds to after-dinner indigestion, these are the most common everyday health complaints of adults. We also address a few more specialized issues, such as a decreasing sense of balance and skin problems, that if handled now, should have minimal impact on you later.

The big message: Long Life living is more than just eating well, exercising, and maintaining a great attitude. It also includes listening to your body, and responding quickly and thoughtfully to what it is telling you. With the quick-healing advice in the pages ahead, you'll have what you need to get the healthy long life you want!

Balance

It happens to *everyone* at one time or another. You get lightheaded, or your foot catches on a loose rug, or you don't spot that hidden patch of ice. Suddenly, you're on the ground, hurting and embarrassed. If only we all could instantly bounce back up like 6-year-olds! Unfortunately, as you age, falling becomes more than just a passing episode barely to be considered; instead, it becomes a serious risk to your health and independence.

"People underestimate how important falls and fall prevention are and what an impact it can have on your life," says Sonia Sehgal, MD, an assistant professor in the department of internal medicine program in geriatrics at the University of California, Irvine. "We have a tendency to think that if you're in a nursing home, yeah, you might fall—but you can be 55, and a fall could be that much more devastating." For instance, one of her patients is a 50-year-old man who fell while putting his kayak on his car. He broke his hip and needed three surgeries.

Trust us when we tell you that a single fall can be more debilitating than even a heart attack. If you fall and break a hip, for instance, you have a 20 to 30 percent greater risk of dying the following year. If you consider that one out of every three people over 65 fall each year, the scope of the damage is pretty considerable.

Overall, falls are the leading cause of injury deaths and disabilities among people 65 and older. Yep, that's right: You're more likely to die from falling in the bathroom than from being in a car accident. That's why balance is part of the fitness pyramid we introduced on page 195.

We don't want you to suddenly become obsessed with falling and balance, but a little mindfulness and some preemptive home adjustments could go a long way toward diminishing this concern now and for decades to come.

To Improve Your Sense of Balance

First, evaluate your balancing ability. It's simple enough to do: See how long you can stand on one foot (make sure there's something stable nearby to grab if you feel yourself start to fall), then switch feet. Next, try it with your eyes closed. Which side of your body balanced better? How did you feel when you closed your eyes (thus removing one source of information from your brain and making balancing more difficult). Still think you don't need to learn how to balance better?

Exercise, exercise, exercise. No matter what you do—walking, strength training, or specific

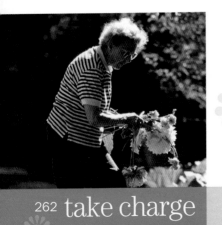

For a senior, a fall can be more debilitating than a heart attack. That's why practicing and focusing on balance is so important.

balance exercises—it will help your balance. One physical activity touted for improving balance is the ancient Chinese martial art called tai chi (you can read more on page xxx). Yoga, dance, hiking, and stretching also challenge your sense of balance, as do sports that emphasize side-to-side movement, like badminton, tennis, soccer, and basketball.

Try an exercise ball. These plastic spheres are ideal for strengthening key parts of your body to prevent falls, and they improve your overall balance as well. Sit on the ball with your feet about hip-width apart on the floor, then do the following exercises.

Hula. Pretend you're balancing a glass of champagne on your head as you shift your hips in a circular motion from right to front and left to back, as if doing the hula. Try not to move your upper body at all. Repeat 5 times in each direction.

Foot lifts. Slowly raise one foot, keeping the other on the floor. Try to maintain your balance and stability by tightening your core (abdomen, chest, and back). Count to 3, then gently return your foot to the floor and raise the other. Repeat 10 times on each side. As you get better at balancing, increase the amount of time each foot is raised.

Knee lifts. Tighten your core, then try raising your knees together without falling backward. Initially, you might try lifting one knee at a time until your balance improves. Repeat 5 times with each knee or 10 times if you're lifting both together.

Get off the beaten path. Take walks frequently on natural surfaces rather than paved sidewalks or paths. A nature path, with its tree roots and rocks, will naturally challenge your sense of balance. The same is true of sand at the beach.

Vibrating Shoes?

In the not-too-distant future, you may be asked to slip on a pair of vibrating shoes to prevent falls. A study published in the British medical journal *Lancet* found that these special shoes, which include a pair of battery-operated insoles that randomly vibrate so slightly you can't even feel it, improved balance in older people. They help boost the messages your nervous system sends to your brain when you walk and turn, enabling you to adjust your posture. Although the shoes aren't available yet, their success in this and other studies means they could be coming to a shoe store near you soon.

Wear shoes that grip the ground. Yes, life sometimes calls for high heels, dress shoes, or best of all, dance shoes. But for everyday life, wear shoes that have the best possible traction. Today, every style of shoe—from sleek work shoes to sandals—is available with rubber soles that are as ground grabbing as hiking shoes.

Take a calcium/magnesium/vitamin D supplement daily. While it won't build bone you've already lost, this mineral/vitamin combination can help slow any future loss. The stronger your bones, the less likely you are to fall and, if you do fall, to seriously injure yourself. Vitamin D also contributes to neuromuscular strength. One analysis of five studies found that supplementing with this vitamin reduced the risk of falls by more than 20 percent.

Review your medications. Get out all of the medications and vitamin, mineral, herb, and other nutritional supplements you're taking—even if you take them only once a week or once a month—and list the names, dosages, and when and how you take them. Then e-mail, fax, or mail the list to your doctor. Ask if any individual medications or supplements (or combinations of them) could contribute to dizziness or balance problems.

Drink up! If you spend most of your time at home, keep a large pitcher filled with ice water or diluted juice in your fridge and be sure you drink all of it—or more—every day. If you're on the road, carry a large refillable water bottle with you. Dehydration, which becomes more common as we age, can contribute to low blood pressure, dizziness, and falls.

Consider hip pads. If your risk of falling is particularly high due to age or infirmity, wear padded cloths on your hips. If you do fall, the pads, which are available at many health supply stores or for order online, reduce the risk of hip fracture by shunting the energy away from the point of impact. In one study, frail women living in their homes who wore hip pads reduced their risk of hip fracture when they fell by nearly 80 percent.

To Reduce Fall Risks at Home

Alarm your pets. A cat weaving in and out between your legs or a dog sneaking up behind you is a fall waiting to happen. Add a small bell or jangling tags to your pet's collar so you're never surprised.

Buy lots of double-sided carpet tape. Use it to prevent area rugs from slipping and sliding. Also put it on the mats in front of the kitchen sink and in the bathroom.

Call an electrician. Ask to have outlets added in rooms where you have electrical cords attached to extension cords. The fewer cords, the less likely you are to trip over one of them. Also ask the electrician to install extra light fixtures in dark areas of your home, such as

hallways, and make sure you have switches at the top *and* bottom of your stairs.

Measure your doorsills. Doorway thresholds should be no more than 1/2 inch high; otherwise, they're tripping hazards. Replacing high thresholds with lower ones is a task any handyman can handle.

Evaluate your stairways. Are the backs of the steps closed in? Are there handrails mounted about waist high on both sides of the staircase? Do the steps have nonskid surfaces? In addition to good lighting, these are all steps (no pun intended) designed to reduce your risk of falling on the stairs.

Visit the flooring shop. If it's time to replace that carpet anyway, consider hard-surface flooring or Berber-style carpeting. Both are less likely to trip you up than most popular deep-pile carpets. Just make sure the flooring isn't slippery. There's even a special kind of hard-surface flooring that's been developed for nursing homes that you might consider for your kitchen or bath. It's designed to provide a firm walking surface, but if you do fall, it reduces the force of impact. It's similar to the type of flooring you might see in a dance or Pilates studio and can be ordered through commercial flooring distributors.

Add extra phones. The closer the phone is, the less likely you are to run to answer it, reducing your risk of tripping and falling.

Check your lighting. Make sure there are outside lights with high-wattage bulbs (75 watts or more) near all entrances and the garage. Put high-wattage bulbs (if allowed) in all the lamps and overhead lights indoors as well.

Remember curb appeal. Not for selling your house, but for making sure you don't trip and fall when entering or leaving it. Steps should be clutter-free, be in good condition, and have non

Why We fall

No one forgets how to walk. But starting as early as our forties, any number of physical factors make us more prone to falls. With time, many of these risks grow considerably. Be most mindful of the following ones.

Lack of exercise. Leg weakness is the greatest risk associated with falls, increasing the risk of tumbles more than fourfold. Weak muscles not only make you prone to falling but also make it more unlikely that you'll break your fall or regain your balance if you start to slip. If you have time for only one activity, make it walking or strength training for your legs.

Vision problems. Maintaining balance is harder when you lose your peripheral vision, but that's what happens in macular degeneration, the most common cause of vision problems as we age. Overall, you're 2 1/2 times more likely to fall if you have vision problems than if you don't.

Medications. Certain medications, including antidepressants, anti-arrhythmia drugs, digoxin (a heart medication), and diuretics, significantly increase your risk of a fall. Plus, if you're taking three or more medications (and many of us are), you're also more likely to fall.

Environmental hazards. Throw rugs, random floor clutter, and overcrowded rooms become minefields as you age. Even wall-to-wall carpeting can be a tripping risk if the sole of your shoe catches in the carpeting. Other potential problems in your home include low lighting, missing or loose handrails on stairs, and lack of handrails in the shower/bath.

Arthritis. If you have arthritis, you're more than twice as likely to fall as someone without the disease. It's not the arthritis itself that increases the risk but the fact that people with the disease often stop exercising, so their muscles get weak. This doesn't have to happen! On page 347, you can read about ways to maintain your strength even if you have arthritis.

Depression. Depression doubles your risk of falling. Possible reasons include not paying attention to your environment, drinking more alcohol and eating less, or medication side effects.

Age. If you're over 80, your risk of falling is double that of someone younger.

Previous falls. If you've fallen before, you're three times more likely to fall again than someone who has never fallen.

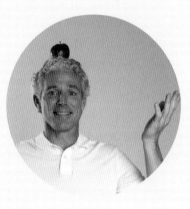

slip surfaces; handrails should be installed and tightly fastened; and leaves, snow, and ice should be removed as soon as they appear. You can also paint the edge of each step a contrasting color to aid in depth perception.

Forget about floor wax. If you must use it, make sure it's the nonskid type.

Attach your reading glasses to a chain around your neck. That way, when you walk upstairs— or anywhere else—you can take them off and let them hang. If you keep them on, your far vision isn't good, so you may misjudge a step; if you take them off and hold them in one hand, you're more likely to lose your balance and fall.

Colds and Flu

How is it possible that you've seen men walk on the moon in your lifetime but no one's come up with a cure for the common cold? Because getting to the moon is *easy* compared to curing colds. Space travel is just a matter of figuring out how to get from one point to another. When it comes to colds, however, researchers have to contend with more than 100 different cold-causing viruses, all constantly changing.

The common cold has been around since the days of ancient Egypt; the famous Greek physician Hippocrates described colds as early as the fifth century BC. Today, adults typically get two to four colds a year. While primarily a nuisance in younger people, in older people, colds can be precursors of more serious diseases, such as bronchitis and viral pneumonia.

The flu isn't much easier to confront. Another ancient illness (the first flu epidemic was recorded in AD 1173), it's also caused by wily viruses that change almost weekly.

Like colds, the flu is much more dangerous in older people than in younger folks. Most of the 36,000 yearly deaths from influenza that occur in the United States are in people over 65. Overall, those 75 and older have the greatest risk of dying from the flu, followed by children under age 4.

Have you gotten in the habit of ignoring minor colds and flu? That could spell trouble as you get older. Take charge of colds and flu today so they'll be nonissues tomorrow.

To Prevent Colds and Flu

Set a timer for 45 minutes, five days a week. That's all the time you need to spend exercising over a year to reduce your risk of colds by more than threefold. And we're talking about moderate exercise, like walking or biking at an intensity level that still enables you to talk. As it turns out, moderate exercise is one of the best ways to prevent viral infections.

Don't worry; be happy. And you'll have fewer colds—even if a researcher happens to squirt some cold virus in your nose. It seems people who are happy, relaxed, and energetic are simply less likely to catch colds, even if they're infected with the virus. Researchers have yet to figure out the link between psychological states and the immune system, but studies confirm it exists.

Wipe down your hotel room. Start packing a mini-bottle of Lysol or some disinfectant wipes in your luggage to rid your room of the previous occupants' germs. When University of Virginia researchers infected volunteers with cold viruses and had them spend the night in a motel room, they found afterward that nearly everything in the room—from the telephone to the light switch, faucets, and TV remote control—was contaminated with the virus. Even if your room has been cleaned, it's a pretty good bet the housekeeper didn't disinfect the phones, light switches, and remote control.

Take some vitamin C. There's a lot of controversy over the benefits of vitamin C when it comes to preventing or treating colds. One thing is pretty clear, though: It won't make much difference in treating colds or reducing their severity or duration. A large Japanese study found, however, that people who took daily doses of vitamin C over five years had many fewer colds than people who skipped the extra C. If you choose to take supplements, take 500 milligrams a day. Participants taking this dosage were a third less likely to have three or more colds during the study than those taking 50 milligrams.

Take 200 IU of vitamin E daily. A study at Tufts University in Boston found that when elderly people supplemented with this dosage for a year, they had significantly fewer colds than those who didn't take supplements. And if they did get colds, the symptoms didn't last as long as they did in people who took placebos.

Swallow a garlic supplement daily. It won't cure the common cold, but it may help prevent it. That's what British researchers found when they gave 146 volunteers either daily garlic capsules or placebos from November through February (the primary cold season). There were 24 colds in the garlic group versus 65 in the placebo group, a significant difference. Plus, the placebo group's colds lasted longer and were more severe than the garlic group's.

Get some sun. Researchers from New York University published a convincing paper in December 2006 suggesting that vitamin D protects against influenza and that lack of vitamin D—correlated with the lack of sunshine in winter—helps explain why winter is peak season for colds and flu. The researchers note that vitamin D is an important component in keeping the immune system from overreacting, thus reducing inflammation and oxidation (which are responsible for cold and flu symptoms). At the same time, vitamin D dramatically stimulates the production of cells that line the respiratory tract and help prevent infection. Spending 20 minutes a day in the sun with your hands, face, and arms exposed puts about 20,000 IU of vitamin D into your body within two days, compared to the 98 IU or so you get from milk.

Carry some hand cleaner. One study of elementary school absenteeism due to infection found that schools that provided gel sanitizer for hand cleaning had absentee rates from infection that were nearly 20 percent lower than those in schools where other hand-cleaning methods were used. Teachers in one school reduced their infection-related illnesses by 10 percent.

Get control of your life. Feeling out of control, whether at work or at home, stresses your immune system to the point where it overexerts and weakens itself, making you more likely to catch a cold. That's what researchers found when they studied more than 200 workers over three months. Even those who had control over their work were more likely to begin sneezing if they lacked confidence or tended to blame themselves when things went wrong.

Wash your hands again and again. We're a world of dirty-handed people, which helps spread cold and flu viruses. One study of 1,000 adults found that 43 percent barely ever washed their hands after coughing or sneezing, 32 percent didn't always wash before eating lunch, and 54 percent didn't wash long enough to effectively remove germs and dislodge dirt. When Columbia University researchers searched for germs on volunteers' hands, they found that washing just once, even with antibacterial soap, did little good in eradicating the culprits. So wash twice, and do it often. The researchers found that after a year

The Etiquette of Sneezing

Don't cover your mouth with your hand when you cough or sneeze. Instead, do what your kids and grandkids have been trained to do: Sneeze or cough into the crook of your elbow. You don't touch your mouth, nose, or eyes with your elbow, nor do you shake hands or smooth a child's hair with it, so you'll be less likely to pass on the germs.

A vaccine *that works*

Should you get a flu shot each year? Based on objective scientific studies, the answer is most certainly yes. One major study of people 65 and older not in nursing homes found getting flu vaccine every year for six years reduced the risk of hospitalization for pneumonia (a common flu-related complication) by 39 percent and of hospitalization for all respiratory conditions by 32 percent. In addition, the risk of being hospitalized for congestive heart failure dropped by 27 percent, and the overall risk of dying dropped by half. The healthier the individual, the greater the risk reduction. Plus, other studies found that the vaccine seems to protect against stroke and against heart attacks in those with preexisting heart disease.

All this protection is probably due to the fact that infections like the flu increase inflammation, which can knock plaque off artery walls and send it into the bloodstream, where it can block vessels to the heart or brain.

Despite these benefits, many older people don't get vaccinated because they believe certain myths about the flu vaccine. Let's set the record straight.

You can't get the flu from injectable flu vaccine.

This form of vaccine is made from inactivated, or dead, viruses, and there is no way they can infect you. The new nasal vaccine (FluMist) is made with weakened versions of live viruses, but it's not approved for use in people over 49 or those with weakened immune systems. Even in studies of FluMist involving hundreds of healthy children and adults, however, there was no evidence that the vaccine itself resulted in the flu. If you get sick after having a flu shot, and even if you get the flu, it's not due to the vaccine but to a virus that differs from those used to make up that year's batch of vaccine.

You can be vaccinated at any time during flu season.

True, the ideal time is a full month before the season peaks, which in North America is usually November. That's because it takes about two weeks for the vaccine to fully activate your immune system. But any time during flu season (October 1 through May 31) is still a good time to be vaccinated.

The mercury in the flu vaccine isn't harmful.

Yes, the vaccine contains tiny amounts of mercury (thimerosal) as a preservative. However, this small amount will not hurt you. Note, too, that with each passing year, more vaccine is prepared without thimerosal as the ability to manufacture this new form increases.

of regular washing, fewer microbes remained on volunteers' hands even after just one wash.

If You're Already Infected

Take time to heal. Too many people try to tough out viral infections. But your body is designed to rest when it gets sick so it can focus all its internal healing resources on fighting the infection. Following your regular daily routine when you're sick denies your immune system the time and energy to focus on healing. Don't feel guilty about it. Just take a day or two off; set yourself up on the couch with your favorite blanket, a book, and plenty to drink; and let your body do the work of making you well.

Suck on zinc lozenges. At the first sniffle, snap up a bag of these lozenges (you can get zinc lollipops now, too) and suck on one every three or four hours for up to six days (don't chew them). Not only have at least two well-designed clinical studies shown that the lozenges can reduce the severity and duration of the common cold, but another study of 66 women between the ages of 60 and 91 who had serious medical conditions found that the lozenges were safe.

Hit the doctor's office at the first sign of fever. If you want to reduce the duration and severity of the flu, get a prescription for an antiviral medication such as oseltamivir (Tamiflu) or zanamivir (Relenza). You must start taking it within 48 hours of your first symptoms. You can also start taking an antiviral drug to protect yourself if someone in your household just got the flu.

Use a sports cream for aching muscles. Viral infections often make your muscles ache. While over-the-counter pain relievers work great, if you're looking for something that won't affect your liver or stomach, try the deep heat of a sports cream like Bengay or Tiger Balm.

Try homeopathic remedies. Homeopathy is a form of healing based on the idea that "like cures like," so the remedies contain minute amounts of the very thing that causes the problem. It sounds outlandish, but numerous studies support the benefits of some remedies, particularly those for colds and flu. For colds, try Zicam. A Cleveland Clinic Foundation study found that people using this nasal gel recovered from their colds three times faster than those taking placebos. Zicam comes in a nasal gel pump, nasal gel swabs, chewable tablets, melt-in-your mouth tablets, and a mist you spray into your mouth.

For the flu, start taking Oscillococcinum, which is prepared from wild duck (these birds often harbor the flu virus). A review of seven studies found the remedy shortened the duration of flu symptoms by about half a day, although it's not a preventive.

Reduce inflammation with Kan Jang. This commercial preparation is a mixture of the herbs *Eleutherococcus senticosus* and *Andrographis paniculata*. Think of it as the new echinacea, since a plethora of studies has found echinacea of little use in preventing viral infections. Kan Jang (available in health food stores) worked more than twice as well as a popular prescription antiviral medicine in preventing flu complications in people exposed to the flu virus. Those taking Kan Jang also had flu symptoms that lasted 6 to 7 days compared to 9 to 10 days in those receiving amantadine. At the first sign of symptoms, take two tablets containing standardized extracts of *Andrographis* (88.8 milligrams) and *Eleutherococcus* (10.0 milligrams) three times a day and continue for 3 to 5 days.

Start cooking. When cold season hits, it's time to make a pot of Grandma's chicken soup. She knew what she was doing when she spooned the steaming broth into your mouth when you were a child. Not only does the steam help open stuffed sinuses, but the antioxidants in the vegetables used to make the soup help reduce the inflammatory response of your immune system to a cold.

Open up clogged sinuses with dinner. In addition to the aforementioned chicken soup, sushi with wasabi, roast beef with horseradish sauce, and spicy chili or curry (Indian food, anyone?) offer other ways to thin mucus and clear your head during a cold.

To Boost Flu Vaccine Effectiveness

The flu vaccine works by introducing your immune system to the flu virus so it can develop an antibody response more quickly when the real thing appears. The older you are, however, the less effective the vaccine. The following can help supercharge your immune system so the vaccine works better.

Meditate. Researchers from the University of Wisconsin found that people who regularly meditate show significant changes in areas of the brain related to the ability to adapt to negative or stressful events. These individuals, they also found, have much stronger responses to the flu vaccine than people who don't exhibit these meditation-related brain changes. Meditation

training classes are available at community hospitals and recreation centers, or check with an alternative healthcare provider.

Go green. Not environmentally green, but algae green. A Canadian study published in one of that country's most prestigious journals found that compared to a placebo, the green algae supplement Respondin significantly boosted immune response to the flu vaccine in people ages 50 to 55. Take 400 milligrams a day for three weeks before your vaccination, then continue this dosage for another week.

Go for a brisk walk just before your vaccination. A study of healthy young adults who boosted their immune systems with a brief bout of exercise or a stressful mental activity prior to getting the flu vaccine found that women, but not men, showed stronger immune responses to the vaccine than those who didn't get the boost. Brief periods of exercise or mental activity provide acute stress, "turning on" the immune system in some way that makes it respond better to the "challenge" the vaccine provides. Even though this study was conducted in young people, the results may also apply to older people, so give it a try!

Spend some time with friends. You've read elsewhere in this book about the health benefits of socializing. Now you can add one more. Researchers from Carnegie Mellon University in Pittsburgh found that lonely first-year students had weaker immune responses to flu shots than did students with more friends.

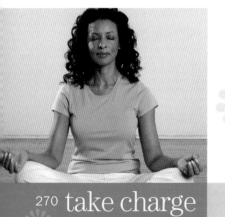

Have a little horseradish or hot sauce with dinner to clear out your sinuses. Who cares that it's not "medicine"? It works!

Dental Problems

Flash a toothy smile, bite into juicy corn on the cob, kiss your sweetheart smack on the lips—when your dental health's tip-top, there's no need to hesitate before enjoying life's little pleasures.

But healthy teeth are more than a social asset. Many of the world's healthiest, most disease-fighting foods are crunchy (think fruits, vegetables, whole grains, and nuts) and require a good set of teeth to eat. When teeth hurt or fall out, your diet goes downhill. A Harvard study of 3,183 men confirms this: Men who lost five or more teeth cut back on exactly these healthy foods.

Healthy gums guard against major health problems, too. A growing stack of research shows that even low-level gum disease revs up your immune system around the clock, fueling the chronic, low-level inflammation that contributes to clogged arteries, high blood sugar, and perhaps even Alzheimer's disease.

We'll be honest. Staying on top of oral health often gets more difficult as we age. Most older people have receding gums, a sign of early gum disease, and half already have periodontitis, or advanced gum disease. Your natural supply of mouth-cleansing saliva also declines with age, and some health conditions and the medicines used to treat them cause lower saliva output. Less saliva is one reason older teeth "grow" a bigger layer of sticky, colorless plaque (a mix of microscopic food particles and bacteria) faster than younger people's teeth do. As if that weren't enough, natural changes in dentin—the bonelike tissue beneath the translucent enamel coating on your teeth—may make your teeth look darker.

"Teeth go through life, too, and they age just like the rest of the body," notes Kenneth Shay, MS, DDS, who heads a major geriatric dental center. "The nerves in older people's teeth are smaller, so their sensitivity is actually less." That's why it may take longer to notice the little twinges that mean a tiny cavity's growing—just one reason you may have more untreated cavities, or worse ones, as you get older. And if you've always been cavity prone, you may find that you're developing new ones in surprising spots, such as underneath or next to existing fillings.

Experts now say that the most cavity-prone age group isn't the under-10 set; it's people over age 65. But there's one positive reason for that: Better oral health means more people are keeping more of their teeth. The fact is, as recently as 1960, two out of three people over age 75 had lost all of their natural teeth! That number has dropped significantly, but still, gum disease and tooth decay have conspired to claim the teeth of about *one in four* older people—and to raise the risk of cavities for the rest of us.

Your best move for reversing—or preventing—the tooth decay, gum disease, bad breath, and dry mouth that accelerate as the years pass? Give your teeth and gums the extra TLC that they—and you—deserve. Here's how.

To Maintain Healthy Teeth and Gums

Brush up your expectations. When Canadian researchers polled older people about the state of their teeth and gums, they got a jaw-dropping shock: Most said their oral health was great, yet 49 percent believed that tooth loss was inevitable with age. "We absolutely can keep our teeth healthy for a lifetime," counters Jack Cottrell, DDS, president of the Canadian Dental Association. "It just looks like attitudes may have to catch up with the new reality."

Faithfully follow the basics. Unless you've been living on a deserted island for the past 30 years, you've heard this a million times: Brush twice a day and floss once a day. There's no better way than that to care for teeth and gums!

Brush along to your egg timer. Two minutes of brushing, with light to medium pressure, is the most effective way to remove the most plaque, say researchers from England's University of Newcastle upon Tyne. Longer and harder isn't better—in fact, it may damage your gums as well as the softer, thinner enamel on the sides of your teeth.

"Although we found that you have to brush your teeth reasonably long and hard to get rid of the harmful plaque that causes dental diseases, our research shows that once you go beyond a certain point, you aren't being any more effective," says lead researcher Peter Heasman, a professor of periodontology at the university. "You could actually be harming your gums and possibly your teeth."

To prevent overzealous brushing, use a soft-bristled toothbrush and hold it like a pencil, moving it in circles rather than up and down. Think "sweeping" rather than "scrubbing."

Invest in a floss holder. A disposable one-use holder or the type you thread with your favorite floss are both good choices if you find you don't have the dexterity to carefully clean between your teeth by grasping the floss with your hands, notes Iowa prosthodontist Patrick Lloyd, DDS. Floss once a day—it will take off plaque and leftover food that a toothbrush can't reach. Be sure to rinse afterward.

Clean your tongue, too. Use your toothbrush or a special tongue scraper to gently remove filmy material from your tongue. In one study of 51 sets of twins by the New York College of Dentistry, twins who added tongue brushing to their tooth-cleaning and flossing routine reduced gum bleeding by 38 percent after just two weeks— and had less bad breath. In contrast, the twins' brothers or sisters who didn't brush their tongues had 4 percent more gum bleeding. Cleaning your tongue helps remove bacteria that take up residence just below the gumline, damaging gums and leading to bigger problems.

"Gingival bleeding and halitosis are often the first signs of poor oral hygiene that may eventually lead to further periodontal problems," says Walter A. Bretz, DDS, PhD, of New York University College of Dentistry and the mentor of the study. "A good way to prevent periodontal disease and tooth decay is through at-home oral hygiene care and routine dental visits."

Rinse in the morning for your gums, at night for your teeth. Studies show that rinsing with an antibacterial mouthwash in the morning can significantly cut your risk of gum disease. But if you've had cavities recently, have unfluoridated water at home, or have dry mouth, you should also consider using fluoride mouthwash at night. Ask your dentist, too, about having fluoride gel treatments two to four times a year to further protect your pearly whites.

Skip soda. Fizzy drinks attack your teeth two ways. First, there's all that sugar for tooth-damaging bacteria to gobble up. Second, both regular and artificially sweetened sodas contain strong acids that erode the protective enamel on your teeth. Most sodas are nearly as acidic as battery acid. The worst ones for your mouth are noncolas, which contain more citric acid, and diet sodas, which may contain phosphoric acid and citric acid. The best bet for healthy teeth:

Sip water or unsweetened iced tea (tea may help guard against gum disease, some research suggests). Gotta have a bubbly drink? Sip soda through a straw to avoid contact with teeth, and have it with meals, since other foods may buffer the acids somewhat.

Chew xylitol-sweetened gum if you're cavity–prone. Xylitol, a sugar alcohol made from substances found in birch trees and other woods, may help lower levels of cavity-producing acids made by bacteria in your mouth, Swedish researchers report. Even if xylitol levels are low, they may help somewhat—and sugar-free gum can also help remove bits of food stuck deep in crevices on the chewing surfaces of your teeth.

Stiff hands? Pad your brush. If arthritis has made your finger joints stiff or painful, gripping your brush long enough to do all the cleaning your teeth need may be a challenge. Try slipping a piece of foam tubing over the end of your toothbrush (you'll find these in a bike shop or large department store). Other options: Try a longer-handled brush to reach the back of your mouth more easily or slip a wide elastic band over your hand and tuck your brush handle underneath it. The band will help hold up the brush so you don't have to grip it as tightly.

Treat bleeding gums as seriously as you would a cut anywhere else. You wouldn't live with a scrape that made your hands bleed every time you washed them, and you shouldn't live with gums that bleed every time you brush or floss. If this is happening to you, first make sure you're faithfully brushing and flossing, then add an anti-gingivitis mouthwash. If bleeding persists, schedule a dental appointment.

Watch for subtle (and not-so-subtle!) signs of gum disease. You may have it if you have any of these symptoms: red, swollen, or tender gums; gums that have pulled away from the teeth; persistent bad breath; pus between the teeth and gums (causing bad breath); loose or separating teeth; a change in the way the teeth fit together; or a change in the fit of partial dentures. You know what to do: Call your dentist.

Schedule dental cleanings and checkups the day before your birthday and again on your "half-birthday." Your smile will be whiter in pictures, and you'll cut your odds of developing gum disease in two ways. First, professional cleanings remove calculus—hardened plaque that can make gums recede—even better than brushing and flossing. Second, your dentist will have a chance to check for signs of gum disease. Schedule appointments even if you have partial dentures, a bridge, dental implants, or a full set of dentures. Your dentist will check your mouth for signs of oral cancer and other problems.

Investigate color changes. Some teeth darken naturally with age, but sometimes darkening

Dental health isn't just about teeth and gums. The state of your mouth affects almost every part of your body in ways scientists are only beginning to understand.

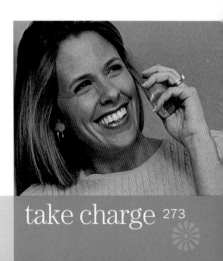

dental problems

teeth can signal more than a cosmetic problem, says prosthodontist Mike McCracken, DMD, of the University of Alabama at Birmingham. "People can have a variety of diseases that they may not be aware of. Big cavities, periodontal disease, some oral cancers, and some medications can cause staining or darkening of the teeth." Whitening treatments are most effective for teeth that have become discolored due to yellowing from age, tobacco, red wine, coffee, or tea.

Turn in earlier—and stop smoking. Japanese factory workers who slept seven to eight hours per night and who didn't smoke cigarettes were less likely to have gum disease than those who snoozed for six hours or less, say researchers. Those who didn't smoke and controlled their stress had better oral health, too. The connection? Lack of sleep, high stress, and smoking all lower immunity, giving infection under the gumline free rein.

To Battle Dry Mouth

Review your meds with your doctor. Drugs that can cause reduced saliva production include antihistamines, decongestants, painkillers, and diuretics. Ask if you can change prescriptions or cut back.

Buy a water bottle with a shoulder strap—then fill it, slip it on, and go! Sipping water throughout the day can help remedy decreased saliva. Tote your own so you've always got a no-cost supply at the ready. Slip the shoulder strap over your head and then under one arm so you're carrying your bottle messenger–style. Simply hooking the strap over your shoulder, as you would a handbag, could lead to neck and back pain.

Taste-test sour, sugar-free hard candies and sugarless gums, then carry your favorite. Sucking on sour candy and chewing both stimulate saliva.

Test-drive the dry-mouth helpers. Artificial saliva products, available as sprays, swabs, and rinses, make your mouth more comfortable. Some even have fluoride or calcium to protect your teeth. Try several (some are flavored with mint or lemon); the best one is the one you'll use most frequently. In addition, ask your dentist about special chewing gums that contain enzymes similar to those in real saliva. Dry-mouth toothpastes may also help; they claim to fight bacteria and soothe gum irritation.

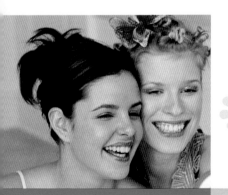

Sodas are highly acidic, with some approaching the levels of battery acid. Imagine the corrosive effect they have on your teeth!

Digestive Problems

The human digestive system operates pretty much like a modern recycling factory. A mishmash of materials comes in, is put on an assembly line, is broken down by force and caustic chemicals, and has the useful ingredients extracted and the waste efficiently released at the end.

It's a system that operates 24 hours a day, nonstop, for decades on end. It warrants our respect, care, and—dare we say?—admiration.

As with any relatively violent mechanical process, pieces and parts of your digestive system occasionally go awry. There are four common breakdowns.

The gates malfunction. Notice that you're burping a bit more or feel pain in your chest after meals? You may have heartburn or its more serious cousin, gastroesophageal reflux disease (GERD). The two typically occur when the valve that's supposed to keep the bottom of the esophagus closed weakens, allowing digestive juices to flow up from the stomach and into the esophagus, sometimes all the way to the back of your throat. Studies find more than half of people 65 and older have heartburn.

Waste backs up. It's nothing to be embarrassed about, but we're all more likely to become constipated as we age. It's not because we're older but because we tend to become less active, follow unhealthier diets, and take more medications. An estimated 41 percent of older people have constipation.

Bad things get into the system. The microbes that cause food poisoning are the obvious ones; they make you sick almost immediately after eating contaminated food. But we're more concerned with a type of bacteria called

Helicobacter pylori, which is the primary cause of ulcers—sores in your stomach and intestines that can cause great pain and possibly blood loss.

The pipes get irritated. As waste passes through the intestines, small amounts sometimes get caught in the crevices, where they can cause infection. Other intestinal issues include diverticulitis, inflammatory bowel disease, and irritable bowel syndrome. All of these require a doctor's care.

Ulcers, heartburn, and constipation are easier to manage on your own. If you've been checked out and your doctor found no underlying medical cause for these digestive issues, start with some simple lifestyle changes. Most of the following steps will not only improve your condition but also help prevent problems from starting or recurring.

To Prevent and Manage Heartburn

Slow down. Most of us eat the way we do everything else—too fast! When you eat too fast, you take in more air with your food, which can distend your stomach and lead to belching—which can also force stomach contents upward. Try this: Take a bite, put your fork down, swallow, talk to your dining companion for a minute or read a page of your book, then pick up your fork and take another bite. A bonus: You'll eat fewer calories because your body has more time to sense fullness, even though you've eaten less food.

Closely monitor your food choices. Although the traditional advice is to cut out certain foods like tomatoes, spicy foods, fried foods, and alcohol if you have heartburn, the evidence just doesn't support it. Instead, learn what foods make *your* stomach burn. Grab a notebook and, over a week's time, list the foods you eat during each meal. Then note any signs of heartburn and how long after eating they occur. Look for patterns, and if you see a suspicious food, cut it out. If your condition improves, you're done; if it doesn't improve after a week, add back that food and cut out a different suspect.

Use gravity. When you're upright, the contents of your stomach stay down, so walk instead of lying around after eating, raise the head of your bed with bricks to keep stomach acid flowing downward, and even consider eating while standing if it helps. This isn't just a folk remedy; Stanford University researchers evaluated more than 2,000 studies on treatments for heartburn or GERD and found that "gravity" solutions worked to prevent that burning feeling.

Lose weight. The closer you are to a "normal" weight, whatever that is for you, the fewer symptoms of heartburn and GERD you'll experience. Why? The primary reason is probably that extra weight increases pressure on your abdomen. Also, overweight people are more likely to develop a hiatal hernia, which occurs when the top part of the stomach protrudes into the abdominal cavity, increasing reflux.

Skip that before-bed soda—or sleeping pill. It's been found that carbonated beverages and the most widely prescribed class of sleeping pills—benzodiazepines like diazepam (Valium) and lorazepam (Ativan)—can lead to heartburn during the night, disrupting your sleep. And no, you don't have to swallow them together to get this result.

Try acupuncture. A study by Australian researchers found that applying very light stimulation to the wrist area with electrical acupoint stimulation (a needleless version of acupuncture) reduced relaxation in the lower esophagus—a contributor to GERD and reflux—by 40 percent during the stimulation compared to no change with a sham procedure.

See a sleep specialist. A sleep specialist for GERD? Yep. It seems that the same treatment used for obstructive sleep apnea, in which you stop breathing multiple times during the night, can help with nocturnal GERD, or severe nighttime heartburn. The treatment is called continuous positive airway pressure (CPAP). You sleep with a mask over your nose that's attached to a machine that delivers pressurized air to maintain an open airway. It appears to work for GERD by increasing pressure in the back of the throat and preventing stomach contents from coming up the esophagus, much the way a blowing fan keeps draperies pinned against a window. Since GERD and obstructive sleep apnea often occur together, that visit to the sleep specialist could be more worthwhile than you think.

Make a doctor's appointment. Persistent backflow of digestive juices can damage the esophagus, possibly leading to a condition called Barrett's esophagus, a potential precursor of esophageal cancer. If your heartburn has moved beyond the usual discomfort and is causing a chronic cough, nausea, vomiting, or wheezing, see your doctor.

To Prevent and Manage Constipation

Fixate on fiber. Eating high-fiber food is one of the seven key choices of Long Life Eating (for more on that, see page 129). One more reason to get more fiber is that it's a magic ingredient when it comes to relieving constipation. Fiber is the indigestible parts of plants. When eaten in whole fruits, vegetables, and grains, it serves as a wick in your stomach, soaking up liquid and creating bulk to make it easier to move stools out of your system. Your goal is 20 to 30 grams a day, which is easy enough to get if you have a breakfast of high-fiber cereal with a cup of strawberries, then have a salad and a cup of beans or brown rice with lunch or dinner.

Bake some muffins. Just mix in 2 teaspoons of psyllium seed or husk for each muffin you're making. This grain is a natural laxative that's great for simple constipation, although it may take a day before you get relief. You can also sprinkle 2 teaspoons of psyllium over cereal or yogurt.

Carry a refillable water bottle. Actually, get two. Fill them halfway with water and freeze. Then pull one out, top it off with water, and carry it with you everywhere. When it's empty, fill it halfway with water again, put it in the freezer, and take out the other bottle. The older people get, the less likely they are to drink enough fluids, and dehydration—however subtle—is a major cause of constipation. It's also extremely common in older adults. That's because age blunts the "thirst response," or your ability to feel thirsty. Plus, the amount of body fluid declines with age, from about 60 percent of body weight in men and 52 percent in women before age 60 to 52 and 46 percent respectively after age 60. Another age-related change occurs in the kidneys, which become less able to concentrate urine, so you lose more liquid overall.

Learn to control the uncontrollable. Get a prescription for biofeedback, a mind/body technique that helps you become aware of and control involuntary processes. One study of 79 adults who had a form of constipation in

The Paint-Card Test

Urine is mostly water plus waste products that have been filtered from the blood by your kidneys. It's naturally a pale yellow color due to excretion of urochrome, a pigment in blood. Since urine changes color easily, it is a good marker of your body's hydration level.

Try this test: Pick up color samples of yellow paint at your local hardware store and use them to assess your level of hydration (or dehydration). Your urine should be as pale as the palest shade of yellow; if it's anywhere near the gold colors, it means you've been shortchanging your body of water.

Note that natural foods rarely affect urine color, though food dyes can have a small effect. Then there are the B-complex vitamins; they have more effect on urine color than almost anything else, turning the shade to a bright, almost neon yellow. Cloudiness or murkiness usually means a urinary tract infection or kidney stone, so see a doctor if your urine is cloudy.

which the muscles used for bowel movements don't work well (particularly common in older people) found the technique worked better than laxatives, diet, and exercise for relieving constipation.

Get evaluated for depression. The links between the brain and the gut are powerful. It's why you often feel nauseated when you're nervous or can't eat when you're stressed. This strong link could be why a British study of 35 women found that those who were anxious, depressed, and having difficulty maintaining intimate relationships were more likely to be constipated than healthier women. The reason? Your mental state affects the function of the nerves linking the brain to the gut. The less arousal in the brain—common with many psychological conditions—the less stimulus to the gut. It could explain why low doses of antidepressants, often prescribed for gastrointestinal conditions like irritable bowel syndrome, are so effective.

Hit the gym. Move, move, move. Physical movement gets other things moving, including your bowels. But the more you sit on the couch or go from car to door to bed to car, the less likely you are to go to the bathroom.

Enjoy mornings. About 30 minutes after waking up, just after that first cup of hot coffee or tea, is the ideal time for a bowel movement, so create a place for it in your schedule. Instead of rushing through your morning, gulping the coffee, and scarfing the bagel, design a new schedule. Wake up, sip the hot drink while perusing the paper, then take your favorite section with you to the bathroom. Keep doing this even if you don't initially have any luck. Remember, you're retraining your system, getting it back on a schedule. Eventually the muscle memory will kick in.

List your medications. Then take the list to your doctor. The following meds can all contribute to or be blamed for constipation: antacids containing aluminum or calcium, anticholinergics, antidepressants, antihistamines, calcium channel blockers, diuretics, iron, narcotics, nonsteroidal anti-inflammatory drugs (NSAIDs), opioids, psychotropic medications, and beta-agonists like dopamine and epinephrine.

To Manage and Prevent Ulcers

Nix the aspirin. Taking aspirin and other nonsteroidal anti-inflammatories, like ibuprofen and naproxen, is one of the primary causes of ulcers not related to *H. pylori*. If you're taking daily aspirin for heart health reasons, talk to your healthcare professional about alternatives.

Swallow some licorice. Not licorice whips, but two tablets of deglycyrrhizinated licorice, available in health food stores. The herbal remedy can improve ulcers caused by NSAIDs and protect against future ulcers. It induces cells in your stomach and intestinal linings to release more mucus, which acts like a coat of armor for your stomach lining and protects it from the damaging effects of stomach acid. Studies find it may be just as good at preventing ulcer recurrence as the prescription medication cimetidine (Tagamet). It may also protect against *H. pylori*. Chew the tablets slowly and thoroughly 30 minutes before meals.

Prime your stomach with a PPI. A daily dose of a proton pump inhibitor like esomeprazole (Nexium) can prevent ulcer formation in people taking over-the-counter NSAIDs as well as prescription pain medications.

Spoon in some yogurt. Live-culture yogurt (available at most food stores) contains probiotics, "good" bacteria that help keep the proper acidic environment in your stomach. Studies find that these friendly bacteria can help your body eradicate *H. pylori*. Eat one 8-ounce container of yogurt a day or take one or two probiotic capsules with each meal and at bedtime for several weeks until the ulcer heals, then continue taking them at night for several months (and keep eating that yogurt!).

Chew on some C. One effect of *H. pylori* and NSAIDs is that they increase oxidative stress in your stomach, leading to inflammation and damaging the lining, thus creating ulcers. So it makes sense that adding a powerful antioxidant like glutathione, found in large amounts in the stomach lining, is a good idea. Your body makes glutathione from vitamin C, so take 500 milligrams of either glutathione or vitamin C three times a day.

Sip some cranberry juice. When 97 people infected with *H. pylori* drank 8.5 ounces of cranberry juice a day for 90 days, the bacteria were completely eradicated in 14 percent of the participants as compared to 5 percent of a placebo group, a statistically significant difference.

Raid the spice cabinet. You're looking for turmeric, a.k.a. *Curcuma longa*, a spice commonly used in Indian dishes. Supplements of this spice reduce stomach acid secretion and protect against ulcers in animal studies. Turmeric works by preventing cells lining the stomach from producing histamine, a chemical that produces stomach acid. This is the same way anti-ulcer drugs like ranitidine (Zantac), famotidine (Pepcid), cimetidine, and nizatidine (Axid) work. You can certainly use more turmeric in food, or you can find supplements in health food stores. Follow the package directions for dosage.

Get a good night's sleep. British researchers monitoring 12 healthy people for 24 hours to check how their digestion worked found higher levels of a protein called TFF2, which is responsible for helping to repair the stomach lining, while the volunteers slept. In fact, levels increased up to 340 times during sleep. In a second study, they found that depriving volunteers of sleep significantly reduced TFF2 levels throughout the day. Sleeping well, the researchers speculated, provides more time for the protein to repair stomach lining damage, helping to prevent ulcers. For more on a good night's sleep, see page 299.

The digestive system works hard— around the clock. Feed it well.

Fatigue

Being tired is such a fact of modern life that it's easy to forget it's not normal. Sure, if you had a late night, just moved into a new house, started a new job, or are ill, you're going to feel tired for a time. But if fatigue is part of your daily life, if no amount of sleep makes a dent in your tiredness, or if fatigue penetrates you to the bone, then it's a real health problem.

This deeper level of fatigue becomes more common as we age. In fact, tiredness is one of the most common complaints primary care physicians hear from their older patients. In one study of 422 relatively healthy people, Danish researchers found that 17 percent of men and 28 percent of women age 75 said they felt tired while doing merely the simple activities of daily living, like getting dressed.

Tiredness is often a biological syndrome related to low energy reserves, less muscle mass, and decreased resistance to stressors, whether environmental or physical. Other times, fatigue is a psychological reaction to social stressors. The antidote in simple cases of chronic tiredness—and this holds for the majority of cases for people young and old—is merely to push yourself to be active, with the goal of rebuilding muscle and resparking your joy and energy for

life. Exercise may make you tired afterward, but it's the best medicine of all for general fatigue and listlessness.

Other times, fatigue is a symptom of a deeper health issue, ranging from the simple, such as an infection, to the serious, such as cancer. Whether it's a symptom or the result of other issues, tiredness predicts future disability and sometimes even death. One study of 429 people found that those who felt tired doing regular daily activities at age 75 were three times more likely to become physically disabled over the next five years than those who didn't experience chronic tiredness.

If you feel chronically tired, take it seriously. Start with a full physical with your healthcare provider, then add one or more of the following strategies.

To Respark Lost Energy

Hit the gym. As we mentioned, loss of muscle strength appears again and again in studies examining the causes of tiredness or chronic fatigue. You must build your energy reserves to

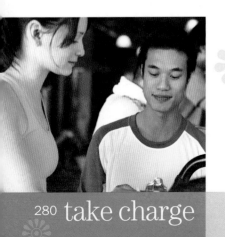

Being tired is not our normal state. If you find yourself out of energy come afternoons or early evenings, you need to remedy the situation.

remedy fatigue, and the best way to do that is by building your muscle strength. It's ideal if you can start with a personal trainer, even for just a couple of sessions, to create a personalized program designed to gradually increase your strength. If that's not possible, look for specialized classes for people who have recently been inactive or just have the gym manager show you the best machines and weights to use. Or turn to page 201 for an introductory strengthening routine.

Get out for a walk. Aerobic exercise is just as important as strength training in alleviating tiredness. Study after study has found that something as simple as a daily walk improves fatigue in cancer patients and people with chronic fatigue syndrome, lupus, and other serious medical conditions.

Turn to your faith. A study of 365 older people with heart disease found that those who used religion and prayer as a way to cope, as well as those who were optimistic and felt they had strong social support, were much less likely to report physical fatigue than those who weren't religious.

Take short naps. Just 10 to 20 minutes. These so-called power naps are indeed powerful at restoring energy levels. Following the nap, wash your face with cold water, then go outside in the sunlight or sit under a bright lamp while you drink a cup of regular tea. These postnap activities, alone or together, will give you more energy than the nap alone.

Swallow a B vitamin supplement. The older you get, the harder it is to absorb vitamin B_{12}, a key energy vitamin, from food. Talk to your doctor about taking a B-complex supplement (it's best to get your Bs together rather than in single supplements since they have a synergistic effect).

Get screened for depression. Feeling fatigued and tired regardless of how much you're sleeping is a primary symptom of depression. Ask your doctor to administer a depression screening test or just answer the following two questions, which studies find are as good as longer screenings at predicting depression.

1. Over the past two weeks, have you felt down, depressed, or hopeless?
2. Over the past two weeks, have you felt little interest or pleasure in doing things?

If you answer yes to these questions, see your doctor for a more complete examination.

Pull out your meds and take them to your doctor. Polypharmacy, or taking multiple medications, is a common cause of tiredness. Ask the doctor if this could be the reason you're so low on energy.

Ask for a blood test. Anemia, or low levels of oxygen-carrying red blood cells, is a major cause of fatigue in older people, occurring in about 11 percent of men and 10 percent of women over 65. A simple blood test can indicate if you're anemic, and a course of prescription-strength iron or other medications can improve anemia within a few weeks.

Go herbal with roseroot. Supplements of *Rhodiola rosea L*, also called Arctic root or roseroot, can improve fatigue. It's considered an adaptogenic herb, meaning it helps strengthen your body systems to better manage stress. The plant is used in traditional medicine to stimulate the nervous system and reduce depression, so it makes sense that it could help with tiredness. Doses of 200 to 600 milligrams a day of an extract standardized to contain 2 to 3 percent rosavins and 0.8 to 1.0 percent salidroside are typical, but check with your doctor first about

When fuel runs low

Fatigue has many causes, some complex. But sometimes we overlook the most obvious reason why we lack energy: We haven't properly fueled ourselves.

Often, lack of energy means nothing more than you are hungry or thirsty. In fact, it is often a better marker that you need something to eat than any sensation emanating from your belly!

With that in mind, here are some tweaks to your food choices and eating patterns that could go a long way towards remedying low energy and daytime fatigue.

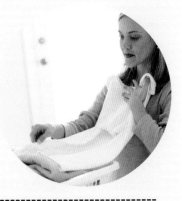

1. EAT OFTEN.

Eating small meals throughout the day, or three meals and two smart snacks, helps keep your blood sugar stable, which fends off fatigue. Try to eat something healthy every three hours; longer than that, and you risk a drop in blood sugar that will effect how you feel.

2. SKIP THE COFFEE...

The caffeine in coffee is a mostly safe and natural stimulant that increases your heart and breathing rate. But its effects wear off, leaving you either craving more or feeling tired again. Many experts now say to *avoid* caffeine if fatigue is an ongoing problem.

3. ...BUT NEVER SKIP BREAKFAST.

You wake up and do your morning routine, and by the time you arrive at the kitchen, 12 hours have passed since your last meal. Even if your stomach doesn't feel hungry, your body is. Eat a small breakfast every day. Studies show that people who eat breakfast concentrate and are more productive than those who don't.

4. KEEP DRINKING WATER.

Water is needed for the basic chemistry of energy in your body. Without enough in your diet, your body has to compensate for it in a way that can sap you of vitality. Drink a glass every two hours or so.

5. EAT SUFFICIENT PROTEIN.

The amino acids in proteins help increase levels of neurotransmitters in your bloodstream that play a major role in mood and alertness. A good rule of thumb is to be sure to have a serving of protein at every meal, including breakfast.

6. CONSUME FEWER SWEETS.

Refined sugar and corn syrup digest quickly and cause nearly instant blood-sugar surges—the well-known "sugar rush" we accuse overactive kids of having, followed by a crash in blood sugar that leaves people without energy. While grownups may not feel sugar-related surges like a child might, they often do suffer from the crash. So skip sodas, cake, cookies; opt for proteins instead.

any possible interactions with other medications you're taking.

Try Siberian ginseng. Another adaptogen, this herb significantly improved symptoms among 45 people with moderate fatigue as compared to a placebo group.

Choose the right antioxidant. One that seems to help people with unexplained chronic fatigue is coenzyme Q10. Certain medications can reduce levels of this important antioxidant in the body, particularly the widely prescribed cholesterol drugs called statins.

Try yoga. You're never too old to start it. This ancient stretching, strengthening, mind/body regimen offers something for everyone, regardless of physical condition. In one survey, 25 percent of people with unexplained fatigue who added yoga to their activities found it improved their fatigue throughout the two-year study period. Try the form called pranayama. It involves breathing techniques and stretching, and in one study, it significantly improved mental and physical energy in people with chronic fatigue.

Women, consider an iron supplement. The appropriate dosage is about just 8 milligrams a day. One study of 144 women who had chronic fatigue found that most had low iron levels, although not low enough to warrant an anemia diagnosis. After one month, levels of fatigue dropped by 29 percent in women taking iron compared to a 13 percent improvement in the placebo group.

Breathe deeply. As we said earlier, cumulative stress could be the culprit behind your fatigue. That's why relaxation breathing may help. In one study of patients who had had stem-cell transplants, those assigned to listen to a tape that instructed them in relaxation breathing for 30 minutes a day for six weeks reported significantly lower levels of fatigue than a group who didn't listen to the tape. It may test your patience at first, but give prolonged deep breathing a try. It's the next best thing to yoga or meditation and requires no training or skill. Merely sit in a comfortable chair, close your eyes, and slowly and fully inhale through your nose, then slowly exhale through your mouth. Keep doing it for 15 minutes. For variation, feel free to add a gentle stretch or move your ankles in circles while performing the deep breathing.

Many things can trigger fatigue. Some are physical, some mental. Be thoroughly honest with yourself when diagnosing the causes of your tiredness.

Joint and Muscle Pain

Twinges. Spasms. Stiffness. Aches. On any given day, the universe of adults who are coping with joint and muscle pain is huge. Half of those over age 65 report having ongoing knee, shoulder, and other joint-related pain. Many more report lower-back pain and some form of significant ongoing muscular discomfort. After coughs and colds, back pain is the most common complaint that sends older people to the doctor.

As the ranks of the aching increase, it may seem that the number of available remedies is shrinking. Several widely used prescription-strength pain pills have been pulled from pharmacy shelves due to the discovery of troubling potential side effects. Even more troubling is that the three most common pain stoppers—aspirin, ibuprofen, and acetaminophen—have all been subjects of serious warnings in recent years.

While nearly one in eight older people still take nonsteroidal anti-inflammatory drugs (NSAIDs)—such as aspirin, ibuprofen, and prescription celecoxib (Celebrex)—more and more research shows that these drugs can be dangerous. Taking aspirin or ibuprofen regularly can raise your risk of gastrointestinal bleeding and ulcers by two to nine times. These drugs can also raise blood pressure and increase your odds of a heart attack, and—perhaps most surprising of all—they may not be all that effective against most joint pain.

The good news: You don't ever have to live with pain. Smart strategies that combine safe ache easers and proven at-home care steps—from ice to heat to gentle exercise, or even getting a new wallet or purse—can cut the pain you're feeling now and lower the odds that it'll ever show up again.

On page 344, we'll tell you how to protect yourself from osteoarthritis and from the inflammation of rheumatoid arthritis and how to cope with damage that's already been done by these chronic conditions. Here, you'll get the lowdown on easing discomfort when otherwise healthy joints, muscles, and backs "act up."

To Relieve Aching Joints

Take acetaminophen first. Easy on your gastrointestinal system, acetaminophen tablets such as Tylenol are safe and effective for ongoing pain, according to a government review of hundreds of pain-relief studies. Your safe dose? Up to 4,000 milligrams per day—taken according to package directions. (One caution: Don't take acetaminophen with combination cold and flu remedies that contain it. An overdose could cause liver damage.)

Make a slow switch from aspirin, naproxen, or ibuprofen. In one study, people who gradually switched from these daily NSAIDs to acetaminophen over three months said they didn't feel any increase in pain during the transition.

Consider NSAIDs for short-term needs. These drugs aren't recommended for people who take a daily low-dose aspirin for heart protection, have stomach ulcers, or are at risk for heart problems. If you don't fit any of those categories, taking an NSAID for a few days, using the lowest dose that works for you, is usually safe and can help reduce the swelling and inflammation of arthritis.

Rub in capsaicin cream. The same compound that lends hot peppers their fiery heat can help manage pain. Store-bought creams such as Zostrix and Capzasin-P irritate nerve endings so much that your brain forgets about the joint pain. Some researchers think capsaicin also uses up a chemical inside nerve cells called substance P, which helps deliver pain signals to the brain. Use it for a week or two to get the most benefits.

Wet heat helps. A "thermographic" heating pad (the type that makes "wet" heat); a hot shower; or even hot, wet towels applied to an achy joint can loosen it up. Do easy stretching exercises as the pain subsides to restore a comfortable range of movement and ease stiffness.

For stronger pain, supplement with glucosamine and chondroitin. Capsules packed with glucosamine (a sugar extracted from shellfish) and chondroitin sulfate (a carbohydrate extracted from animal cartilage) cut joint pain by 20 percent or more in a landmark study of 1,583 women and men with arthritis. Nearly 80 percent of those with moderate to severe arthritis got some relief. Experts aren't sure how the two supplements work, but they know that both substances are found naturally in human cartilage.

Walk, don't run; swim, don't play basketball. Low-impact activities with smooth movements can keep joints flexible, functional, and pain-free. Sports and exercises like stretching, swimming, water aerobics, cycling, walking on a treadmill or outside, and playing golf fit the bill. Those that require quick, high-impact jumps, twists, and turns—such as tennis, basketball, racquetball, and baseball—don't.

Strengthen your support system. Strong muscles take stress off joints and relieve pain. In a 2002 study of people with joint pain, performing strengthening exercises three times a week for 16 weeks brought pain relief as powerful as that from prescription drugs. You don't need a gym membership or fancy weight machine at home; folks in this study used inexpensive elastic bands. Bonus: If you've tried a new, joint-lubricating procedure called viscosupplementation, be sure to exercise as well—the combo cut pain in half in one study.

Lose weight. Dropping just 11 pounds could cut your risk of developing arthritis in half and reduce pain at least that much. For every pound you lose, your knees are subjected to 4 pounds less pressure with every step you take, or about 4,800 pounds less every time you walk a mile.

Pop fish-oil capsules. Omega-3 fatty acids—the "good fats" found in fish such as salmon and in fish-oil capsules—helped people with arthritis ease pain and stiffness in more than 15 well-designed research studies. Volunteers were also able to cut back on prescription and over-the-counter painkillers. Fish oil may help with back pain, too. However, in some studies, the dosage was as high as 5,000 milligrams of omega-3s. That's a lot of daily pills, so talk to your doctor first, and never take fish-oil capsules without a medical consultation if you're taking blood thinners.

Give acupressure a try. This ancient Chinese healing art uses thumb and fingertip pressure to stimulate the flow of energy within the body. It works better than physical therapy at easing lower-back pain, according to a recent Taiwanese study of 129 women and men with chronic pain. For the study, 64 volunteers had six acupressure sessions, and 65 had physical therapy. When researchers checked up on them six months later, the acupressure group had 89 percent less pain and disability than the other group. They took fewer days off from work or school, too.

Zap it. Buzzing your body with low-level electricity while you sleep sounds like science fiction, but a new arthritis treatment does just that. In studies, the device—known in some countries as the BioniCare Bio-1000—cut knee pain and stiffness in half after four weeks of use. Among people with osteoarthritis whose doctors recommended total knee replacement surgery, 65 percent of those who used the device for four years were able to avoid the operation, compared to 7 percent of those who didn't use it, report Johns Hopkins University researchers. In animal studies, electrical pulses stimulated the growth of cartilage, the tough, spongy material that cushions joint bones. The device must be worn for 6 to 10 hours every day—usually while you sleep or relax—for best results. Talk to your doctor if you want to learn more.

To Relieve Muscle Pain

Take a walk—and swing your arms. Experts have a name for the general hurt you feel the day after you overexert yourself: delayed-onset muscle soreness, or DOMS. It turns out that if you were a little overzealous playing, working, exercising, or even gardening, the best remedy the day after is to get moving again. Staying active works the painful chemical by-products of overexertion out of your muscle tissue and keeps muscle fibers flexible so they can't tighten up and stay sore longer. Light exercise helps sore muscles heal so you'll have less pain next time.

Ice down painful strains and sprains. Keep a cold pack, a 1-pound package of frozen corn or peas, or several paper cups filled with a few inches of water in the freezer. If it's been less than 48 hours since your injury, rub the ice in a cup over the sore muscle or ice it down by wrapping the frozen veggies or cold pack in a clean kitchen towel and placing it over the area. Cold compresses reduce swelling and inflammation and relieve pain. Apply for 10 minutes, remove for 10 minutes, then apply for another 10; this strategy helps protect older, thinner skin from being damaged by the ice. But skip the process if you have blood-flow issues, diabetes, or Raynaud's syndrome or if you are highly sensitive to cold.

Stretch and prop. If all you have is mild soreness, we've already told you that movement and light exercise are the right remedies. But more severe pain is your body's signal to stop moving around or putting weight on an injured muscle. If you sense that your soreness crosses that line, stay off your feet or avoid using an injured arm for the first day or so. If you've injured a muscle in a hip or leg, keep it raised above groin level with pillows or folded blankets. This helps your body reabsorb fluid sent into the area and reduces swelling. Make sure an injured arm is supported, not hanging down, for the same reasons.

After two to three days, add homemade heat. Warmth relaxes tight, sore muscles and relieves pain. Fill an old knee sock or long tube sock three-quarters full of raw white rice, tie off the open end tightly with a rubber band, and microwave it for 2 minutes. Lay it over a sore spot or use it to gently massage a healing muscle that feels tight. This do-it-yourself hot pack is reusable and works for muscle cramps as well. Add cinnamon sticks and cloves or dried lavender buds for a spicy scent.

Stash stick-on heating pads in your medicine cabinet and glove compartment. Single-use heat wraps and patches that adhere to your skin or clothes at a sore spot are great for fast relief—and they come in shapes and sizes that fit particular high-ache areas perfectly. Inside are chemicals that warm up when the package is opened and they're exposed to air. The low-level heat is safe to use for up to eight hours, sometimes longer.

Or soak it. Sink into a warm tub, Jacuzzi, or whirlpool and add 15 drops of relaxing lavender essential oil or muscle-warming ginger essential oil to the water along with 1/2 cup of Epsom salts or Dead Sea salts. (This is great for muscle cramps, too.)

Treat yourself to a rubdown. Try this on a warm muscle a few days after an injury: Rub the length of the muscle, moving from the point farthest from your heart toward the point closest to your heart. Research shows that postexercise and postinjury massage can reduce pain and speed healing. It can reduce inflammation, too.

Listen to your body. Never push through pain or fatigue. The truth is, tired, stressed muscles are injury prone. Pay attention when your arms or legs feel fatigued or your back feels tight. These are signs that it's time to rest and relax. Pushing too hard could lead to cramps and pulled muscles.

Check your "D" supply. A vitamin D deficiency can cause muscle weakness, aches, pains, and even balance problems. Skin produces D in the presence of sunlight, but older skin makes less— and virtually everyone (of any age) living north of an imaginary line running between Baltimore and San Francisco can't get enough from sunshine, anyway—the rays are too weak. Older people need at least 600 to 800 IU of vitamin D per day, and some experts say 1,000 IU would be even smarter. You can't get that much every day from food, so add up the amount in your multi and take a supplement to cover any shortfall.

Muscle cramps? Fight 'em with this breakfast bowlful. Low levels of potassium, calcium, and magnesium—which act as message-carrying electrolytes in your body—can raise your odds of having sudden, painful muscle cramps. Get more of all three important minerals by spooning up some whole-grain cereal with milk and sliced banana at breakfast and by taking a multivitamin. And drink plenty of water throughout the day, since cramping can also be a sign of dehydration.

To Reduce Back Pain

Get up and move. Once, experts (as well as know-it-all relatives) said that bed rest was best for bad backs. Not anymore. Study after study shows that movement helps keep muscles supple and boosts circulation, bringing oxygen and nutrients to heal strained spots. Don't expect to play tennis tomorrow; do expect that after a brief rest, you'll rise and go about as much of your daily routine as possible, taking it as easy as you need to.

Pain is inevitable. Chronic, debilitating pain is not. No matter what your age, health, or situation, there are always solutions to treating ongoing pain.

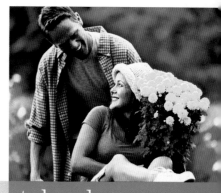

hot *or* cold?

Confused about when to use ice or heat on a muscle injury? Here's what you need to know.

Ice

When Within 48 hours of a sudden injury or the reinjury of a chronic problem spot.

How Ice cubes in a sealable bag, a bag of frozen peas or corn, or a freezer pack made for icing injuries. Wrap in a small towel to avoid damaging skin.

How long Up to 10 minutes at a time, but stop sooner if your skin turns pink. Typically, you can reapply about 10 minutes after the end of the previous icing session.

Key effects Curtails swelling and reduces pain.

Warning Don't use ice if you have circulation problems or easily damaged skin.

Heat

When More than 48 hours after a sudden injury or before starting an activity that may hurt a weak, frequently injured area. (Heat loosens up tight, injury-prone muscles.) Also good for arthritic joints.

How Use a heating pad set on low, a washcloth dipped in warm water, a single-use heat pack available at drugstores and designed for specific areas like your neck or lower back, or a reusable microwavable hot pack.

How long 20 minutes at a time.

Key effect Draws blood to the area for nourishment, healing, and muscle relaxation.

Warning If the heat causes pain, immediately remove it from your skin to prevent damage. The heat should feel comfortable and pleasant, not scalding.

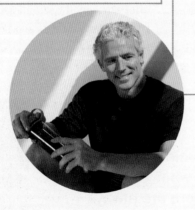

Then stretch and strengthen. Add stretching and gentle strengthening exercises, too. After a few weeks, start doing easy abdominal exercises like those in our three Long Life fitness routines (pages 198). These strengthen your core—the "inner corset" of muscles that steady your spine. (Go easy on back exercises, though. One study found that walking provided more relief.) Aim to exercise for a half hour five days a week—whether you walk, swim, or do aerobics or another activity you like.

Find time for relaxing stretches such as yoga. Many of us unconsciously hold years of tension in our upper and lower backs. There's some evidence that mental stress can cause physical stress that could push back muscles past the tipping point, leading to pain. If chronic stress is tensing you up, you need regular doses of healing stretches. Yoga is the perfect form, but regular, slow stretching will work fine, too. Better yet, don't let anger, frustration, and other strong emotions affect your physical well-being.

Walk while you talk on the phone. In one University of California, Los Angeles, study of 681 people with lower-back pain, those who walked briskly for three hours a week felt better physically and mentally, while those who performed regular back exercises had more pain. Movement of any kind improves the flow of oxygen and nutrients to muscles and redistributes the gel inside the shock-absorbing disks that cushion your vertebrae. In contrast, sitting allows the gel to squash to one side or the other, leaving you with uneven cushioning between the joints of your spine.

If you're sitting, take a stretch break every 20 minutes. Sitting still for hours deprives your back muscles of oxygen and nutrients, allowing the disks between your vertebrae to bulge if you're not using perfect posture. Over time,

muscles grow tight, and a bulging disk can press on nerves, causing pain.

Use a commonsense approach to pain relievers. The same advice we gave for using NSAIDs for joint pain holds true for back pain.

Lift smarter. Instead of using your back as a crane, bend your knees, pick up the object, and then stand up. And get help moving heavy objects—another person or two, or something like a cart, a two-wheeled hand truck, or a dolly or wheelbarrow will all work.

Reconsider the myth of the firm mattress. Spanish back-pain sufferers who slept on medium-firm mattresses for 90 nights cut their morning aches more than those who snoozed on firm beds. Beds with a bit of "give" seem to support and cushion stiffer muscles and joints better than harder, less yielding mattresses—especially for people with lower-back pain.

Uncross your legs. Love to cross your legs? There's a surprising reason why this sitting position feels so relaxing: Studies show it literally puts muscles in your back and abdomen into "sleep" mode, decreasing electrical activity, says physical therapist Evan Johnson, PT, DPT, an assistant professor of clinical physical therapy at Columbia University Medical Center. The problem: Muscles that should be supporting your back are now off-duty, leaving your spine literally "hanging" on various muscles and ligaments. Over time, this stretches some and tightens others, setting the stage for the day when the tiniest move—bending to tie your shoe or reaching for the breakfast cereal at the back of a shelf—will lead to painful back spasms.

Instead, plant both feet flat on the floor when sitting for a long time. Make sure your hips are slightly higher than your knees (you may need a wedge-shaped seat cushion to achieve this) to keep your abdominal and back muscles active and perfectly positioned to support a well-aligned spine.

Women, lighten your purses. Oversize handbags, often made with heavy quilted leather and decorated with equally weighty chain handles, are great for carrying everything under the sun—but experts find that they can weigh 7 to 10 pounds. At that weight, these over-the-shoulder suitcases throw off your back's finely balanced architecture. You hike up one shoulder, putting stress on your neck, upper back, and shoulders, which leads to not only upper-back pain but also a stiff neck.

A better fashion move: Invest in a small, lightweight handbag just large enough for a small wallet, cell phone, lipstick, tissues, and car keys (and while you're at it, pare down your key ring to the essentials). A backpack or messenger-style bag distributes the weight better than a traditional shoulder bag.

Men, lighten your wallets. In fact, consider swapping an overstuffed wallet for a money clip—and carry it in a front pocket. Sitting on a big wallet in your back pocket can irritate the sciatic nerve that runs from your lower back through your buttocks and down your leg. The result: a burning sensation that just won't quit. To remedy this, put your wallet on a diet—get rid of bank receipts, out-of-date insurance cards, and store discount cards (put 'em on your key ring). Switch from a thick leather wallet to one made of the new breed of thin, flexible fabric, or use a money clip. Cheapskate trick: Use a thick rubber band or a binder clip to hold your bills, driver's license, and credit cards together.

Switch from old-fashioned high heels to high-style flats. Walking in heels is like walking downhill all day—you have to lean back to avoid the feeling that you're falling forward, a move that compresses the disks in your lower back. When Pennsylvania State University engineers compared muscle tightness in five women wearing flats, medium-height heels, or stilettos, they discovered that the higher the heel, the more the women's lower-back muscles tightened up. Save your back by switching to shoes with heels that are less than an inch high. Look for a snug, firm heel counter—the part of the shoe that supports the sides and back of your heel. This gives you better foot control while walking and actually helps support your arch.

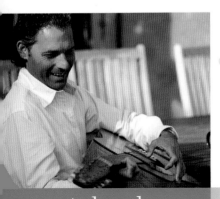

Sometimes, the remedy to back pain is as easy as adjusting how we sit, what we carry, or where we sleep.

Peripheral Artery Disease

Millions shrug off the problem as merely part of the aging process, but despite its name, there's nothing "peripheral" or unimportant about it.

Up to 30 percent of aging women and men develop the aches, pains, and risks of peripheral artery disease (PAD), a circulation problem that some dramatically describe as "angina of the legs"—clogged arteries that cause sharp pain when you move and even, in later stages, when you lie down to rest. Your legs and feet may grow cold, numb, or even discolored. You may develop sores that won't heal (due to reduced blood flow and a lack of oxygen and nutrients to mend the tissue and fight infection). The long-range risks: Once PAD becomes painful, your odds of having a fatal heart attack or stroke within 10 years rise to nearly 50 percent.

"If someone has PAD, there are two issues," says vascular surgeon James Stanley, MD, a director of the University of Michigan Cardiovascular Center: "What happens to your leg, and what happens to your life."

A slow, progressive disorder of blood vessels throughout the body, PAD is the most common form of peripheral vascular disease (PVD)—narrowing of arteries and veins that disrupts the natural function of blood vessels and even parts of the lymphatic system anywhere outside the heart (hence the name "peripheral"). Other health conditions that fall under the PVD umbrella include intermittent claudication (a special designation for PAD leg pain), deep-vein thrombosis, varicose veins, and chronic venous insufficiency.

Most often, PVD and PAD are heavily influenced by what you eat, how much you exercise, how well you guard your health, and whether you smoke. You no doubt know that all of these lifestyle factors can help keep arteries in your heart clear and help control blood pressure. But did you ever stop to wonder how healthy living—or its opposite—may affect the miles of blood vessels that supply every cell in your body with oxygen and nutrients?

Most of us don't—until the day when a stroll from the front door to the car makes our legs ache. It's an early warning signal for PAD, and one that should be heeded. "It's like gray hair—you don't just get it on one side of your head," says Dr. Stanley. "So if you've got this kind of blockage in your leg, you're going to have it other places."

Just one in four people with PAD know it—and tell their doctors. Half haven't experienced the most classic red alerts yet, such as a strange foot sore that won't heal or tight, aching fatigue in the muscles of the thigh, buttocks, or calves that's grown worse over the past couple of months or years. You may not be able to walk long distances—or even a few blocks. Many who've felt these funny aches never tell the doctor, and often, those who do don't get the urgent head-to-toe care they need to stop PVD in its tracks before it's too late.

You need more than pain relief if you have PVD. Fortunately, all the lifestyle steps that protect your heart can slow, stop, or even reverse this all-over artery clogging so you can walk where you want, when you want and cut your risk of heart attack and stroke. You may also need medication—but don't wait for your doctor to offer. In one shocking university study of 553 people with PVD, only those who'd had heart problems in the past got all the cholesterol- and blood pressure–lowering medications they needed—even though every person in the study was at high risk.

If you've had unexplained leg pain for at least a week, see your doctor. If you know you have PVD, PAD, or other related circulation problems—or would like to avoid them—the following steps can help.

To Beat Peripheral Artery Disease

Stop smoking. The best strategy for successful quitting? A combination of nicotine replacement products, a prescription antidepressant, and counseling. It's worth it. In one study, smokers with PAD who kicked the habit doubled or even tripled their pain-free walking distance. In another, 16 percent of smokers who didn't quit went on to develop severe PAD in just a few years, compared with none of those who quit. Ditching the cigarettes also lowers your risk of amputation (about 4 percent of people with PAD eventually require this grisly procedure) and cut your odds of having a heart attack or stroke.

Walk, walk, walk! We know it hurts. But this is one time when pushing yourself a little (but not too much!) does yield real benefits. That's because after quitting smoking, exercise is the most powerful move you can make to cut the pain and immobility PAD can cause—and to reverse the artery clogging that makes it worse.

Exercise works its magic by lowering levels of inflammation in the bloodstream, making artery walls more flexible, and improving the way muscles use oxygen. It may even trigger the growth of new blood vessels to deliver oxygen and nutrients to hungry muscles.

If you have access to a medical center that offers exercise programs for people with PAD, give it a whirl—you'll get personal attention and plenty of motivation. In one study, people in a supervised walking program nearly tripled their pain-free walking time!

Home exercise is just as effective if you stick with it, so why not find a walking buddy in your neighborhood and get started? In one Northwestern University study of 417 men and women with PAD leg pain, those who walked for at least 30 minutes three times a week saw no worsening of their symptoms, but those who didn't walk at all or walked for less than a total of 90 minutes per week did. Be patient; it may take six months or more to see dramatic benefits. And if you can walk longer than 30 minutes, do so. Some experts say that hour-long sessions ultimately provide more pain relief.

Make all your dairy foods fat-free. Fight clogged arteries by getting rid of the building material for gunky plaque: LDL cholesterol. The body uses saturated fats to build cholesterol particles, and we get most of the saturated fats in our diets from milk, cheese, ice cream, and yogurt. Promise, right now, that you'll buy only dairy products labeled "skim" or "fat-free." (Love margarine? Look for brands that contain neither saturated fats nor artery-blocking trans fats.)

Invest in sharp kitchen shears—and use them! It's far easier to trim away globs of fat clinging to pork chops, chicken breasts, and steaks with scissors than with a knife. Kitchen shears needn't be expensive; just be sure they're sharp so the job's fast and easy. Cutting fat off meat (and removing skin from poultry) will subtract another substantial source of saturated fat from your diet—a move your arteries will love.

Evening munchies? Snack on walnuts, not ice cream. Enjoying a small handful of these nutty nuggets every evening seems luxurious, but the good fats in these yummy morsels have a unique ability (rare among foods) to raise your HDL cholesterol. You could see a 2- to 3-point rise in HDL that will cut your risk of heart attacks and strokes by up to 18 percent.

Double up with two servings of veggies and one serving of cut fruit every day. Compounds found in fruits and veggies can help prevent the artery clogging that causes PAD and worsens it. How? Antioxidants shield particles of "bad" LDL cholesterol from oxidation by rogue oxygen molecules called free radicals. Oxidized LDL starts the chain of biochemical events that leads to the formation of gunky, blood vessel–narrowing plaque in artery walls.

Sip orange juice at breakfast and crunch a spinach salad at lunch. Nothing's easier than grabbing a carton of 100 percent orange juice and a bag of prewashed spinach leaves at the supermarket. Both are rich sources of folate, a B vitamin that helps lower high levels of heart-threatening homocysteine in people with PAD. And both supply vitamin C—an inflammation-fighting antioxidant that seems to be depleted swiftly in the bodies of people with more severe PAD, say researchers from University Hospital in Ghent, Belgium.

Try compression stockings for faulty vein valves. If you have varicose veins or a condition called chronic venous insufficiency, faulty valves in the veins in your legs allow blood to pool in your legs instead of being pushed back to your heart. One comfort solution: Prescription compression stockings. These elastic stockings squeeze veins and prevent excess blood from flowing backward and stretching out weakened blood vessels. Worn regularly, the specially made stockings can ease pain, prevent more swollen veins from developing, and even help sores heal.

Part of the elixir of long life is frequent, pleasurable walks.

5 Must-Ask Questions for Your Doctor

1 Should I take aspirin or an anti-clotting drug? Low-dose aspirin could cut some of your extra risk of heart disease and even stroke, and that's why the American College of Chest Physicians recommends a daily low-dose tablet for people with PAD. But aspirin raises your odds of developing a stomach ulcer or gastrointestinal bleeding. If you've had problems with these in the past, or if you already take other pain relievers every day (such as ibuprofen or a prescription nonsteroidal anti-inflammatory drug), consider an anti-clotting drug that doesn't pose gastrointestinal risks.

2 Can you help me lower my blood pressure? If your blood pressure remains above healthy levels despite several months of improved eating, exercise, and even weight loss, ask your doctor whether it's time to add blood pressure–lowering drugs to reduce your chances of a heart attack or stroke.

3 What else can I do to slash my "bad" LDL and boost my "good" HDL? Your new cholesterol target: Get your LDL below 100 mg/dl and keep your HDL above 50 mg/dl for women and 40 mg/dl for men. Each 1-point drop in LDL and each 1-point rise in HDL will cut your heart risk by 3 percent. If diet and exercise changes haven't rebalanced your blood fats enough, ask your doctor about LDL-lowering statin drugs and HDL-raising drugs such as prescription-strength niacin. In one study, people with PAD who took a statin not only cut heart risk, they also had less leg pain.

4 How are my triglycerides? Too-high levels of this blood fat also raise heart attack and stroke risk. Cutting out refined carbohydrates (a hallmark of the Long Life Eating approach) can bring them in line. But if your triglycerides still top 150 mg/dl (the recommended target for people with PAD), ask your doctor whether a statin or other drug could help.

5 How's my blood sugar? A scary fact: People with diabetes who have PAD are six times more likely to develop dangerous skin infections and twice as likely to have PAD-related leg pain even when they're resting. If you have diabetes, keeping your blood sugar at healthy levels around the clock can lower your odds for these big problems. If you don't, getting regular blood sugar checks (as often as your doctor recommends) can help you catch prediabetes early, in time to slow the development of full-blown diabetes by years—perhaps decades. (For more ways to control blood sugar, turn to Part 4.)

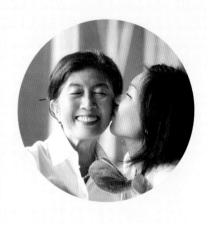

Skin Problems

Say the words *skin* and *age,* and you probably think about wrinkles. Listen up—forget about wrinkles. Normal, age-related wrinkles do you no harm. You are beautiful with them; don't let advertising, plastic surgeons, or shallow, vain neighbors convince you otherwise. Years of sun exposure, not discovering moisturizer until your thirties, and a persistent rosy flush on your face—*these* are the skin issues that adults over 40 should be most concerned with.

Consider this: When you're young, your top layer of skin typically turns over every 26 to 42 days. Beginning at around age 30, that turnover rate slows. By your eighties, your skin takes 50 percent longer to renew itself. "And that's a problem," says Wendy E. Roberts, MD, an assistant clinical professor of medicine at Loma Linda University Medical School in California. "Now you have this protective part of the epidermis just hanging around, and it's impaired in function."

That in turn leads to a whole host of skin-related problems, including dryness and a greater susceptibility to irritation. It also means that dead skin cells stay on the surface longer, giving your skin a dull appearance and rough texture. That dryness and flaking can also make your skin itchy, sometimes resulting in red, scaly patches of eczema. Plus, your oil glands produce less oil, also contributing to dryness.

Your skin also thins with age, with one study finding that women over 65 had lost about 20 percent of their skin thickness. This is why skin becomes more sensitive to creams and oils with age. Just a little permeates the skin more completely and may lead to the itchiness and rashes of contact dermatitis.

This time of life is also when the sunbathing of your youth returns to haunt you. Any time the sun hits your skin, it creates an inflammatory reaction that breaks down collagen—the binding material in your skin—as well as elastin fibers. That's why people who spent a lot of time in the sun when they were younger have that leathery look. It's also why they may find themselves visiting the dermatologist every few months to have skin cancers removed.

Aging also delivers two other skin challenges.

Shingles is a painful skin condition in which the nerves just under the skin become inflamed. It's caused by the chickenpox virus, which has lain dormant in your system all these years just waiting for your immune system to weaken. About 20 percent of people 60 and older who get shingles are left with a painful condition called postherpetic neuralgia.

Rosacea starts out looking like blushing or ordinary skin redness, but eventually, tiny pimples and very noticeable blood vessels may appear, particularly on your nose and cheeks. Again, blame that early sun damage, in part, for this condition. "The baby boomers were the first people to get out there in the sun," says Dr. Roberts. "They've sunned their whole lives, and this—rosacea and other skin problems—is what they're seeing."

While these last two conditions require medical treatment, usually in the form of laser therapy and/or prescription medications, there are certain lifestyle steps you can take either alone or as an add-on to your doctor's care.

To Manage Dry, Itchy Skin

Skip the soap. If your skin is showing signs of aging, then your days of using soap are probably over—most soaps are simply too drying for older skin. You may be able to get away with a milder soap, says Joel Schlessinger, MD, president of the American Society of Cosmetic Dermatology and Aesthetic Surgery, but many popular bar soaps are too strong for older skin. Instead, choose a moisturizing body wash for showering and a moisturizing cleanser for face-washing at the sink.

Slather on the moisturizer. Forget fancy ingredients and $60-an-ounce treatments; just look for a drugstore moisturizer especially formulated for dry skin, says Dr. Roberts. She directs her patients to petroleum-based cream products. Try one that includes SPF 15 sunscreen so you can attack two problems with one emollient. Moisturize at least twice a day—when you first step out of the shower, before your skin is completely dry (the moisturizer will form a film over your skin, locking in liquid), and again before you go to bed after cleansing your face with a moisturizing cleanser.

Hydrate the air. It makes sense that dry air is bad for dry skin, and the air in your home is driest in the winter. So moisturize the air and your skin with a humidifier. You can have a humidifier installed as part of your heating system or use portable humidifiers. Another way to put more moisture into the air in winter is to hang just-washed clothes to dry in the house. A final spin in the dryer helps remove any stiffness and wrinkles.

Stick to nonsmoking bars and restaurants. Secondhand smoke harms your skin nearly as much as smoking cigarettes yourself. Luckily, it's getting easier to avoid as more cities and even countries ban indoor smoking.

Exfoliate at least weekly. Exfoliation is the process of removing dead cells from the skin's surface and revealing "younger," fresher skin below. It helps get rid of that dull look aging can bring, shrink the appearance of large pores, and remove any flakiness from dry skin. Typically, you use a liquid exfoliant to do the job. But if these are too harsh for your skin, try a cleanser with 10 percent alpha-hydroxy acids (AHA), naturally occurring acids that act as exfoliators. If you use products with AHAs, look for over-the-counter brands with glycolic acid, which seems to penetrate the skin best.

Wear gloves. Not for warmth, but for skin protection. Use rubber gloves for washing dishes, doing housework, and handling household cleaners. Even better, switch to gentler, "green" cleaners that aren't made with harsh chemicals, or use natural ingredients like vinegar for cleaning. But still wear the gloves!

Take your vitamins. At 400 IU or more (check with your doctor regarding dosage), vitamin E can help reduce inflammation and soothe itching. One study of 96 people found significant improvement or complete remission of atopic dermatitis in 62 percent of those taking the vitamin. Dr. Roberts also recommends that her patients take 500 milligrams of vitamin C daily. Both E and C are powerful antioxidants that can protect the skin from further oxidative damage.

Take a warm bath. Add 10 drops of chamomile oil to bathwater, then soak for 10 minutes. Other bath additions to help itchy skin include oatmeal and geranium, hyssop, peppermint, and myrrh essential oils (use 10 drops of one type). Don't forget to slather on the moisturizer afterward, and make sure the water is warm, not hot. Hot water tends to dry out skin.

Swallow some evening primrose. Several studies find taking this omega-3 fatty acid significantly reduces itching and rash related to dry skin, most likely by increasing levels of anti-inflammatory chemicals in the blood. Take four 500-milligram capsules twice a day until your condition improves.

To Manage Rosacea

Cool off flare-ups. When the redness of rosacea appears, combine several drops of soothing herbal oils like rose, lavender, and chamomile in a basin of cool water. Soak a washcloth in the liquid and lay it over your face for 10 minutes. Repeat as necessary. These herbs are often used to reduce skin irritation.

Breathe deeply. Stress is a common trigger for rosacea, so practicing stress-reducing deep breathing can help avoid flare-ups. Learn to breathe from your stomach, so that each breath in is deep enough to expand your abdomen, while each breath out lowers it. When you start to feel the blood rising in your face, practice this form of breathing for three minutes, ideally with your eyes closed.

Swallow some fish oil. Fish-oil supplements are rich in anti-inflammatory omega-3 fatty acids. Since rosacea is related to inflammation, these inflammation dampers can help reduce flare-ups. Take 1,500 milligrams or less twice a day. You can also try 500 milligrams of evening primrose oil three times a day.

Use green-tinted makeup. The green helps cover the red. This won't get rid of your rosacea, but it will keep people from asking if you've gotten too much sun lately.

Skip the alcohol. Take this test: After a glass of wine or gin and tonic, look at your face in the mirror. Is it as pink as a glass of rosé? Alcohol dilates blood vessels, and since facial blood vessels are so close to the skin, you get the telltale flush of rosacea.

Watch your diet. Spicy foods, hot liquids, and even aged cheeses can trigger a rosacea flare-up.

Try hypnosis. Several studies reported in medical journals found that hypnosis can help patients learn to control the flushing of rosacea.

Test for *Helicobacter pylori.* This bacterium is the primary cause of stomach ulcers. However, a growing body of evidence suggests it may also be linked to rosacea. In one study of 44 patients with rosacea and *H. pylori* infection, completely eradicating the bacteria in 29 of them led to complete or significant improvement in rosacea for 19 patients, or 65 percent.

Talk to your doctor about intense pulse light (IPL). Just two or three sessions of this therapy

When it comes to skin, don't confuse beauty with health. Focus on caring for your skin from both the inside and outside.

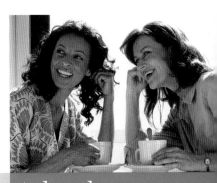

can make a huge difference in your rosacea, says Dr. Roberts. A full treatment should cost between $300 and $600 and may be covered by insurance.

To Manage Shingles

Start an antiviral. At the first sign of shingles, get a prescription for an antiviral medication like acyclovir (Zovirax), which was approved for the treatment of herpes viral infections almost two decades ago. Studies find that taking this or other antiviral medicines early can prevent the lingering pain that often occurs after a shingles outbreak.

Spread on hot pepper. It may sound counterintuitive, but capsaicin, the ingredient that gives peppers their fiery taste, works wonders at reducing nerve irritation and pain. You can find capsaicin creams and ointments (0.025% or 0.075%) in drugstores. The compound works by depleting a chemical called substance P from the nerves in the skin, short-circuiting the transmission of pain signals from the nerves to the brain. Apply it several times a day and wash your hands after each application.

Ice yourself down. When the pain is bad, apply an ice pack wrapped in a small towel to the affected area for 10 minutes, take it off for 10 minutes, and then reapply for another 10.

Take an antihistamine. Some people have terrible itching with shingles. If you experience itching, try an over-the-counter antihistamine like oral diphenhydramine (Benadryl). Cool baths can also help.

Wrap yourself in plastic. Putting on clothes over the blisters of shingles can be incredibly painful. Try covering the area with plastic wrap so your clothes slide over the affected skin.

Get vaccinated. A shingles vaccine was approved in the United States in 2006. In clinical studies, it prevented shingles in half of those over 60 on whom it was tested and reduced pain in those who developed the disease. It is *not* recommended for people with weakened immune systems; those taking drugs like steroids that affect the immune system or receiving cancer treatment such as radiation or chemotherapy; or those with a history of cancer affecting the bone marrow or lymphatic system, such as leukemia or lymphoma.

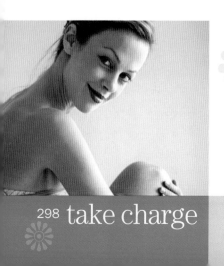

Yes, there are diseases of the skin. Yes, they can be managed. No, they need not affect your life or appearance.

Sleep Problems

Insomnia—annoying, exhausting, and mysterious—becomes a sadly common experience as we age. Sleep patterns change radically after age 55, when your body clock resets itself and levels of important sleep hormones drop. Diseases, medications, everyday habits, and even your evening bedtime routine play important roles as well.

The good news: While you can't reverse natural and inevitable sleep changes, you don't have to settle for wide-awake nights or dog-tired days.

"I'm convinced that sleep doesn't have to be a problem for older people," says Michael V. Vitiello, PhD, a professor and senior scientist in the Sleep Research Group at the University of Washington in Seattle. "In my studies of healthy, active women and men in their seventies and eighties, I've found that while their sleeping patterns change, they still find ways to get enough rest so that they can lead the lives they want to lead. Yes, they do need more time to fall asleep than when they were younger. They wake up more often and for longer periods of time at night. And they may wake much earlier in the morning. But they've found ways to get enough sleep to feel refreshed."

Their secrets to overcoming—or sidestepping—the extra insomnia risks that come with the passing years? Everything from exercising in sunlight and saying no to an after-dinner cocktail to working with their doctors to minimize the effects of health issues and medications on their sleep schedules. "If you're feeling tired during the day and can't do the things you'd like to do or need to do, it's time to do something about your sleep," Dr. Vitiello says. "Getting older doesn't have to mean living with insomnia and exhaustion. There's plenty you can do about it."

Your first step? Understanding and accommodating the way your body and mind sleep now. "The truth is, sleep changes don't happen suddenly. They start gradually in your thirties, but you may not notice them until you're older or retired or until other factors get in the way," Dr. Vitiello says.

To Adjust to Sleep-Pattern Changes

Accept them. It's crucial to understand that the timing and quality of your sleep does change over time. Just as you will never have the body shape and weight of 30 years earlier, you will not have the sleep patterns you once had. Be sensitive to the changes. Are you tired earlier or more sensitive to morning light? Monitoring changes and adjusting to them is half the battle.

Tired at 8 p.m.? Turn in. Lower levels of melatonin, the hormone that helps control your sleeping and waking cycles, are one reason you may feel sleepier early in the evening than you used to. Just accept the change and go to bed earlier. "Your need for seven to eight hours of sleep per night hasn't changed," Dr. Vitiello notes. "Don't miss a chance to get it."

Can't drop off to sleep in an instant? Be patient—you'll get there. Taking longer to fall asleep is a natural part of aging. "Older people may need 20 minutes or more to fall asleep, while younger people may only need 5 to 10 minutes," he notes. (Read on for ways to feel sleepier at bedtime and to tell your brain it's time to doze.)

Waking up three or four times a night is normal now. Once asleep, older people go through the cycles of sleep more quickly than younger people—and wake up between cycles more frequently. Researchers suspect that lower levels of growth hormone in your system may help explain why you spend less time in the deepest, most restorative sleep stage, called Stage Four by researchers.

Wide awake at 5 a.m.? Get up! Your body clock may have shifted to an early-to-bed, early-to-rise schedule. Turning in earlier will help ensure that early wakeups aren't a rude awakening.

Consider daytime naps. Napping is a controversial solution for people struggling with insomnia. "Two studies in older people show that a short daytime nap doesn't have much impact on nighttime sleep," Dr. Vitiello says. But if you find that a 30- to 45-minute afternoon nap keeps you awake too long at night, it may not be right for you. "You may have to decide which matters most—using the nap to feel more awake and functional all day or trying to get all your sleep in one stretch at night," he says. "Whichever you choose, what matters is regularity—if you're going to nap, do it at about the same time every day to train your body and mind."

To Improve Your Nightly Sleep

Reserve your bed for sex and sleep. "Don't watch TV in bed and don't pay bills in bed," Dr. Vitiello says. "You don't want to start linking your bed with activities that keep you awake or that cause worry."

Create a clutter-free sanctuary. Your brain deserves the balm of a soothing, organized, pleasant environment, free of worrisome reminders like baskets of laundry that needs to be folded, stacks of magazines to be sorted, or bills to be paid. Consider painting the walls a soothing color, too. How about sage green or a luminous, pale purple-blue?

Block the light. Moonlight, street lights, late sunsets, and early dawns can all interfere with the circadian rhythm changes you need to fall asleep. "Here in Seattle, daylight comes at 4 a.m. in the summer and stays till 10 p.m., so I need heavy shades or curtains to keep my bedroom dark enough for good sleep," notes Dr. Vitiello.

Nestle on a new pillow. If yours is more than six months old, or if you wake up in the morning with a sore neck and shoulders or a stuffy nose, it may be time for new head support. What's best? It depends on you, but here are some pointers.

• Neck pain? Go for a thinner pillow or look for a special "neck pillow." In one Swedish study, a neck pillow—rectangular with a depression in the middle—enhanced sleep. The ideal neck pillow is soft and not too thick.

• Always turning your pillow over to find the cooler side? Invest in natural cool. Natural fibers—and natural-fiber pillowcases—stay cooler. In studies, "cool pillows"—some were water-filled, and others used a mix of sodium sulfate and ceramic fibers—enhanced sleep.

• Stuffy or allergy-prone? Go hypoallergenic—and invest in an allergen-reducing pillow cover, too.

Move your bed. Outside walls and windows in your bedroom mean more noise. Locating your sleeping spot along an inside wall could improve things, a Spanish study suggests.

Turn your digital clock to the wall. "One of my biggest pet peeves is the invention of the digital clock with a big, luminous display, because it can make you think you've got a sleep problem when you don't," Dr. Vitiello says. How? You may wake for a moment at 2 a.m., drift back to sleep, then wake again at 2:30—and think you've been awake the whole time. "It's annoying and leads to anxiety and arousal," he says. "Just turn the clock around. The alarm will still wake you up in the morning."

Keep bedroom reading to a minimum. A few minutes of relaxing reading is a perfectly fine presleep ritual. But if you get in the habit of reading in bed for a long time, or if the only time you read is at night in bed, that's a problem. You should do any prolonged reading in a chair in another room during waking hours.

Splurge on new pajamas. Yes, your old nightgown or boxers are still in good condition, but if they're not completely comfy, you deserve better. Invest in 100 percent cotton pajamas for cool comfort or cozy flannels for cold winter nights.

And slip on some toe-toasting socks. Got cold feet? Wear warm socks to bed. Researchers at the Psychiatric University Clinic in Basel,

Sick and tired

Without question, bad health affects how you sleep.

When the National Sleep Foundation asked older people to rate the quality of their slumber, they found that those with four or more medical conditions were five times more likely to be sleepy during the day and four times more likely to say they slept poorly than people with no major health concerns. "If you can't sleep and you have health conditions, your doctor should treat both problems at the same time for best results," says Sonia Ancoli-Israel, PhD, director of the sleep disorders clinic at the Veterans Affairs San Diego Healthcare System. Here are examples of health conditions known to affect sleep.

Pain. A bad back, an arthritic knee, a pulled shoulder muscle, heartburn—any type of ongoing pain has the power to keep you awake or pull you out of a deep sleep. Talk with your doctor about pain treatments that can ensure you get a proper night's rest. Also review your prescriptions with your doc—codeine, demerol, morphine, and steroids can disturb your sleep, as can migraine relievers that contain caffeine.

Allergies. People with allergic rhinitis—the most common form of allergies resulting from ubiquitous dust, pollen, and animal dander—are much more likely to experience insomnia, wake up during the night, snore, and feel fatigued when they do wake up. The French researchers who discovered this also found that those with allergic rhinitis are more likely to sleep fewer hours, take longer to fall asleep, and feel sleepy during the day than those without the condition.

Gastroesophageal reflux disease (GERD). Pennsylvania State University researchers found a significant relationship between GERD, a particularly severe form of heartburn, and daytime sleepiness, insomnia, and poor sleep quality.

How to Fix a Snorer

Bedding down with a chronic snorer is bad for your sleep and worse for your hearing. Loud snorers can generate 80 decibels of noise, as loud as rush-hour traffic, report researchers from Queen's University in Kingston, Ontario—and their bed partners suffered hearing loss as a result. If you can't or won't sleep in separate rooms, try these remedies.

- Store-bought rubber earplugs can screen out about 32 decibels, which is often enough to let you fall asleep.

- An audiologist can make you custom-fitted ear protectors that filter more noise. They're expensive but worth it.

- A white noise machine, which creates a steady, soothing layer of sound, can help mask the snoring.

- Present your partner with a box of anti-snoring strips, which work by pulling the nostrils open wider. A Swedish study found they significantly reduced snoring.

- If all else fails, ask your mate to make an appointment at a sleep center. He or she may be a candidate for a test called polysomnography, which detects sleep apnea.

Switzerland, found that when blood vessels in the feet dilate late in the evening, the body can effectively cool down and get ready for sleep. Putting on socks can help make the blood vessels widen and radiate heat.

Scent your sheets with lavender. Place a single drop of lavender essential oil on your pillow or spray your sheets with lavender water before you turn in. Studies at the University of Leicester in England and the Smell and Taste Research Center in Chicago found that this soothing botanical works as well as sleeping pills for quelling insomnia and tension.

Or infuse your bedroom with jasmine. Other studies suggest that a faint jasmine aroma may work better than lavender for helping you drift into peaceful sleep and stay more alert the following day. Try a scented oil stick or place a few drops of jasmine essential oil in a cup of hot water by your bed.

Interview your partner. Ask whether you stop breathing, jiggle your legs, or wiggle your body while you sleep. Millions of people have obstructive sleep apnea, which causes brief interruptions in breathing all through the night and which over time can raise your odds of developing high blood pressure and heart disease. Wiggly legs or thrashing in your sleep could also be signs of restless legs syndrome or another movement disorder. "If there's clear evidence of a medical problem, it's smart to cut to the chase and ask your doctor for a referral to a sleep clinic," Dr. Vitiello suggests. "An evaluation and treatment could make all the difference and improve not just your sleep but also your health."

Kick Fluffy and Fido out of your oasis. A 2002 study found that one in five pet owners sleep with their pets—or more accurately, *don't* sleep, because their pets are on the bed or in the room. It could be that sneeze-provoking kitty dander, those midnight potty runs to the backyard, or the patter of little Labradoodle feet, but the study found something more incriminating: 21 percent of the dogs and 7 percent of the cats snored!

To Live a Sleep-Friendly Lifestyle

Take a walk after lunch, then read the paper on the patio. Exercise cuts stress, and getting exercise in the sun can help keep your body's circadian rhythms calibrated. You need about two hours of daily exposure to bright sunlight to help your body stay in sync. If you can't get outdoors, consider buying a light box—a fixture that radiates light that mimics the brightness and wavelengths of natural sunlight.

Or try tai chi on the lawn. In China, people rise at dawn to perform this series of ancient, gentle, dancelike movements in local parks. The sleep bonus: Tai chi beat a low-impact exercise class for improving sleep in a study of 118 women and men ages 60 to 92 conducted at the Oregon Research Institute. People who did tai chi three times a week for six months fell asleep 18 minutes faster and slept 48 minutes longer each night than other exercisers.

Schedule worry time during the day, in the kitchen! We're not kidding. If your mind is accustomed to revving up sleep-robbing anxiety in bed, retrain your brain by moving your worry session to another place and time. Try midmorning at the kitchen table—pour a mug of chamomile tea (a natural soother) with honey, grab a notebook and pen, and write out your worries, Dr. Vitiello suggests. This will clear your mind and break the association between bed, night, and worry. "If thoughts keep popping up, keep a notebook by your bed and write them down so you can think about them during the day," he says.

Make herbal tea or water your drink of choice after lunchtime. Nix coffee as well as other caffeine sources like chocolate; colas and other soft drinks; and black, green, or white tea. Even small amounts of caffeine may keep you up late, and older people may be more sensitive to it. Caffeine blocks a brain chemical called adenosine that helps us feel drowsy and fall asleep, and the effect may last longer in older people, whose livers don't filter caffeine as effectively. Instead, sip some chamomile tea, which contains ingredients proven to calm the nervous system and, at bedtime, can induce sleep.

Instead of an evening cocktail, have a glass of wine with an early supper. Drinking before bed

The quality of your sleep is closely related to the quality of your waking hours. Live happily and actively, and sleep will come more easily.

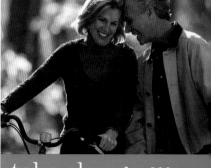

Sleep in a Pill

Sleep aids are among the most prescribed medications today, and for good reason—they are a good short-term option for insomnia, particularly if it's linked to issues like stress or anxiety. But remember—your primary remedies for chronic bad sleep are lifestyle changes and fixing the underlying causes. Vow to never rely on pills alone to solve your sleep problems!

If your doctor does recommend medication, it should be the lowest effective dose, prescribed to be taken two to four times a week for no longer than four weeks. When it's time to stop taking the medication, work with your doctor to gradually reduce the dosage so you don't have a "rebound" bout of insomnia. Finally, ask your doctor whether the pill he recommends will make you drowsy the next day; several do.

The story isn't as positive with nonprescription sleep drugs. Most over-the-counter sleep remedies contain the active ingredient diphenhydramine, an antihistamine that makes you drowsy. Not only can it cause daytime drowsiness, especially in the morning, it can also make urination difficult and even cause confusion or delirium, especially in people over age 65. "Older people shouldn't take these drugs at all. The side effects can be very worrisome," notes Sonia Ancoli-Israel, PhD, director of the Sleep Disorders Clinic at the Veterans Affairs San Diego Healthcare System.

If you think you need sleeping pills, it's a sign you should see your doctor about your sleep problems. But don't be surprised if the prescription isn't for a pill but rather for cognitive behavioral therapy, a mind-over-body approach to the problem that's been proven to work better than prescription sleep drugs in older people.

may help you fall asleep, but as the alcohol wears off, you're likely to have light, easily broken sleep. If you enjoy a drink, have one with supper a few hours before bed.

Drink more water during the day and less in the evening. If you have diabetes, an enlarged prostate, incontinence, or even garden-variety "tiny bladder syndrome" (the bladder shrinks with age), you may get up frequently to urinate, then have trouble falling back to sleep. Try drinking more water during the day so you don't feel thirsty in the hour or so before you turn in. That way, you may ensure fewer slumber interruptions without risking dehydration.

To Soothe Yourself Before Bed

Soften the mood. An hour before bedtime, switch on the answering machine, turn off the television or computer, pull on your softest PJs, and cue up your favorite relaxing sounds. In one recent University of Nevada, Reno, study of 52 women over age 70, those who listened to quiet music fell asleep faster and had fewer middle-of-the night awakenings than before they started scheduling listening time. The best music? Whatever soothes you, whether it's Frank Sinatra, the Bee Gees, mellow jazz, or classical Debussy.

Try progressive relaxation. Sit in a comfortable chair with both feet on the floor or lie on the sofa or your bed. Inhale and exhale naturally. After a few minutes, systematically tighten a muscle group as you inhale, then relax it completely as you exhale. Progressively loosen and tighten both feet, your lower legs, and upper legs, then work your way up to your back, arms, neck, shoulders, and even your face.

Then continue to breathe naturally, feeling any remaining tension ebb away. Ahh!

Next, combine progressive relaxation with music. When 60 women and men with sleep problems listened to soft, slow music while they performed a relaxation exercise, their heart-beats and breathing rates slowed—and they slept better and longer. "Music is pleasant and safe," notes researcher Marion Good, a professor at Frances Payne Bolton School of Nursing at Case Western Reserve University in Ohio. "It's easy to use and does not cause side effects."

Soak in a hot bath. Immersing yourself in warm water an hour or two before bed helps blood vessels dilate so your body can release heat—part of the natural cooling down that precedes sleep.

Take a supplement with 500 milligrams of calcium and 300 milligrams of magnesium. Magnesium is a natural sedative—even a slight shortfall can leave you lying in bed with your eyes wide open—while calcium helps regulate muscle movements. Getting plenty of both minerals can cut your risk of nighttime leg cramps. Take a supplement right before bed.

Enjoy a sleepytime snack. Have a handful of walnuts, a banana, or a glass of milk—all rich sources of the sleep-inducing amino acid tryptophan. (Bananas also pack melatonin, the sleep hormone.) If incontinence or frequent bathroom visits aren't a problem, have a glass of water—but not juice. In one study, people who drank juice just before bed became extra-alert due to the high sugar content of their drinks and needed an extra 20 to 30 minutes to fall asleep.

Take antacids right after dinner, not before bed. Antacids contain aluminum, which appears to interfere with sleep.

Make your presleep rituals soothing and joyful.

Urinary Problems

Sometimes you just gotta go. And it seems that the older you get, the more often this happens—with or without your conscious control. We're talking about something most people are loath to discuss, even with their doctors: urinary incontinence.

As many as 30 percent of people over 65 have one or more of the three forms of urinary incontinence. Although women are far more likely than men to experience incontinence, by age 80, the gender disparity disappears. Urinary incontinence is not just an embarrassment; it can affect your entire quality of life, leading you to cut out activities and friends you love and even changing the way you feel about yourself.

But here's the thing: Leaking urine and sudden strong urges to urinate are not conditions you have to live with simply because you're getting older. There are excellent medical and lifestyle treatments for incontinence. The first step, however, is admitting you have a problem and contacting your healthcare professional.

Together, the two of you need to figure out what type of incontinence you have. There are three main types—urge, stress, and overflow—although you can have more than one at a time, in which case it's called mixed incontinence.

Stress incontinence. With this form of incontinence, you involuntarily leak urine when you laugh, run, sneeze, cough, or otherwise exert yourself. This is by far the most common form in women because of its relation to childbirth. If the pelvic floor muscles (which hold everything in your reproductive area in place) become weak, stretched, or otherwise damaged during pregnancy or labor, stress incontinence often occurs. But men aren't off the hook! Stress incontinence is often their cross to bear after prostate surgery.

Overflow incontinence. This is the second most common form in men. It occurs when something blocks the urethra, the tube leading from the bladder to the outside of the body. In men, the blockage is most often caused by an enlarged prostate, medically known as benign prostatic hyperplasia (BPH). With BPH, your prostate pinches the urethra closed like a clothespin pinches a garden hose. Pressure builds until urine finally leaks out without your voluntary assistance. Don't be embarrassed about BPH: It's the most common health problem in men 60 and older.

Urge incontinence. In this form of incontinence, the urge to go strikes as suddenly as a summer storm—and often with similar flooding. Urge incontinence can occur if you have a central nervous system condition like Alzheimer's or Parkinson's disease or have had a stroke. It may also be related to increased sensitivity of your bladder muscles to a brain chemical called acetylcholine, which stimulates the bladder into action.

Treatments include medication, surgery, or behavioral therapies like exercises and bladder retraining. Lifestyle and behavior changes are more effective overall than the medical options, but they may take longer to work and require more effort on your part, and they may not provide a complete "cure." Here's how to get started.

To Reduce Incontinence

Go into training. One of the best treatments for urge or stress incontinence is performing pelvic floor muscle exercises called Kegels. The beauty of these exercises is that they can be done anywhere, nearly anytime, and you never have to break a sweat. Start by pulling in or squeezing your pelvic muscles as if you were trying to stop the flow of urine or keep from passing gas. Count to 10 as you hold the contraction, relax, and repeat. That's it! Try to perform at least three sets of 10 contractions a day. Start out lying down, then once you're good at them, perform your Kegels while standing in line, driving, sitting in church—you get the idea. In one study comparing Kegels with medication, participants who did Kegels saw their epsiodes of incontinence drop by 81 percent, compared to a 69 percent drop in patients taking prescription medication. The combination of medication plus Kegels, however, works best for urge incontinence.

Check your meds. Certain medications can induce incontinence, including many diuretics, asthma drugs, alpha blockers, narcotic pain relievers, anticholinergics, calcium channel blockers, and ACE inhibitors. If you aren't sure which types of medicines you take, ask your doctor for help.

Women, consider estrogen. Sometimes incontinence in middle-aged or older women is related to low levels of estrogen. This hormone plays a role in the strength and overall health of the muscles that control the bladder as well as the bladder and urethra themselves. Talk to your healthcare professional about using vaginal estrogen. Because the estrogen is inserted into the vagina via a cream or tablet, very little gets into your bloodstream, but enough gets to the urinary tract to help reduce incontinence. One study found that 58 percent of women receiving topical estrogen to the vaginal area three times a week had significantly fewer episodes of urge incontinence than a placebo group.

What the Doctor Will Say

If you want a doctor to solve your urinary incontinence problems, you're facing either prescription drugs or surgery, depending on the type of incontinence you have.

Urge incontinence. Several prescription drugs can prevent the bladder from contracting, keeping urine where it belongs until you deliberately choose to release it. Studies find that these medications can reduce the number of incontinence episodes by up to 70 percent, curing the condition altogether in about 20 percent of people.

Stress incontinence. In women, surgery to tighten and strengthen the pelvic floor muscles, followed by pelvic floor muscle exercises, can reduce incontinence episodes by between 88 and 94 percent. In men, however, surgical treatments may be less successful, with studies finding an improvement range of between 36 and 95 percent. A major study comparing a minimally invasive form of surgery (in which a sling is used to hold up the urethra) to the more traditional procedure (in which the urethra and bladder are stitched to the pelvic wall) found the sling was much more effective in relieving stress incontinence.

Overflow incontinence. The only real treatment for overflow incontinence is to treat whatever is blocking the urethra. In men, this usually means medication for an enlarged prostate.

Also check out these options. If pelvic exercises aren't doing it for you, you may want to consider a prosthetic device to help prevent incontinence. There are several, including an adhesive foam patch you put over the urethral opening, a balloonlike catheter device you insert into the urethra, a silicon device that sticks to the top of the urethral opening like a

When Embarrassment Calls

I have stress incontinence but I'm embarrassed to tell my doctor about it. How can I get the medical treatment I need if I can't even discuss it in a face-to-face examination?

Join the crowd. More than half of all women with stress incontinence don't share their symptoms with their doctor, and by the time they're diagnosed, most have suffered with this condition for at least four years, studies show. Often, they don't bring it up because they don't think anything can be done, assuming it's a normal part of aging. But incontinence is *not* a normal part of aging and there are numerous treatments available to improve it. Instead of starting from scratch during an office visit, write your doctor an e-mail or letter outlining your concerns and your symptoms. Include a schedule of all your bathroom usage and incontinence issues over a few days' time. Then make your appointment. When you turn up, your doctor can ask you any questions not answered in your letter, and then the two of you can discuss treatment options.

suction cup, and vaginal devices designed to support the neck of the bladder.

Get on a schedule. With this approach, you work out a urination schedule with your doctor. Initially, you urinate every hour or two whether you need to go or not, then gradually reduce the frequency to train your bladder to hold urine. This approach is best for urge incontinence, with studies finding it more effective than the major medication prescribed for the condition.

Take a seat. A special chair called an extracorporeal magnetic innervation chair has been approved by the US government for the treatment of stress incontinence. When you sit in the chair, a low-intensity magnetic field strengthens your pelvic floor muscles.

Get mildly shocked. Your doctor can prescribe electrical stimulation, in which an electric current is applied directly to the pelvic floor, causing the muscles to contract and strengthening them.

Get lightly stuck. Acupuncture appears to be a safe, effective treatment for urge incontinence, reducing symptoms in four to six weeks of treatment. However, the relief is likely to be short term, and you may need additional follow-up treatments.

Lose a few pounds. If you're overweight or obese, there's more pressure on the neck of the bladder, increasing the risk of incontinence. Losing weight can help.

Skip the tea. We're not sure why, but tea drinkers seem more likely to experience incontinence than coffee drinkers. Although it's obviously not due to the caffeine, researchers aren't sure what causes it.

Stub the butts. Several studies have found a very strong link between smoking and incontinence, particularly heavy smoking.

enlarged prostate *That Man Thing*

Guys, are you noticing that it's taking a bit longer these days to, well, go? Finding yourself checking for the nearest bathroom like you used to check for attractive women? Producing a urine stream that's weaker than your sense of humor? Don't be embarrassed. Every other man your age is probably having the same problem.

Technically, you're dealing with benign pros-tatic hyperplasia (BPH), commonly known as an enlarged prostate. It's the most common health problem in men 60 and older. The prostate, in case you didn't already know, is the gland that creates and releases the fluid that makes up much of your semen. The gland surrounds the ure-thra, the thin tube that carries urine from your bladder to outside your body. As you age, your prostate gets larger (kind of like your ears, and no, we don't know why that happens), pressing on the urethra and, like a clamp on a garden hose, turning a stream into a trickle.

You can go the medication/surgery route for a remedy, but you might be able to handle yourself by doing the following.

Stop drinking—at least before you go to bed. Set the alarm on your watch for two hours before your normal bed-time. That's your signal to go dry so you can sleep through the night.

Go decaffeinated. Okay, one cup of coffee in the morn-ing is fine. But after that, ask for decaf. And check the caf-feinated tea, chocolate, and aspirin at the door, too. Caffeine is a natural diuretic.

Check your pills. If you're taking diuretics for high blood pressure or heart failure, talk to your doctor. A lower dose or even a different medication could help reduce your fre-quent trips to the loo. Along those same lines, nix the decongestants and antihista-mines. An unintended effect of these meds is to tighten the band of muscles around the urethra, making it harder to go.

Don't wait. Don't try to hold it in. Hit the can at the first urge so you don't overstretch your bladder.

Follow a heart-healthy lifestyle. The same things that increase your risk of heart disease—being overweight, lack of exercise, high blood pressure, high cholesterol, and diabetes—also increase your risk of BPH and make your symptoms worse. For specific recommendations on avoiding heart disease or diabetes, check out our suggestions on pages 314 and 361.

Try saw palmetto. An analy-sis of 21 clinical trials involving more than 3,000 men conclud-ed that the herb worked better than a placebo at improving symptoms of enlarged prostate and inadequate urinary flow and worked about as well as a wide-ly prescribed medication. Follow package directions for dosing.

Preventing the Diseases
of Aging

Get the Most from Your
Health Care

Screening Smarts

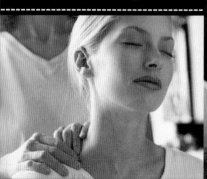

Protecting
Future Health

Each of us has the capacity to avoid the diseases of aging.

It just takes a little preventive medicine—usually in the form of active,

mindful living. Here's your guide.

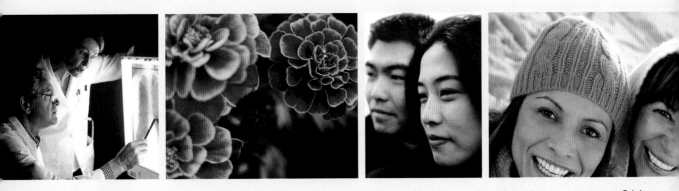

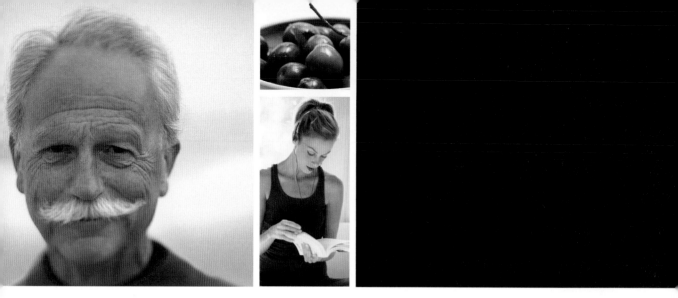

Preventing the Diseases of Aging

When it comes to the reasons why people die, we are entering what some consider a "third age." It is a fascinating tale and a wonderful development.

For most of history, viruses, bacteria, or injuries were mankind's main causes of death. This is the "first age," and it continued well into the 20th century. But with the discovery of vaccines, antibiotics, and general medical knowledge regarding how to fix a broken body, we began to control many killer diseases and repair what once would have been fatal injuries. And as a result, this "first age" ended, and average life spans began to rise incredibly fast in modern countries over the past 100 years.

This newfound expertise in combating disease and injury was a huge leap forward. What was still ignored or misunderstood, however, was the science of *good* health. Many of us—including doctors—smoked, overindulged with alcohol, ate fatty foods, embraced the emerging comforts of modern life (such as television), and didn't think at all about exercise. The result was the "second age," spanning much of the past

preventing

60 years, in which heart disease and cancer rates grew to epidemic proportions and replaced viruses and bacteria as the leading causes of death in modern nations.

But something amazing has happened in just the past two decades. Researchers figured out what makes a heart go wrong, and how to fix it. We even began to understand and successfully treat cancer. Today, a diagnosis of either condition carries with it a greater measure of hope and recovery than ever before. And along the way, we discovered how nutrition, exercise, stress, and compulsive habits like smoking and drinking affect our bodies and cause disease.

Welcome then to the "third age," in which we are living longer and healthier than ever before. But with this new era has come a new crop of health problems that threaten to rob our senior years of vitality and happiness. Generally, these are conditions caused by wear and tear. They are the natural outcomes of a long life, often led without health in mind.

For example, arthritis is frequently due to years of abuse to your joints. Diabetes, in many cases, is the result of years of poor eating and the gradual breakdown of the energy-transfer process within the cells in your body. Vision and hearing problems are often due to decades of overuse and abuse. Osteoporosis is a long, gradual decline in bone density; it, too, is a disease far more of the old than the young. And chronic pain, including back pain, is often an unwelcome side effect of a life long lived.

The goal: to take good enough care of your body that one part doesn't wear out ahead of the others.

Living Long Life

Just because you are living longer doesn't mean that you are destined to suffer from these diseases and conditions of aging. For one component of the "third age" of health is an unprecedented understanding of the underlying causes of good health. Fifteen years ago, issues like chronic inflammation weren't understood. Today, we know that a perpetually on-attack immune system is a major cause of age-related disease. We also didn't know the subtleties of "good" cholesterol or the complex chemistry changes in your body that is caused by stress and relaxation or the power of micronutrients in our food to fight age-related disease and decline.

With all this new understanding, we are on the verge of achieving not just long life, but long health. But—and this is a major but—it is up to you. Doctors and the health-care system cannot deliver long health; it doesn't come in a pill. Only you can make it happen.

Forgive this auto analogy, but it makes the point well: What makes one car break down at 75,000 miles for one owner, and the same model of car last 150,000 miles for a different owner? That's easy: regular maintenance, smart usage, and constant loving care by the second owner.

It's no different for your body.

This final section of this book delves into the causes of 10 of the most common diseases and conditions of aging. More important, it provides the newest methods for preventing their onslaught. Many of these preventive measures are surprising and easily achieved. So take action!

Heart Attacks and Strokes

Once, doctors believed that the biggest risk factor for heart attacks and strokes was getting old. Conditions like high blood pressure, out-of-balance cholesterol levels, and high levels of blood fats called triglycerides were seen as unfortunate, yet normal, parts of the aging process.

But that was then, and this is now. The evidence today is overwhelming: Making healthy lifestyle changes—as simple as an after-dinner stroll, a tropical-fruit dessert, a night out laughing with your best friends, even a glass of fine wine—can powerfully reverse those three threats and others that are the underlying causes of heart attacks and strokes.

That's the happy conclusion of hundreds, even thousands, of medical studies conducted around the world. And it holds true for people of all ages and health levels—whether you have arteries that are in tip-top shape, are taking medications to control somewhat problematic blood pressure or cholesterol levels, or have already had one heart attack or stroke and want to avoid a second.

You've no doubt heard the dire warnings already: Heart attacks and strokes kill or alter the lives of more older people than any other health problem. And the cause of the damage sounds so simple, so *possible*: A clot comes loose in your bloodstream, stopping the flow of blood and oxygen to vulnerable heart muscle or brain cells. A clot can change your life in a matter of seconds.

But here's the news you need to know: Making small, healthy changes *at any age* can dramatically lower your risk for a life-altering clot. When researchers at the Medical Universi-ty of South Carolina, in Charleston, tracked 15,708 women and men for six years, those who practiced four basic heart- and brain-healthy lifestyle habits were 35 percent less likely to have cardiovascular disease and 40 percent less likely to die from any cause. Most of the volunteers were in their fifties and sixties—and some had turned 70 by the end of the study. Their healthy habits included eating at least five fruits and vegetables daily, exercising at least 2.5 hours per week, maintaining a healthy weight, and not smoking. It's never too late to start, concludes lead researcher Dana E. King, MD, an associate professor of family medicine at the university.

"People who newly adopt a healthy lifestyle experience a *prompt* benefit of lower rates of cardiovascular disease and mortality," he says. "We call this the turning back the clock study. The benefits were dramatic and immediate, even at age 65."

When it comes to the heart, most of us do need to work at turning back the clock in our later years. At least half of all older adults have out-of-balance cholesterol levels, and 90 percent of us will develop high blood pressure in older age, experts say. These and other threats team up to fill artery walls with heart- and brain-threatening plaque, and to make blood vessels stiff and prone to damage that leads to clots.

The Seven evils

Current science points to the following closely connected health conditions as primary causes or indicators of future heart attacks and strokes.

1 Body fat:
New research reveals that an excess of visceral fat around your internal organs greatly increases your chances of heart disease. Interestingly, hip, thigh, and butt fat are more benign when it comes to your heart; a pot belly or wide waist is the real danger signal.

2 Cholesterol:
Excessive amounts of "bad" LDL cholesterol in your bloodstream provide the foundation for plaque to build up on artery walls. A shortage of "good" HDL cholesterol is equally problematic.

3 Triglycerides:
These are a type of fat cell found in your bloodstream. They have an important function, but an excess amount acts much like bad cholesterol.

4 Blood pressure:
Compare a raging river to a gently flowing river. High blood pressure creates the former in your arteries; that makes dislodging a clot far more likely.

5 C-reactive protein:
This is an immune-system chemical that is created in response to inflammation. An excess amount in your bloodstream appears to contribute to the creation of plaque.

6 Insulin resistance:
Insulin signals each cell of your body to absorb fuel (in the form of blood sugar). When cells reject insulin, it builds up in the bloodstream, causing a chain reaction of unhealthy events for your arteries.

7 Homocysteine:
This is an amino acid created when your body breaks down proteins in your diet. High levels in your bloodstream have proven to be a remarkably good predictor of future heart disease.

Controlling, reversing, or preventing these dangerous conditions can dramatically lower your odds for big problems: If everyone with high blood pressure got their condition under control, for example, the number of strokes would be cut nearly in half. And adopting healthier habits could cut your odds for heart attack by up to 82 percent.

The key? Don't rely on drugs or surgery alone. Make these healthy—and enjoyable—steps the foundation of your personal heart and brain protection plan.

Cholesterol: The New Thinking

If you're used to automatically thinking that cholesterol is bad for you, here's news: At healthy levels, this natural substance isn't a demon at all. Your body uses this soft, waxy material every day to build cell membranes and to produce sex hormones, vitamin D, and fat-digesting bile acids.

But modern-day cholesterol levels are out of balance—and it's not simply a matter of too much. We eat too many "bad fats"—saturated fats and artificial trans-fatty acids that raise levels of heart-threatening LDL cholesterol. We consume too little of the "good fats"—the unsaturated fats and omega-3 fatty acids found in foods like canola oil, nuts, and fish—that protect levels of "good" HDL cholesterol. And we skip exercise, the key to keeping LDLs lower and HDLs higher.

The result? Not just dangerously high cholesterol but also dangerously out-of-balance levels of good HDLs and bad LDLs. The latest research on heart health shows that ignoring this balance, by focusing solely on lowering your cholesterol, can lead to trouble. Cutting-edge cardiologists are finding that the higher your HDLs *and* the lower your LDLs, essentially, the closer you can come to the "natural" cholesterol balance humans were meant to have. It's the most powerful way to lower your risk for clogged arteries, heart attacks, and strokes. At the same time, maintaining healthy levels of another important, though less well-known, blood fat called triglycerides, is important, too.

9 Ways to Lower LDLs

Tiny, spherical LDL particles are your body's cholesterol delivery trucks, bringing liquefied cholesterol directly to cells. But when too many LDLs crowd your blood (thanks to a diet high in saturated fat, overweight, inactivity, and sometimes, to your genes), extra particles burrow into the delicate lining of artery walls. Free radicals—rogue oxygen molecules from cigarette smoking, digestion, or aging—damage the LDLs. A pool of fatty, gunky plaque builds up in the artery wall. If it ruptures, it will cause a blood clot that could lead to a heart attack or a stroke.

Put simply, high LDLs raise your risk for a heart attack or stroke. Low levels reduce your risk. For every 1-point drop in LDLs (which are measured in milligrams per deciliter of blood, or mg/dl), heart risk falls 2 percent. The safety zone: Experts now believe that most people should shoot for a number lower than 100 mg/dl—especially if you have heart risks such as diabetes, high blood pressure, or a family history or personal history of heart disease, or if you smoke.

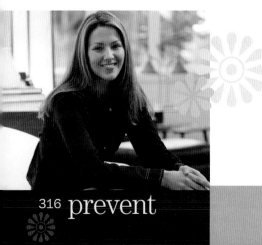

The goal no longer is to just lower your overall cholesterol count. Instead, it is to get the two main types in proper balance.

Researchers at the Cleveland Clinic have found that pushing LDL levels below 100 mg/dl halted the progression of heart disease and cut mortality rates by 28 percent. "We stopped heart disease in its tracks," the researchers say. While they used statin drugs, you can take powerful lifestyle steps to cut your LDLs significantly—whether or not you also use medications. Here are nine great tips to start.

Cut trans fats out of your diet. Eat chopped veggies instead of snack crackers, and fruit instead of boxed cookies or store-bought cakes and pastries. Choose margarines that clearly state on the label that they contain no trans fats, too. Why? Trans fats are worse for your heart than saturated fats because they boost levels of "bad" LDL cholesterol and decrease "good" HDL cholesterol. Avoiding these processed fats could cut your heart attack risk by 55 percent, studies show.

Keep your slow-cooker on the counter—and use it! Eating leaner cuts of meat can cut your LDLs because you're getting less cholesterol-raising saturated fat in every bite. Low-fat meats can be tough; cooking them in a slow-cooker is an easy way to tenderize without adding gobs of fat.

Make your own salad dressing. Use olive oil and vinegar or lemon juice, spices, and crushed garlic. You'll get more cholesterol-lowering unsaturated fat and avoid the trans fats and saturated fats swimming in most bottled dressings—especially the creamy types!

Sit down to a steaming bowl of oatmeal most mornings. Oats are packed with a soluble fiber called beta glucan that whisks excess cholesterol out of your body. Having 1 1/2 cups of oatmeal on a regular basis could lower your LDLs by 12 to 24 percent.

Have a pear or a grapefruit half every morning. Both fruits are rich in pectin, another soluble fiber that helps lower LDLs. Other great pectin sources are apples and all types of berries. Grapefruit contains a substance that can interfere with the absorption of many medicines, so check with your doctor before making it a regular part of your morning.

Devote 10 minutes a day to resistance-training exercises. Women who did 45 to 50 minutes of muscle-building resistance training exercises three times a week lowered their LDL levels by 14 percent. Can't do that much? Just 10 minutes a day of the easy exercises developed for the Long Life Health plan—or just doing sit-ups, leg lifts, and hip extensions—will help.

Eat six small meals per day. You'll get there if you follow the Long Life Eating approach. In a large British study, people who "grazed" throughout the day had lower cholesterol levels than those who ate big meals twice a day. The difference was big enough to give the small-meal aficionados a 10 to 20 percent reduction in risk for heart disease.

Add a half-teaspoon of cinnamon to your coffee before brewing. Pakistani researchers have found that this amount (about 6 grams) reduced LDL levels 30 percent in people with type 2 diabetes.

Avoid saturated-fat traps. Your body uses saturated fats to produce LDLs. Overeating foods like cheesecake, cheeseburgers, premium ice cream, and steaks provides way too much raw material for producing this heart-threatening stuff. A better plan: Always stop and think before saying "yes" to the foods heavy with animal fat. Ask yourself: What could I have instead? The answer might be a fruit salad, a plain burger (or even better, a piece of grilled chicken or fish), or a small helping of low-fat or fat-free frozen dessert such as sorbet or reduced-fat frozen yogurt.

LDL Cholesterol by the Numbers

LDL Level (mg/dl)	Heart and Brain Protection
Under 100	Optimal
100–129	Near optimal
130–159	Borderline high
160–189	High
190 and above	Very high

6 Ways to Raise HDLs

HDL, or "high-density lipoprotein" cholesterol is the body's LDL cholesterol clean-up crew, actually fusing with the bad type of cholesterol and carrying it to the liver for disposal. New evidence suggests that HDLs also act as antioxidants, shielding LDLs from the type of damage that makes it promote plaque.

Long ignored by doctors, HDL is the newest heart-protection factor to receive serious attention from progressive researchers. "Every 1-point rise in HDLs reduces your risk for a fatal heart attack by 3 percent," says Johns Hopkins University cardiologist Roger Blumenthal, MD, director of the university's Ciccarone Preventive Cardiology Center. "That's as potent as a 1-point drop in LDLs. For too long, doctors only emphasized cutting LDLs. Now we know how to raise HDLs and that it has heart-protecting benefits. It's time to take action."

The new thinking: Higher is better. Women after menopause should aim for levels of 50 mg/dl or higher, while men should aim for at least 40 mg/dl. Here are some ways to move your measure higher.

Quit smoking. Kicking the cigarette habit can raise your HDLs about 4 points.

Enjoy one alcoholic drink per day. A glass of wine with dinner could increase your good cholesterol by 4 points. But skip this step if you also have high triglycerides—alcohol can make them soar and would cancel out the benefits.

Snack on walnuts or pecans. You'll enhance your HDL level by 2 to 3 points if you regularly snack on a small handful of walnut halves or pecans, report researchers from Shiraz University of Medical Sciences in Iran and from Loma Linda University in California.

Achieve a healthier weight. If your doctor approves of your weight-loss plans, gradually moving to a healthy weight could raise your HDLs by 1 point for every 6 1/2 pounds you lose, experts say.

Walk briskly, three times per week. You can raise your HDLs by 1 to 4 points with a fast-paced stroll (just vigorous enough that conversation is a little difficult) for a half-hour on Monday, Wednesday, and Friday, Johns Hopkins University cardiologists say.

Avoid a fat-free lifestyle. You read that right. Your body needs some fat to help maintain its HDL level. Choose "good" monounsaturated fats, found in olive and canola oils, and omega-3 fatty acids, found in fish, walnuts, and fish-oil capsules, to help your body keep HDLs on an even keel.

HDL Cholesterol by the Numbers

HDL Level (mg/dl)	Heart and Brain Protection
Less than 40	Low (risky)
40–59	Average
60 and higher	High (protective)

5 Ways to Reduce Triglycerides

Triglycerides seem innocuous: They link to excess blood sugars from the food you eat and whisk them to fat cells for long-term storage. But when levels are high, triglycerides can also become the raw material for LDLs, making them another dangerous actor in the heart-disease drama. Newer studies suggest that triglycerides alone can predict a heart's risk, by encouraging atherosclerosis—and may be twice as dangerous for women as they are for men.

Smoking, drinking, eating too many refined carbs (including sugar or corn syrup), and being overweight can all elevate triglycerides. These additional strategies can help you keep your triglycerides within a healthy range.

Have a "natural" whole-grain at dinner every night. Try brown rice, whole-wheat couscous, barley, even quinoa. Simply choosing whole grains instead of the refined type could cut your risk of heart attack by 30 percent.

Enjoy Mother Nature's desserts. We're talking about fruit—fresh, frozen (without syrup), canned in its own juice, or dried (provided it's not sugar-coated). Yes, fruit has fructose, but in smaller quantities than high-fructose corn syrup has. And, fruit brings you a wealth of fiber, vitamins, minerals, and a host of antioxidants. Have a piece for dessert most evenings.

Avoid "liquid candy." Skip high-sugar sodas, processed fruit juices, and sweetened iced teas. Switch to seltzer with a splash of orange juice or lemon, plain water, or, if you just love soda, try the diet version.

Take your reading glasses to the supermarket. Even applesauce, stewed tomatoes, and pasta sauce may contain corn syrup. Usually, there's a syrup-free version right next to it on the shelf.

When to Get Help

If your cholesterol and triglyceride numbers are only slightly elevated, talk with your doctor about giving lifestyle changes a try for about six months. After six months, ask for another blood test to check levels. If your HDLs are still low or your LDLs and/or triglycerides are still high, ask about medications such as cholesterol-lowering statins and drugs that can raise HDLs, such as prescription-grade niacin.

Set a drink limit. The limit for women is one drink; for men, two. If your triglyceride level is in the healthy range, the one/two-drink rule is fine. If your triglycerides are high, cut out alcohol, since it can actually raise triglyceride levels. Even small amounts can send levels soaring in some people.

Triglycerides by the Numbers

Triglyceride Level (mg/dl)	Heart and Brain Protection
Under 100	Ideal
100–149	Normal
150–199	Borderline high
200–499	High
500 and above	Extremely risky

Supplements

Your Heart Will Love

These safe, well-chosen nutritional supplements repair and protect your heart in ways that go beyond a healthy lifestyle. Adding them to your personal long life prescription could add even more healthy years to your heart.

Fish Oil

Two heart-friendly omega-3 fatty acids—eicosapentaenoic acid (EPA) and docosahexaenoic acid (DHA)—found in fish-oil capsules can cut heart attack risk by 73 percent. Fish oil stabilizes dangerous artery plaque so that it's less likely to burst and trigger the formation of heart- and brain-threatening blood clots. These oils can also cut triglycerides by 30 to 40 percent. And fish oil helps keep hearts beating in a regular rhythm, cutting the odds for out-of-rhythm beats that can trigger strokes and sudden cardiac death.

HOW TO TAKE IT:

Experts suggest getting a total of 1,000 to 2,000 milligrams of EPA plus DHA—though less-conservative experts suggest twice as much may be better. How many capsules? Read the label; it varies by brand. Take it with food, and talk with your doctor if you have a bleeding disorder or take an anticoagulant drug such as warfarin.

Soluble Fiber

Soluble fiber—found naturally in foods like oatmeal, barley, beans, and many fruits—forms a thick, cholesterol-trapping gel in your digestive system. Get enough and you could lower your "bad" LDL cholesterol by 5 percent—enough to reduce heart disease risk by 10 to 15 percent. While we need at least 8 grams per day—and up to 25 grams if you have elevated cholesterol, most of us barely take in 4 grams—about the amount in a bowl of oatmeal and a handful of strawberries. That's where a soluble fiber supplement comes in.

Niacin

Megadoses of this B vitamin can raise your "good" HDL cholesterol by a respectable 15 to 35 percent, while lowering triglycerides 20 to 50 percent. But this supplement should only be taken as a prescription drug. The side effects of high-dose niacin include severe, painful facial flushing and potential liver damage.

HOW TO TAKE IT:

Fiber supplements come as flavored powder you mix with water, as capsules, and even as wafers. Soluble fiber supplements can be made from ground psyllium seed (the most extensively researched fiber supplement for cutting cholesterol), from beta glucan (the same fiber in oatmeal, and also from fibers called inulin, methylcellulose, and polycarbophil). Aim for 7 to 10 grams of soluble fiber from supplements per day—and take half in the morning, half at night. Always drink a full glass of water with your fiber. Check the product you choose; each supplement contains a different fiber content.

HOW TO TAKE IT:

If you have low HDLs and high triglycerides, talk with your doctor about a timed-release, prescription-strength niacin supplement. Some are formulated to reduce flushing and go easy on your liver.

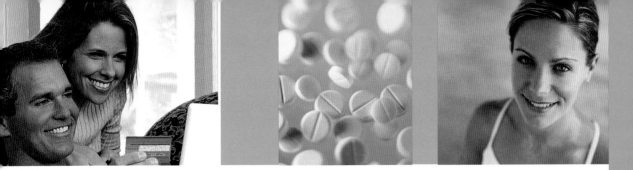

Aspirin

Aspirin's pain-soothing, inflammation-cooling active ingredient—acetylsalicylic acid—is also a potent heart-protector that works by cutting clot risk. A daily, low-dose aspirin can cut your risks of a heart attack by a huge 33 percent. But new evidence suggests that the benefits are far greater for men than for women.

HOW TO TAKE IT:

Talk with your doctor. Generally, the recommended dose is 81 milligrams per day—often, about the amount in a children's aspirin. Higher doses don't offer more protection. In fact, doses over 100 milligrams per day can double your risk for gastrointestinal (GI) bleeding. Take it with a meal to cut bleeding risk. If you take the pain reliever ibuprofen, wait two hours before taking aspirin: Ibuprofen can interfere with aspirin's heart-protective powers.

Coenzyme Q10

Found in every cell in the body, coenzyme Q10 (CoQ10) boosts the effectiveness of enzymes that help cells produce energy. Getting sufficient CoQ10 ensures that heart muscle cells will pump efficiently; it can also cut symptoms of heart failure and shield cells from free-radical damage. It may help lower blood pressure, too. If you take a cholesterol-lowering statin, ask your doctor about adding CoQ10 daily; statins can block production of this enzyme by the liver.

HOW TO TAKE IT:

100 milligrams per day. For best absorption, look for capsules or tablets with CoQ10 in an oil base. Take it with a meal containing a fat, such as salad dressing or peanut butter, to further enhance absorption.

Phytosterols

Found naturally in soy beans, rice bran, and wheat germ, plant sterols and stanols—known collectively as phytosterols—block the absorption of cholesterol from the food you eat. Now, these ingenious substances are available in capsules and in special cholesterol-lowering margarines. A daily phytosterol supplement can lower your "bad" LDLs by 13 to 21 mg/dl—a reduction that cuts heart risk up to 21 percent.

HOW TO TAKE IT:

Experts recommend 2 to 3 grams per day—equivalent to 2 to 3 tablespoons of phytosterol-enriched margarine—to lower high LDL cholesterol levels. They are also available in pill form. Since phytosterols could block absorption of beta-carotene, get an extra serving of beta-carotene-rich foods every day (such as carrots, sweet potatoes, and yellow squash)—and eat it at a meal when you're not using a phytosterol supplement for better absorption.

High Blood Pressure: The New Thinking

As mentioned, doctors once shrugged off high blood pressure in their older patients as a normal sign of aging—a medical lapse that some believe has contributed to the high rates of heart attacks and strokes in people over age 55.

Today, all that has changed. While your odds for high blood pressure do rise with every passing birthday—experts estimate that 90 percent of us will have elevated pressure at some point after age 55—lowering it has never been easier.

Why bother? High blood pressure, also known as hypertension, is a silent killer that plays a role in 75 percent of heart attacks and strokes. When modern living and genetics team up to stiffen artery linings, blood pressure increases. This faster, harder flow of blood damages blood vessel walls, making it easier for heart-threatening plaque to form. At the same time, the extra pressure can cause plaque buildups to break off; these are the clots that kill. When clots block the arteries that feed fuel and oxygen to your heart, that's a heart attack. When clots block the blood vessels to your brain, that's a stroke. And when they block the vessels to your abdomen, that's an abdominal aortic aneurysm.

Scary stuff, yet there's more. High blood pressure can also enlarge and weaken your heart, and even damage your eyes and kidneys.

Lowering your blood pressure can cut your odds for major health problems significantly: stroke, by 30 percent; heart attack, by 23 percent; heart failure, by 55 percent; dementia risk, by 50 percent. At the same time, it can prevent or delay kidney damage and guard your eyes against vision loss brought on by severe hypertension.

The new thinking about high blood pressure is that lower is always better. The standard advice to keep blood pressure readings below 140/90 isn't good enough, experts now say. (The first number represents systolic pressure, the force of blood against artery walls during a heartbeat; the second number represents diastolic pressure, which measures pressure when the heart is relaxed between beats. Both numbers are expressed as mm/HG, or millimeters of mercury.) Now, a healthy blood pressure should be lower than 120/80. You're considered to have prehypertension if your systolic reading is between 120 and 139 or your diastolic reading is between 80 and 89.

Damage to arteries actually begins at blood pressure levels that doctors once considered optimal, even stellar. Evidence gathered from 61 blood pressure studies reveals that for most adults, risk of death from heart disease and stroke begin to rise when blood pressure is as low as 115/75. After that, death risk doubles for every 20-point rise in systolic pressure and every 10-point rise in diastolic pressure. On the

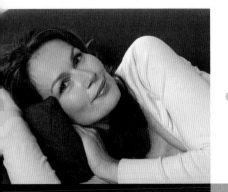

Again and again, research confirms that high blood pressure is a major health risk, and that lower levels are almost always better.

flip side, lowering your blood pressure could actually help unclog your arteries, a surprising study from the Cleveland Clinic has found.

The good news: "It's worth taking all the small steps you can to cut your risk," notes blood pressure researcher Haiou Yang, PhD, a scientist at the University of California, Irvine's Center for Occupational and Environmental Health.

13 Steps to Better Blood Pressure

Even if you take drugs for blood pressure, adding these healthy steps can lower your blood pressure even farther—and allow you to get the most benefit from the lowest dose of medication possible.

Make reduced-sodium products your first choice. Cutting your sodium intake by just 300 mg (the amount in about two slices of processed cheese) reduces systolic pressure by 2 to 4 points, and diastolic pressure by 1 to 2 points. Cut more sodium, and your pressure drops even lower. Processed foods, not a salt-shaker, are the biggest source of excess sodium in our diets. You'll find more tips on ways to reduce your sodium intake on page 160, but here are a few to get you started. Omit salt from recipes; fill your saltshaker with a salt substitute; rinse canned beans and canned vegetables thoroughly twice before cooking; select frozen entrées with less than 5 percent of the daily value for sodium in each serving; and give unsalted or reduced-salt pretzels, chips, and condiments a try. Read the labels on over-the-counter remedies careful-ly—some, such as antacids, can be surprisingly high in sodium. Your pharmacist can help you find lower-sodium options.

Fast Clot-Buster

If you or someone you're with has sudden heart attack symptoms, have them thoroughly chew and swallow one regular-strength aspirin tablet immediately. Chewing delivers aspirin's clot-stopping powers to your bloodstream in just 5 minutes; in contrast, swallowing the aspirin whole delays clot-stoppers for 12 crucial minutes.

Quit smoking. Yes, you've read this advice in most every part of this book, and have heard it for years. And for so many reasons! Here's the blood pressure reason: The nicotine in tobacco constricts blood vessels, immediately raising the pressure within them.

Have a banana, melon slice, or handful of dried apricots every day. All are rich in potassium, nicknamed the *un*salt by experts because of its ability to keep blood pressure down. Other high-potassium foods include spinach, lima beans, sweet potatoes, and avocados.

Snack on soy nuts. An ounce of crunchy roasted soybeans cut systolic blood pressure readings by 10 points in one study. Look for unsalted varieties in your supermarket or health food store.

Sprinkle 2 tablespoons of ground flaxseeds on your morning cereal. Then mix 2 tablespoons into your spaghetti sauce, yogurt, or sprinkle on a salad later in the day. This could lower systolic pressure significantly, one study found. The secret ingredient? Probably the omega-3 fatty acids in flax.

Take tea tomorrow morning (and afternoon) instead of coffee. For every cup of tea you drink in a day (up to four), your systolic blood pressure could fall by 2 points and your diastolic pressure could drop by 1 point, an Australian study suggests.

Stroll four times a day. Exercise cut systolic pressure by 5 points and diastolic pressure by 3 points in a University of Illinois study of 21 women and men. But volunteers who took four brisk 10-minute walks a day kept blood pressure low for a whopping 11 hours, versus 7 hours for those who exercised for 40 continuous minutes once a day. Frequent activity keeps artery walls more fit and flexible.

Avoid overuse of pain relievers. Cut back on nonsteroidal anti-inflammatory drugs (NSAIDs), like ibuprofen. Studies show that these popular pain relievers can raise your blood pressure if you take them frequently.

Go whole grain. Switch from white to whole-wheat bread, from white to brown rice, from low-fiber to high-fiber barley, or refined to whole-wheat cereals, and you could cut your systolic pressure 3 to 7 points and your diastolic pressure by 5 to 6 points, says a new study of 25 overweight women and men from the U.S. Department of Agriculture's Human Nutrition Research Center in Beltsville, Maryland.

Buy a home blood pressure monitor. A study presented at a recent European Society of Hypertension conference found that people who checked their blood pressures at home had lower blood pressure readings than those whose only checks were at the doctor's office. Relying on your doctor's tests alone misses nine percent of high blood pressure cases, another study has found. When you are shopping for a monitor, make sure the cuff is the right size (ask your doctor or pharmacist what size you need); be sure you can read the numbers on the monitor and hear heartbeats if it uses a stethoscope; and take the monitor to your doctor's office to compare results with their professional model.

Go home earlier. If you're working at a job—whether it's paid employment or a busy volunteer position or simply watching your grandchildren—plan to start leaving on time more often. Working more than 41 to 50 hours per week raised hypertension risk by 17 percent, according to a University of California, Irvine, study of the health records of 24,205 California residents. Putting in 51 to 60 hours upped risk by 29 percent. Being a workaholic raises your stress and prevents you from getting enough sleep, exercise, and healthy meals, says study author Dr. Yang. It also makes quitting smoking even more difficult.

Turn off your cell phone—and forget about it. When 20 British students were asked to talk about their cell phones to researchers, their systolic blood pressure jumped 8 points—a sign that having a ringing phone in your pocket or purse is stressful. After the students gave up their phones for three days, the same exercise increased blood pressure just 3 points. Silence, it seems, is healthy, says lead researcher David Sheffield, PhD, of the Staffordshire University in England.

Rediscover (low-fat) milk. Around the world, milk consumption is dropping as we sip more sodas and other sweetened soft drinks. But milk and other dairy products are important for blood pressure control because they contain calcium, which helps regulate fluid levels in the bloodstream.

Blood Pressure by the Numbers

Blood Pressure (mm/Hg)	Heart and Brain Protection
115/75	Ideal
Below 120/80	Healthy
120–139/80–89	Warning! Prehypertensive
140/90 and higher	Danger! Hypertension

Three Other Risk Factors

Keeping tabs on blood pressure and cholesterol is a lot like shampooing your hair but skipping the conditioner: The job's half-done. Your numbers look okay, so you assume your heart is safe. But is it?

New evidence reveals that little-known threats could still be setting you up for big trouble. Yet your doctor may never mention these hidden risks; he or she may underestimate the danger, or not even know about them yet.

"I don't stop with cholesterol and blood pressure when I assess heart health," says Alexandra J. Lansky, MD, director of the Women's Cardiovascular Health Initiative at Lenox Hill Hospital in New York City. "Knowing *all* your risks could save your life."

The reassuring news: Taking control can be as easy as snacking on walnuts (instead of processed snack foods) or taking your multivitamin every day. Here's what you need to know about these important risk factors.

RISK 1: C-Reactive Protein

This chemical is produced in the liver when some part of your body is inflamed. Consistently high levels of C-reactive protein, or CRP, can raise your risk of heart disease even if your cholesterol readings are healthy, report researchers at the Center for Cardiovascular Disease Prevention at the Brigham and Women's Hospital in Boston. High CRP is a warning signal that plaque is building up in artery walls.

So what causes high levels of CRP? Mostly, low-grade infections in your body, such as gum disease, and other ongoing irritants that keep your immune system constantly doing battle. This is the "chronic inflammation" problem

Check Your Pulse

An estimated 1 in every 200 adults has an irregular heartbeat, which doctors call atrial fibrillation (AF). Up to 15 percent of people with AF suffer ischemic strokes each year—and often, they're severe strokes.

In AF, unsteady heartbeats allow blood to pool and form tiny clots in the heart. When a strong beat pushes these along to the brain, the risk of stroke rises four to six times higher than normal.

Finding, and fixing, AF could cut your risk for a stroke by 60 percent. To check for an irregular heartbeat, find your pulse at your neck or wrist with the flat pad of your fingertip. Once you detect the beat, repeat the rhythm out loud: dum-dum-dum-dum. If what you get is more like dum-dum-da-dum or some other variation, talk with your doctor about whether you have AF and what to do. Top AF treatments are electrical stimuli to regulate heartbeat (called cardioversion) and clot-preventing medications such as aspirin or warfarin.

that is increasingly being talked about in health circles.

What's your CRP level? To find out, ask your doctor for a *high-sensitivity* CRP test the next time you're getting a blood sugar or cholesterol check. If numbers seem high (the measurement is milligrams of CRP per deciliter of blood, or mg/dl), get a retest in two weeks. A cold or flu could skew your reading because inflammation levels will be temporarily high.

Here are three top ways to tame your CRP.

Make all your sandwiches on whole-grain bread. A study from the Centers for Disease Control and Prevention in Atlanta shows that getting 32 grams of fiber per day could slash CRP levels by half. You'll get there if you also

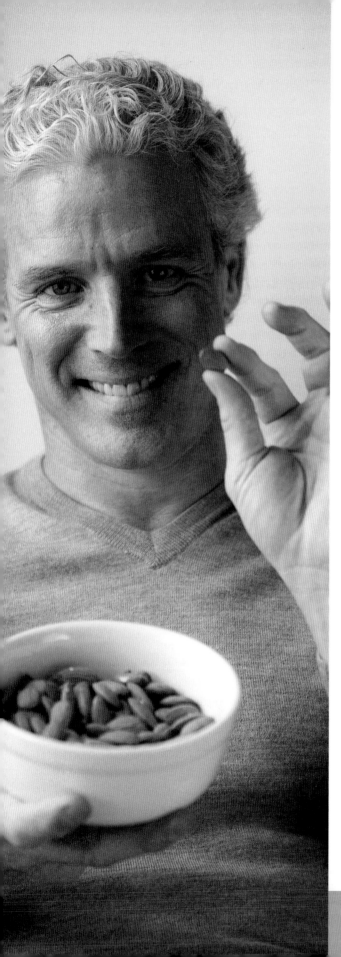

choose high-fiber cereals, beans and lentils, and whole-grain pasta.

Snack on a handful of walnuts instead of a candy bar. Rich in fiber and "good" omega-3 fatty acids, these nuts slash CRP levels and cut heart risk.

Brush, floss, and rinse every day. Even tiny pockets of gum disease increase inflammation levels throughout your body, raising your odds for heart attacks and even strokes. Studies show that pampering your gums by brushing carefully, flossing well, then rinsing with a gum-protecting mouthwash are important steps that not only brighten your smile, but also protect your cardiovascular system.

C-Reactive Protein by the Numbers

CRP (mg/dl)	Heart and Brain Protection
Below 1	Optimal
1 to 3	Average
Above 3	High risk

RISK 2: Metabolic Syndrome

For at least one in four adults, inactivity and overeating lead to high insulin levels—your body's attempt to force muscle cells to absorb blood sugar. The danger: High insulin levels in your bloodstream can double to quadruple heart attack and stroke risk. New research links metabolic syndrome—the phrase doctors use for when insulin and related body chemicals are out of balance—with a 2.5 times higher risk for clogged arteries.

Do you have metabolic syndrome? There's no blood check for this dangerous condition, but a series of tiny warning signs reveals your risk. The big danger is that each of these warning signs is small enough to shrug off. But together, they predict big trouble.

If you have signs of metabolic syndrome, be sure to ask your doctor for a fasting blood sugar check for diabetes; people with metabolic syndrome have about a 30 percent chance for developing major blood sugar problems, which also raise your risk for heart attack and stroke.

Virtually every healthy eating and exercise tip in this book will help reduce your chances of getting metabolic syndrome. But here are three steps that are guaranteed to help make a difference.

Get 30 minutes of exercise per day. Exercise forces muscle cells to take up extra blood sugar and also makes them more sensitive to insulin.

Trim belly fat. Eat whole grains, fruits and veggies, and exercise—these strategies can shrink dangerous abdominal fat, the kind that wraps itself around your internal organs and raises your odds for metabolic syndrome.

Eat snack food from farms, not factories. For example, choose a piece of fruit over cookies. High-sugar, low-fiber processed sweets send your blood sugar levels soaring and trigger the release of loads of insulin in order to bring levels down. Over time, a high-sugar diet taxes your body's ability to control blood sugar, especially if you're overweight or inactive.

Metabolic Syndrome by the Numbers

You're likely to have metabolic syndrome if you have three of these:

- A waistline bigger than 35 inches
- Triglycerides over 150 mg/dl
- Blood pressure above 130/85
- HDL cholesterol below 50

RISK 3: Homocysteine

Evidence suggests that too much of this amino acid—created naturally when your body digests meat—damages the inner lining of arteries and promotes blood clotting. A Norwegian study of 587 women and men found that heart-related death risk was eight times greater when homocysteine was elevated. A 10 percent increase in blood homocysteine levels increases the risk of heart disease by 10 to 15 percent.

Take your multivitamin. A multi supplying 100 percent of the Daily Value for folic acid, vitamin B_6, and vitamin B_{12} can cut homocysteine levels by 32 percent, say Harvard researchers.

Have an orange at breakfast and a spinach-and-cherry-tomato salad with lunch. Citrus fruits, tomatoes, and spinach are all great sources of folic acid, which breaks down homocysteine in the body.

Snack on low-fat, unsweetened yogurt. People who have dairy products regularly had homocysteine levels 15 percent lower than those who avoided yogurt and milk, studies show.

Stir-fry peppers and broccoli for dinner tonight. In a study of 6,000 people, those who ate the most peppers (red, yellow, green, or hot peppers) and the most cabbage, broccoli, and cauliflower had homocysteine levels 16.5 percent lower than people who didn't eat these healthy veggies on a regular basis.

Homocysteine by the Numbers

Homocysteine (umol/L)	Heart and Brain Protection
Under 10	Optimal
10–12	Dangerous
Above 12	Doubled risk for heart attack or stroke

Cancer

If you live long enough, you will get cancer. It's just how we're built. Cancer, for all the fear it invokes, is not some foreign thing that invades your body, like a virus or bacteria. Cancer is simply your own cells run amok. It develops when the built-in mechanisms designed to destroy damaged cells fail or become overwhelmed by the extent of the damaged cells.

And so those damaged or cancerous cells keep doing what cells do—multiplying. Unlike normal cells, however, they don't have an "off" switch. So they divide and divide and divide. In the process, they use up valuable blood, oxygen, and nutrients that healthy cells need. Eventually, the proliferation of cancer cells makes it impossible for healthy cells to survive.

These cancer cells are pretty smart. They are able, in many instances, to disguise themselves to evade detection by the immune system. They also mutate to resist the poisons designed to root them out. And sometimes, they lay dormant for years until something—biochemical stress, its own genetic siren song—triggers them into action again.

The connection between cancer and age? Mathematics. The older you are, the longer your cells have been dividing. The greater the number of divisions, the greater the likelihood that some mistakes will occur. The more mistakes that occur, the greater the likelihood that one of those "mistake" cells will survive and become a cancer. That's why 77 percent of all cancers are diagnosed in those 55 and older. And it's why until about 100 years ago—when the average lifespan in developed countries finally passed the 50-year mark—cancer was relatively rare. Today, it's the leading cause of death in developed countries,

with one in three people dying from some form of cancer.

But here's the thing: About two-thirds of all cancers could be prevented—if people stopped smoking, ate better, and exercised.

Your job, then, is to arm yourself with all known (and suspected) weapons to reduce the probability that cellular mistakes will occur and increase the likelihood that if they do occur, the systems designed to correct or destroy them work. That means reducing the production of free radicals, increasing the availability of antioxidants to fight off free radicals, and stemming the tide of inflammation.

Best Ways to Prevent Cancer

At a cellular level, all cancers are similar. But what makes cancer so challenging is that it can develop in many places within your body, each based on different triggers and causes.

What does this mean? Excessive sun is the top cause of the cellular damage that leads to skin cancer, but has less effect on the inside of your body. Your digestive system directly encounters many toxins and chemicals in your food that ultimately can cause cancer to develop in your

Top 5 Cancer myths

Researchers from the American Cancer Society decided to find out just how much everyday folks know about the disease. What they found might surprise you. More than 25 percent of the 1,000 people surveyed believed the following statements were true. If you thought they were true, too, beware: Lack of knowledge about cancer is itself a risk factor for developing cancer!

1 **The risk of dying from cancer is increasing.** Not true in modern countries. In fact, the risk of dying is decreasing as we get better at diagnosing and treating cancer. Not only that, but the risk of developing certain cancers is also declining as people quit smoking and take other lifestyle steps to reduce their cancer risk.

2 **Pollution is a greater risk factor for lung cancer than smoking.** Nope. While high levels of pollution can increase the risk of lung cancer, the increase is minuscule compared to smoking.

3 **Physical injuries later in life cause cancer.** Huh? Not really. It's genetic changes, not physical injuries, that cause most cancers.

4 **Electronic devices like cell phones cause cancer.** Hardly. In fact, numerous studies have debunked the link between cell phones and brain cancer, and between microwave ovens and cancer.

5 **How you live when you're young has little effect on your risk of cancer later.** Uh, one word here: Sunburn. A single serious sunburn in your teens can set you up for melanoma, the most serious form of skin cancer, 30 years later. Smoking for even a year creates genetic damages in lung tissue cells that can trigger cancerous cells decades later. In fact, some studies are now finding that the seeds of cancer could be sown in the womb—based on what your mother did when she was pregnant with you.

stomach, esophagus, or intestines, but might have less impact elsewhere in your body.

That is to say that one set of preventive measures cannot effectively battle all cancer forms. Identified here are the top five (see page 332) that you should heartily apply to your life; they are the closest you can come to a total cancer-prevention plan. Plus, many of the other healthy-lifestyle tips presented throughout this book help battle cancer. In addition, it is important for you to try many of the following. These are preventive measures that, in recent studies, have truly shown significant benefit. In each case, the type of cancers for which the action is best suited is revealed.

Sip some tea. Real tea—not herbal tea—contains powerful antioxidants called catechins that help protect proteins and cellular DNA from oxidative damage that can lead to cells becoming cancerous. In laboratory studies, catechins stop tumors from growing and protect healthy cells from damage. And in population studies, researchers find that people who are regular tea-drinkers have half the risk of developing some cancers as those who don't drink the liquid at all, or who drink it less frequently.

BEST FOR: **STOMACH AND ESOPHAGEAL CANCER**

Switch to olive oil. You already know about this fat's famous potential for reducing heart disease; now we learn that it's also a great way to elude cancer. In late 2006, researchers from five European countries concluded that olive oil alone may account for the significant difference in cancer rates between Southern and Northern Europeans. They tracked a marker of oxidative damage in volunteers who got about 1/4 cup of olive oil daily for three weeks. At the start of the trial, the marker was found in much higher rates among Northern Europeans than in Southern Europeans. By the end of the trial, however, levels of this marker had dropped considerably in the Northern Europeans. The researchers aren't sure which antioxidant compound in olive oil is responsible for the benefit, but they're on track to find out.

BEST FOR: **ALL CANCERS**

Supplement with vitamin D and catch some rays. Several studies find that the sunshine vitamin reduces the risk of numerous cancers. But while you can get vitamin D from supplements and food sources, it takes sunlight to activate the vitamin, which collects in your skin.

In one study, researchers followed 1,179 postmenopausal women for four years. Half took 1,400 to 1,500 milligrams of calcium alone, and half took the calcium along with 1,100 internatioanl units (IU) of vitamin D. Those getting the calcium/D supplement had a 30 percent lower risk of developing any type of cancer during the four years than those receiving just calcium.

Other studies found that women with vitamin D levels of more than 800 IU a day from diet or supplements had a 19 percent lower breast cancer risk than those getting less than 400 IU. Studies also find that people in sunny climates are far less likely to develop solid tumors like stomach, colorectal, liver, gallbladder, pancreatic, lung, and prostate cancers than those from northern climates.

Bottom line: The more steady, continuous exposure to the sun (not sunburn!), the less likely you are to develop many cancers. Exceptions include lip and mouth cancers, and non-Hodgkins lymphoma, suggesting that you still need to protect exposed areas with sunscreen. One reason for vitamin D's benefits may be its ability to limit cell division and to help insure that when cells do divide, they don't differ significantly from other cells of their type.

BEST FOR: **MOST SOLID TUMORS (SUCH AS BREAST, PROSTATE, PANCREATIC, COLORECTAL, LUNG, STOMACH, LIVER, AND GALLBLADDER)**

Follow a cancer-preventing diet. The link between cancer and nutrition is so powerful, there is even a medical journal devoted just to that topic: *Nutrition and Cancer.* So in addition to substituting olive oil for other fats, as mentioned above, and loading up on tomatoes, as mentioned below, get plenty of these other foods.

- **Apples.** Apples are packed with quercetin, an antioxidant shown to reduce the risk of numerous cancers, particularly lung cancer. One study of more than 77,000 women found just one apple a day reduced the risk of lung cancer by 21 percent, regardless of smoking status. Meanwhile, experiments in the laboratory showed that quercetin prevents lung cancer cells from multiplying.

- **Raspberries.** Black raspberries, seeds and all, have 40 percent more antioxidants than blueberries and strawberries. Inject rats with a compound to cause colon cancer, then feed them a diet rich in raspberries and they develop 80 percent fewer tumors than rats who didn't get the fruit (but who did get the cancer-causing chemical). Freeze-dried black raspberries also kept another set of rats from developing mouth and esophageal cancers.

- **Cruciferous vegetables.** These include broccoli, cauliflower, Brussels sprouts, and even cabbage-based dishes like sauerkraut and coleslaw. Men who ate three or more 1/2-cup servings of these veggies a week reduced their risk of prostate cancer by 41 percent, compared to men who ate less in one major study. Steam the vegetables slightly and drizzle on a little olive oil to get the most benefits.

- **Garlic and onions.** These two flavoring vegetables are jammed with cancer-destroying chemicals. Get 16 servings a week of onions (1/2 cup raw, chopped onion equals one serving) and 22 servings a week of garlic (one clove equals one serving) and your risk of oral, esophageal, colorectal, laryngeal, ovarian, breast, and prostate cancers drops precipitously.

The protective effect from both vegetables stem from the same compounds that give each their distinctive odors: organosulfur compounds. These compounds do many things: They influence enzymes that activate and detoxify carcinogens; they prevent DNA from bonding to cancer-causing substances; they are great at scavenging up free radicals in your bloodstream; and they support the immune system, among other benefits. One hint: Either use garlic raw or let it sit for 10 minutes after chopping; otherwise, heat destroys the cancer-protecting enzymes.

BEST FOR: **NEARLY ALL CANCERS**

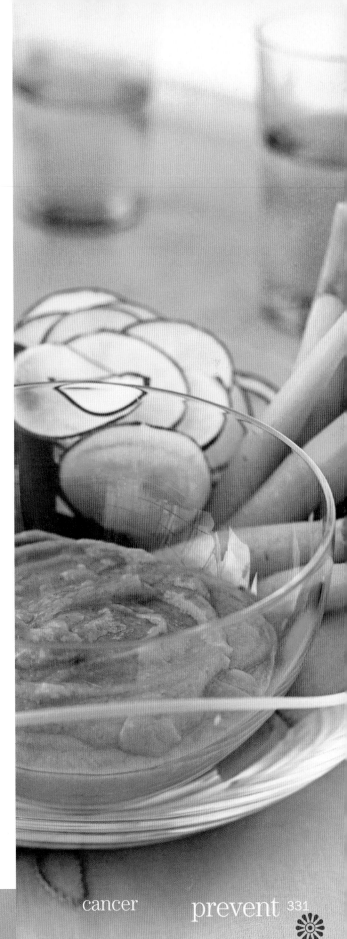

Top 5 Ways to Prevent Cancer

1. Stop smoking. Boring, redundant information you've heard a thousand times before. But consider this: If you smoke, you are 23 times more likely to develop lung cancer than someone who doesn't smoke. Compare that to a woman who had a first-degree relative (mother, sister, or daughter) diagnosed with breast cancer; her overall risk is only twice that of a woman with no first-degree relative diagnosed with breast cancer. Yet what do women tend to worry most about? Breast cancer.

2. Cut back on the alcohol. Drinking beyond healthy levels (generally, one serving a day) is a major cause of breast, bladder, stomach, esophageal, liver, and colon cancers, among others. Scientists suspect the link may be due to the effects of acetaldehyde, a suspected carcinogen that forms as the body metabolizes alcohol. This compound reacts with natural compounds that are required for cell growth. This reaction can cause DNA damage to cells, which can, in turn, lead to malfunctioning cell division.

3. Lose weight. About one in three cancers are the result of poor diet and being overweight, particularly breast, colon, rectal, stomach, prostate, and pancreatic cancers. When you're overweight, your body produces more estrogen—linked to breast, ovarian, and uterine cancers; and more insulin, which can increase inflammation and free-radical damage.

4. Eat right. In addition to getting seven to nine servings a day of fruits and vegetables, studies find that diets low in red meat and high in whole grains also result in lower levels of various cancers.

5. Get moving. Physical activity not only helps you maintain a healthy weight but also it reduces the percentage of body fat and helps your muscles better use insulin, reducing insulin blood levels and free-radical production. Specific studies find that regular physical activity can slash the risk of bowel cancer by half, the risk of uterine cancer by a third, as well as significantly reduce the risk of ovarian, breast, and colon cancers.

Have sex. No, we're not kidding. An eight-year study of 29,342 men ages 46 to 81 found that the more orgasms the men had, the lower their risk of prostate cancer. Specifically, those who had at least 21 orgasms per month slashed their risk of the disease by a third, compared to those who only had four to seven a month. The mechanism at work here? The prostate makes semen; the more you ejaculate, the more potentially cancerous cells you're getting rid of (and no, they won't hurt your partner). If you don't have a partner, or one who isn't willing, don't worry. The benefit comes from ejaculating, which, as you no doubt know, doesn't require a partner.
BEST FOR: **PROSTATE CANCER**

Spoon on some tomato sauce. Lycopene, an important antioxidant in tomatoes, pack a heck of an anti-cancer wallop. Just 10 tomatoes a week reduces the risk of prostate cancer by a third and the risk of breast cancer up to 50 percent. The thing is, you get way more lycopene if the tomatoes are cooked, which releases more of the chemical. Even just gently heating a chopped tomato will up the content.
BEST FOR: **PROSTATE, BREAST, AND ESOPHAGEAL CANCER**

Drink water like a thirsty camel. The more water you drink, the more you dilute toxins in food and other liquids, reducing their damaging effects on your colon and bladder. One major study found that just six 8-ounce glasses of water every day slashed the risk of bladder cancer in half in men; while another found a 45 percent reduced risk of colon cancer in women who drank a lot of water throughout the day. To avoid a huge pile of plastic bottles, keep a pitcher of filtered water in your fridge at home and at work, and make sure you empty it at least once, preferably twice, a day.
BEST FOR: **COLON AND BLADDER CANCER.**

Chronic Pain

Slam your finger in the car door and it hurts. No, it *really* hurts. But after a few minutes and an application of ice, the pain recedes to a dull throb. By tomorrow, only the bruise remains to remind you of the incident. You've just experienced acute pain—pain related to a specific cause, like a burn, bump, or broken bone.

But for 4 out of 10 adults age 65 and older, pain isn't linked to a specific cause, and it doesn't go away. They're suffering from chronic pain, which becomes more common with age.

Acute pain occurs when electrical signals from the damaged tissue travel to the brain in a process called nociception. You don't actually feel the pain until the signal hits the brain. But with chronic pain, you may experience the pain even without an obvious reason. That's because your nervous system begins generating its own electrical signals—irrespective of any injury. Those messages travel to the brain and activate pain centers in a kind of feedback loop from the brain to the nerves and back again that's become stuck in the "on" position.

This is no small thing. Chronic pain significantly affects the quality of your life, increasing your risk of depression, keeping you from the health-enhancing benefits of socializing, and disrupting your sleep. It can even affect your cognitive functioning, including memory and learning ability.

Chronic pain becomes more common with age mostly because of the decades of wear and tear on your body. After five or six decades of active living, you naturally become more likely to experience ongoing pain from arthritis, worn joints, or weakened bones. And if you have certain chronic health conditions like diabetes, you can develop neuropathies—or nerve pain—that are the result of decades of damage to nerve cells (in the case of diabetes, from high blood sugar levels). Back pain is particularly common with age (up to half of all those age 65 and older cope with it daily), due largely to mechanics: The bones and muscles that bear so much of the burden of keeping you upright also are the primary guardians of your largest nerves.

Then there is disease-related pain. Older people are more likely than their younger counterparts to experience pain related to chronic health conditions such as coronary artery disease, Alzheimer's, chronic obstructive pulmonary disorder (COPD), and Parkinson's. As the chronic condition impacts your ability to remain physically active, the pain increases. The more you hurt, the less you move and socialize, making both the chronic condition and your pain worse in a debilitating downward cycle.

That is the harsh side of the pain discussion. There is a positive side as well. Over the past decade, the medical world has made huge strides not only in understanding pain and its remedies but also in how to help communicate with patients regarding pain. The latter point is important; it wasn't long ago that pain was seen as a side issue to other health problems, either to be coped with or dealt with via strong painkillers—many of which have proven to have serious side effects.

Today, intelligent, multifaceted pain management is the norm, with pain specialists often available to you, particularly if the pain is part of a larger health issue.

The message: no one, NO ONE, need to suffer in silence from chronic pain.

Managing Pain the Smart Way

It would be great to give you the perfect mix of tips to guarantee that you won't ever face chronic pain, but it's not possible. There is just too wide a range of causes, from disease to injury to old-fashioned wear and tear.

While we have to acknowledge that pain becomes more prevalent with age, there are effective ways to minimize it, and in some cases, erase it. And so, here you are: Eleven proven, smart ways to control ongoing pain. If you're already taking pain relievers, these tips may allow you to use less medication, or to forgo it altogether.

Hit the stationary bike. You can also try the treadmill. Studies show that exercise can be a powerful antidote to pain. There are many reasons: Strong muscles take pressure off joints; exercise washes your body with nourishing oxygen and nutrients, and it also releases feel-good brain chemicals that provide relaxation and relief. The key is to go for more than 10 minutes—shorter bouts don't seem to help. In fact, nearly any type of physical exercise will significantly improve your pain—as long as you stick with it (even after you start feeling better).

Say "ohhmmm." Okay, you don't really have to chant, but meditating can do more for low back pain in older adults than any over-the-counter drug. In a study published in the journal *Pain*, 37 adults age 65 and older either joined a mindfulness-based meditation program that met weekly for eight weeks, or were wait-listed for the program (the control group). Those meditating significantly improved their scores on an objective pain scale and upped their activity levels compared to the control group. Another study found that people who listened to a seven-minute tape that helped them relax, focus on the images their pain elicited, and then change those images with their mind described their pain as "more tolerable" or "easier to control" than a control group. This type of guided imagery can be learned in a class or through tapes available online and in most health food stores.

Sign on for biofeedback. Biofeedback teaches you to control involuntary reactions, voluntarily. For instance, instead of tensing

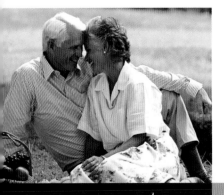

Not every pain can be diagnosed or explained. But *all* pain can be reduced and managed. You owe it to yourself to do so.

when you feel pain, which can make the pain worse, you learn to relax, which stems the release of pain-inducing stress hormones. In one study, 17 participants between the ages of 55 and 78 learned to use biofeedback to relax their muscles and breathe more slowly and deeply. Not only did their pain improve, but they were able to elicit certain physiological changes that contributed to the decrease in pain. For instance, their skin temperature increased, indicating more blood flow to the painful area, which helps clear away toxins and inflammatory chemicals that may be adding to the hurt.

Join a group. It doesn't matter what the group does—tear apart the latest best-seller or the latest political leader (figuratively, of course)—as long as you're interacting with other people. Studies find that older people who keep busy and engaged, including maintaining a strong social network, have significantly less chronic pain than those without.

Become a student of pain management. Ask your doctor for information about educational classes for people with chronic pain. Simply learning the whys and wherefores of your pain can significantly improve it! These programs typically include information about the causes of pain, pain assessment, medications, and nondrug approaches. You might also want to bring a family member along so they can better understand your experiences and the most effective approaches.

See a therapist. Cognitive behavioral therapy teaches you to avoid negative thinking and self-defeating behavior (i.e., I hurt too much to take a walk), and provides positive reinforcement for achieving your goals (i.e., taking that walk!). It also teaches you coping skills for better managing pain. You should see results in just 6 to 15

Assessing Pain

Pain is so subjective that it's often difficult to describe to other people, including doctors. It's also impossible to measure—there is no "pain" chemical or virus you can test for. So doctors often rely on simple rating systems as a way to determine the intensity of your pain. They often are as easy as rating your pain on a scale from 1 to 10, or picking a drawing of a face that best portrays the pain level (they range from smiling happily to crazy grimacing).

Another way doctors monitor pain is through nonverbal indicators, such as these.

Vocal complaints: moans, gasps, sighs, or exclamations

Facial expressions: such as grimaces, winces, clenched teeth, furrowed brows, or narrowed eyes

Bracing movements: clutching a railing or grabbing a body part

Rubbing movements: massaging the affected area

sessions. Ask your doctor to recommend someone experienced in working with pain patients.

Follow an anti-inflammatory diet. Chronic inflammation is often the culprit behind chronic pain, particularly with conditions such as rheumatoid arthritis. And the cause of much of the inflammation in your arteries and the rest of your body is from free radicals, those destructive molecules that damage cells. An anti-inflammatory diet has two main components: lots of antioxidants to neutralize free radicals in your bloodstream, and plenty of healthy fats like olive oil to reduce inflammation. So what do you eat?

- One to two vegetable and/or fruit servings with each meal (even breakfast)
- Some form of fatty fish (salmon, tuna, anchovies) at least once a week

- A daily helping of soy—edamame (soybeans), a cup of soy milk, tofu cubes, even soy-based frozen desserts are all good options

- Flaxseeds sprinkled over salads and yogurt and mixed into sauces

- Olive oil as your primary cooking and salad-dressing oil

- Foods like asparagus, avocado, and walnuts

And here's what to limit or remove entirely from your diet:

- Fats like butter, corn and vegetable oil, and shortening

- Red meats high in saturated fats

- "Simple" carbs, particularly those high in sugar and low in fiber, like candy, doughnuts, cakes, and sodas

Munch some cherries. Cherries are high in anti-inflammatory anthocyanins, plant-based chemicals that give the fruit its dark red color. Some studies find that these chemicals can reduce the pain of arthritis and gout, as well as swelling and inflammation.

Have a sweet. This contradicts our advice for an anti-inflammatory diet, but during times in which pain is an issue, sweet foods (think dark chocolate) can stimulate the release of pain-relieving endorphins in the brain. That's why newborns often get sugar water to suck on during painful procedures, such as collecting blood from their heels.

Obviously, you can't sit around all day eating chocolate truffles, but letting one melt slowly in your mouth when the pain gets really bad can help you relax and tolerate it until other remedies kick in.

Try chiropractic. The evidence behind the use of chiropractic care for certain painful conditions such as back and neck pain is irrefutable. Not only do numerous studies show it is effective but also it is more cost-effective than physical therapy or traditional doctor visits and pain medication—an important consideration if you're living on a fixed income.

Consider acupuncture. This ancient healing practice in which very thin needles, pressure, or electricity are used to stimulate certain parts of your body, called meridians, has entered the mainstream when it comes to pain management. Acupuncture stimulates the release of feel-good endorphins into your spinal fluid, where they serve as a kind of buffer to prevent pain signals from reaching your brain. Acupuncture has been used successfully with few, if any, side effects to treat back pain, neck pain, osteoarthritis, fibromyalgia, and generalized pain. One German study even found that it was more effective than massage for neck pain. One caveat: You may need repeat treatments if your pain is chronic.

3 Pain Enhancers to Avoid

Yes, there are things you might be doing that inadvertently make your pain worse. Here are the biggest culprits:

Sedentary living. When you hurt, the last thing you want to do is move. But that's exactly what you must do. As stated before, studies find that regular, moderate exercise not only benefits pain from osteoarthritis and other conditions, but may help prevent it. For instance, strengthening your core muscles through sit-ups and other similar activities can prevent or improve back pain, just as strengthening your quadriceps, or thigh muscles, through squats and similar movements can relieve knee pain. Exercise can even help with the pain of neuropathy, common in people with diabetes, by making your muscle cells more receptive to insulin and reducing the damaging effects of high blood sugar on nerve cells and blood vessels.

Fear. If your doctor has prescribed medication to help you manage your pain, use it as suggested. Don't wait until the pain is so severe you can't stand it. By then, the medication probably won't help. Taking your medication at the first sign of breakthrough pain provides much greater relief. Many people avoid prescription pain drugs because they fear becoming addicted. Given the news stories of the past few years, everyone is keenly aware of painkiller addiction issues, and most doctors will avoid giving you something that could be addicting, unless absolutely necessary. Also, while you may grow tolerant to some pain relievers, needing higher doses does not mean that you are addicted to them. In any case, do not be shy about discussing any misgivings you have about medications with your doctor.

Depression. Slightly more than half of chronic pain patients seen in pain clinics also have major depression, and low doses of antidepressants are often prescribed to treat chronic pain. The linkage may come from brain chemicals like serotonin, dopamine, and norepinephrine, which play a role in both conditions. That doesn't mean that the two conditions are one and the same; thus, it's important that your doctor treat your depression *and* your chronic pain so you can find relief from both, rather than just treating one and hoping the other improves.

A Habit Worth Breaking

Next time you have a headache or your arthritis flares, stop before you swallow those mainstay medicines of pain relief: **ibuprofen** or **aspirin**. Older people have been systematically excluded from most clinical studies on nonsteroidal anti-inflammatory drugs (NSAIDs), the category of drug under which ibuprofen and aspirin fall. As it turns out, older people are most likely to experience one of NSAIDs' few troublesome side effects—stomach bleeding. The risk of **gastrointestinal (GI) bleeding** in the general population is about 1 percent; for those age 60 and older, it's 3 to 4 percent; and for those with a history of GI bleeding, it's about 9 percent.

If you need medication to control your pain, you may wish to start with acetaminophen, which is milder on most people's digestive systems. If prescription-grade relief is necessary, you may be better off with opioids like codeine and morphine, low-dose corticosteroid therapy, or antidepressants or anticonvulsants, depending on the type of pain you're experiencing. One caveat: If your doctor prescribes narcotic pain relievers, make sure you take the smallest possible dose. Older people tend to be more sensitive to the effects of these drugs, getting stronger and longer pain relief on much smaller doses than younger individuals.

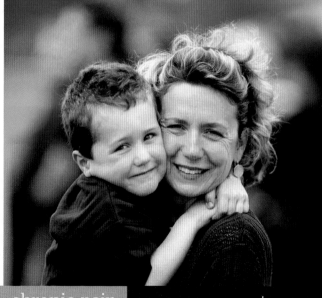

Memory Problems

You've misplaced your car keys, lost your cell phone in the laundry, and can't recall the name of that interesting new book club member. You listened to the weather report this morning but … will you need a sun hat or an umbrella this afternoon? And did your doctor want you to take that new medicine twice a day—or once every other day?

Stereotypes would have you believe that memory loss is a part of growing old. In one survey of older people, it was ranked as the most-feared health problem—even ahead of cancer, heart disease, and diabetes. It's no wonder: Until recently, the conventional wisdom said that memory glitches and fuzzy thinking couldn't be prevented—let alone fixed. Scientists thought that brain cells simply died out, never to be replaced. And what's more frightening to envision than an old version of ourselves, physically healthy but with greatly diminished memories and mental skills?

But today, the story is far more positive—and fascinating. New research shows that the brain can grow new neurons and stronger, more prolific connections between brain cells at any age—and all it takes is a little physical and mental exercise to make it happen.

New Thinking about Memory

In study after study, researchers are discovering that a wide variety of brain "fertilizers"—from exercise to good fats in your diet, from brain-training exercises to simply socializing more often with the neighbors—can promote the development of healthy, new connections between brain cells and even spur the growth of *new* brain cells. In turn, these stronger connections and fresh new neurons may prevent or even reverse age-related memory lapses and sharpen thinking skills. Keeping your brain well-"fertilized" may even lower your risk for major problems like dementia and Alzheimer's disease.

The truth is that we all need this kind of "fertilizer" more and more with every passing decade. For while it's easy to blame memory lapses, concentration problems, and slowed-down thinking on a bad night's sleep or on stress, aging itself *does* affect the human brain. Experts at the Keck Center for Integrative Neurosciences at the University of California, San Francisco, say that the changes start in your thirties and by age 60, your brain takes in information two to three times slower than a 20-year-old brain—so the information you store in memory is two to three times less sharp and detailed. By age 80, you may be five to eight times slower.

If you're concerned about sudden changes in memory or thinking skills—or are worried that memory problems are interfering with your ability to live your everyday life—see your doctor. Other factors that can affect memory include medication side effects (especially from sleeping pills), medical problems such as thyroid disorders or depression, dehydration, a nutritional deficiency, or a head injury. (See "When to Get Help").

For most people, gradual mental decline can be stopped and reversed. If you'd like to sharpen your memory and thinking skills to avoid losses, or reverse minor problems, these 16 strategies are proven winners. Be prepared for a surprise: The first several tips are all about controlling other health issues that once were considered independent of brain function, but in recent years have proven to have a big effect on your thinking skills.

Balance your cholesterol. A growing stack of evidence links high levels of "bad" LDL cholesterol and low levels of "good" HDL cholesterol with memory problems. The same steps that protect against heart attack and stroke guard your little gray cells, too. In one Harvard University study of 4,081 women age 65 and older, those with the highest levels of "good" HDL cholesterol had the highest scores on tests of memory and thinking skills. And in another study of 1,037 older women, those with the highest levels of "bad" LDLs were twice as likely to have memory problems as those with the lowest levels.

Pampering your cardiovascular system—with all the steps outlined earlier—keeps large and small blood vessels in your brain more flexible and free of artery-clogging plaque. This helps guard against vascular dementia—loss of memory and thinking skills that develops when brain cells simply don't receive the oxygen and blood sugar they need to function properly.

Tame high blood pressure. Some doctors have long feared that treating high blood pressure in older people could lead to problems with memory and thinking. But the opposite is actually the case. In a study that tracked 848 men from middle age to old age, researchers at the Pacific Health Research Institute in Honolulu

When to Get Help

Be sure to see your doctor if you have these warning signs of more serious memory loss.

- A sudden or significant decline in your ability to remember facts or assigned tasks
- Repeating phrases or stories in the same conversation
- Trouble making choices or handling money
- Not being able to keep track of what happens each day
- Asking the same questions over and over again
- Getting lost in places you know well
- Not being able to follow directions
- Getting very confused about time, people, and places
- Not taking care of yourself—eating poorly, not bathing, or being unsafe

found that those whose blood pressures were under control the longest were 60 percent less likely to develop dementia than those whose blood pressures were out of control.

Untamed blood pressure damages blood vessels in the brain, leading to the formation of tiny blood clots that starve brain cells of the nutrition and oxygen they need.

Control your blood sugar. Diabetes doubles your odds for memory problems later in life. Experts aren't sure why, but there is some evidence that the chronic inflammation that can help trigger type 2 diabetes can also contribute to the buildup of brain tangles and plaques linked to Alzheimer's disease. Your brain Rx: The same lifestyle steps that lower your blood sugar—a healthy high-fiber, low-sugar diet plus exercise and stress relief—are good for your brain, too.

Maintain a healthy weight. Extra pounds dimmed brain power in a study from the Toulouse University Hospital and the National Institute of Health and Medical Research in France. Researchers checked the body mass index (BMI) and thinking skills of 2,223 women and men, ages 32 to 62, twice over five years. People with high BMIs scored lower on memory tests and had bigger mental declines from the beginning until the end of the study. The cause could be reduced blood flow to the brain.

Sweat a little. People who exercised three or more times a week were 30 to 40 percent less likely to develop dementia than those who were active less often, says a study of 1,740 Seattle-area residents, age 65 and older. Study volunteers walked, hiked, swam, lifted weights, stretched, and did aerobics or other activities for as little as 15 minutes at a time, but the benefits were big.

What's happening? Lab studies show that exercise boosts production of a wonder chemical called brain-derived neurotrophic factor (BDNF)—a sort of cell fertilizer that encourages nerve cells in the brain to multiply, get stronger, and become more resistant to damage and disease. Some studies even suggest that exercise can make brain cells that are already damaged healthier.

Take depression seriously. Low mood, lack of interest in everyday activities, and lack of pleasure are warning signs of depression. But in

Help Your Brain remember

Creating a strong memory is like taking a good vacation photograph: You have to focus, capture the image, and then store it so that you can easily retrieve it again later. Here's how to work with your brain's natural information-processing and storage machinery to improve your memory.

Focus on one thing (or person) at a time.
No multitasking! Your brain needs at least eight seconds of focused attention to "process" information and send it successfully into long-term storage.

Find—and use—your natural "learning style."
You're a visual learner if you tend to say "see what I mean" in conversation or if you look at the pictures or diagrams most when assembling something (such as a toy or piece of furniture). You're an auditory learner if you prefer verbal or written instructions. Use your natural style when learning new info to send your brain the strongest signals possible.

Rehearse.
Hoping to remember the names of the five new people you met at the party yesterday? Practice them tonight, and again tomorrow morning, as you recall their faces. Brain scientists call this spaced rehearsal and say that it refreshes memory more effectively than trying to hastily recall the names five minutes before your next meeting.

older people, depression is often misdiagnosed as dementia and can be virtually ignored. If you or a loved one has any signs of depression, regardless of their age, alert the doctor and demand help. You deserve to feel well and to think clearly!

Schedule a daily "relaxation appointment" with yourself. Best time to do it: mid-afternoon, when natural body rhythms are likely making you feel like taking a break. Try 10 minutes of yoga, a cup of herbal tea and a good book, a leisurely stroll with a friend, or some hands-on time with your favorite hobby. Relaxation can lower levels of the stress hormone cortisol; unchecked, it can damage a brain area called the hippocampus, which is involved with processing information and storing memories. Cortisol can damage the hippocampus if the stress is unrelieved.

Get the sleep you need. Your brain needs sleep in order to organize and store information in memory so that you can retrieve and use it again, studies show. If you're tired during the day, it will be even more difficult to concentrate and remember important things. Sleep patterns do change with age—read all about how to get a refreshing night's sleep on page 299.

Sip cocoa. When researchers at the University of Nottingham in England scanned the brains of 16 women who'd just finished mugs of specially-processed hot cocoa, they found that blood flow to some brain regions rose—and stayed high for two to three hours. In their cups: CocoaVia, a hot chocolate produced by candymaker Mars that's rich in flavonols, antioxidants also shown to improve blood flow to the heart. A piece of dark chocolate might do the trick as well.

Eat fish three times a week. Higher blood levels of an omega-3 fatty acid called docosa-hexanoic acid (DHA)—found in fatty fish like

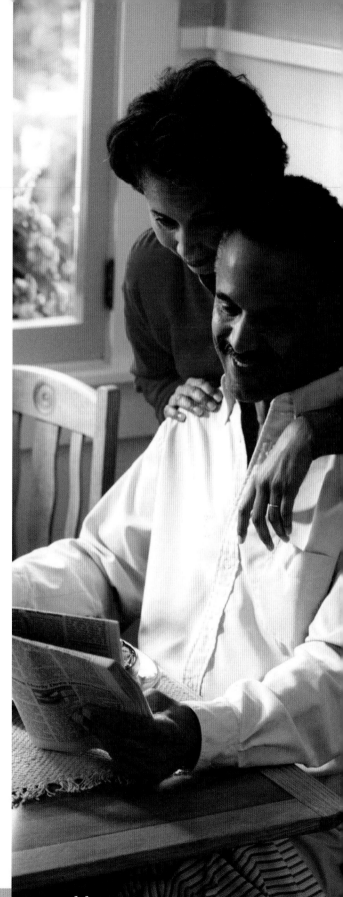

salmon, sardines, and mackerel—cut dementia risk by 47 percent in a 2006 study of 899 older women and men conducted by Tufts University in Boston.

Eating three fish entrées a week led to the highest DHA levels, but if you hate fin food, try fish-oil capsules. A 2006 Swedish study found that taking them cut the rate of mental decline in people with mild Alzheimer's disease.

Sip 100 percent juice. A daily glass of fruit or veggie juice lowered odds for Alzheimer's disease by a whopping 76 percent in a 2006 study of 1,836 women and men, conducted by researchers from Vanderbilt University School of Medicine in Nashville. Antioxidants called polyphenols, which are in rich supply in 100 percent apple, grape, and citrus juices, protect the brain.

Have berries at breakfast. Compounds in black currants and boysenberries seem to block cell damage that leads to Alzheimer's disease, say researchers at the Horticulture and Food Research Institute of New Zealand. But other berries are equally rich in cell-protecting antioxidants. While a healthy diet may not ever cure Alzheimer's, scientists say it could delay its onset or even prevent it from happening in the first place.

Dine on beans 'n' greens ... and broccoli and whole grains. All are rich in folic acid, a B vitamin that improved memory and information-processing speed in a 2007 study of 819 women and men conducted by researchers at the Wageningen University in the Netherlands.

Enjoy a glass of red wine. A glass for women, up to two for men, may cut your risk for Alzheimer's disease and dementia. The reason? Experts suspect that compounds in red wine improve blood flow and cut your odds for blood clots—the same reasons that a moderate amount of alcohol can be good for your heart. But take it easy—overdoing it damages brain cells.

Visit, call, write, or e-mail friends and family every day. Spending time with family and friends, volunteering, or joining a group helps stimulate your memory, concentration, and mental processing. One study showed that regular socializing cut dementia risk by 42 percent. When researchers from Chicago's Rush University Medical Center delved into the brains of 89 Chicago-area residents who had been dementia-free, they found something surprising: They actually had the brain plaques and "tangles" associated with Alzheimer's disease, yet they had had no signs of memory loss or thinking problems. Having a strong social network, the researchers say, seems to strengthen brain pathways that protect thinking skills.

Play brain games. Do something you love—today, tomorrow, and every day. In a study of 469 healthy people over age 75, researchers from Albert Einstein College of Medicine in New York found that those who often played board games, read books and magazines, played a musical instrument, or did crossword puzzles were less likely to develop dementia than those who rarely did these things.

There are also dozens of books and computer games on the market with special mental exercises that promise to make your brain younger. There's some scientific evidence that these may work, but experts say you probably don't need a special game to fine-tune your skills. Just try to challenge your brain in as many different ways as possible: Learn a new language or a new musical instrument; if you're a whiz at crossword puzzles, cross-train with math problems such as Sudoku; if you're a math whiz, take up crossword puzzles. Try an intricate new hobby, and find daily ways to wake up your brain cells:

Take a new route to the supermarket, comb your hair with your nondominant hand, or eat breakfast for lunch.

3 Memory-Robbers to Avoid

These three things contribute mightily to declining mental function.

Tobacco. Smoking cigarettes or cigars constricts important arteries that deliver oxygen to your brain. It raises your odds for stroke and for vascular dementia—inadequate blood flow to brain cells—and doubles the chances that you'll develop Alzheimer's disease.

Endless hours of TV. In one Case Western Reserve University study in Ohio, TV-watchers had a higher risk for dementia. The more TV, the higher the odds. Even a high-minded documentary doesn't stimulate thought and brain connections the way that talking with friends, pursuing hobbies, learning new things, and even playing games can.

Head injuries. Skip the roller coaster and other brain-jarring thrill rides: There's evidence that high-speed amusement-park rides that whip your head from side to side or up and down may cause minor bleeding inside the brain. Experts also suggest that you wear a helmet if you bike or ski, always buckle your seat belt in the car, and keep your home clear of obstructions and slippery spots that could lead to a fall. Any injury to your brain changes blood flow patterns, affects cellular connections, and can contribute to a decline in memory function.

Try Something New

Have you ever gotten dressed with your eyes closed? Turned all the photos on your desk upside-down for the day? Brushed your teeth with your nondominant hand? Or woken up to the smell of vanilla or oregano instead of the usual aroma of coffee?

Surprising your brain with these unfamiliar experiences could help stimulate underused nerve cells in parts of the brain linked to memory and abstract thought, says Duke University Medical Center neurobiology professor Lawrence Katz, PhD. Nerve cells in these key areas tend to shrink with age, reducing the brain's ability to process new information and to retrieve old data.

Dr. Katz suggests trying daily "**neurobics**"—aerobics for the brain. These fun exercises use your senses and force you to think in new ways. Research shows that this kind of brain stimulation prompts the release of neurotrophins, fertilizer-like chemicals that encourage the growth of bigger, more-complex dendrites—the branches that nerve cells use to transmit, receive, and process information.

More neurobics to try: Search for your house keys in your purse, using only your fingers (don't look!). Take a new route to a familiar place. Reverse the order of stops you make in your local supermarket. Type an e-mail or letter with one hand. Dance to music with an unusual beat. Figure out how to say words or sentences backward, or play other creative word games. One fun one: See how long a sentence you can make using words that all start with the same letter or two letters (try "cr" and "st" to start!).

Arthritis

A guy walks into his doctor's office. The doctor asks "What's wrong?"

"It's my left knee," the patient says. "It hurts when I walk."

"Well, you're 70," says the doctor. "That's what happens as you get older."

"But doc," the patient says, "my right knee is the same age, and it feels fine!"

The message? Arthritis is not an inevitable consequence of getting older, nor should it be treated that way. These days, even teenagers, particularly superathletes spending more time on the soccer field than in the classroom, are turning up with arthritis—and they're certainly not old.

Yet one in four patients seen by primary care physicians are there because of musculoskeletal problems; and among those over 65, the most common complaint is osteoarthritis. The condition affects 50 percent of those 65 and older, and up to 85 percent of those 75 and older.

Osteoarthritis results from microscopic damage in the structure and makeup of cartilage—the soft slippery tissue that covers the ends of bones in a joint. When cartilage is healthy, your bones glide smoothly over one another, the cartilage acting as a kind of shock absorber for movement. But when you have osteoarthritis, that surface layer of cartilage has worn down, allowing the bones to rub together. The result? Pain, swelling, and loss of motion. Over time, bone spurs called osteophytes might grow on the edges of the joint, and bits of bone or cartilage can even break off and float inside the joint space, increasing the pain.

Over the past 20 years, researchers have discovered that the underlying causes of many diseases are different than what we had once thought, and that's true, too, with osteoporosis.

In this case, scientists now suspect that the damage lies with cells that help maintain normal cartilage, called chondrocytes. Genetics and wear and tear contribute to chondrocyte damage, impacting their ability to maintain healthy cartilage. In particular, injury and biomechanical stress (that is, how you walk and move) are tough on chondrocytes. With each injury, additional blood and oxygen rush into the area to help repair the damage. This creates oxidative damage, accelerating chondrocyte death and leading to osteoarthritis.

As little as 20 years ago, doctors primarily treated arthritis with medication and rest. Today, they're more likely to prescribe a set of isometric exercises and a 20-minute walk than any type of pill. A comprehensive treatment plan also includes nutritional advice, relaxation, and nonmedical methods of pain relief.

The following provides you with some of the latest thinking on how to prevent osteoarthritis or, if you already have it, reduce the pain and disability without reaching for drugs.

Best Ways to Prevent Arthritis

Focus on your weight. There's no mincing around with words here: If you're overweight, you're much more likely to develop arthritis, particularly of the knees, probably because the weight puts extra stress on weight-bearing joints, eventually damaging the cartilage. Lose just 1 pound, and you put 4 fewer pounds of pressure on your knees, according to a study from Wake Forest University researchers in Winston-Salem, North Carolina.

The researchers also found that even a 10 percent weight loss can significantly improve overall function. While losing pounds is important, studies also suggest that reducing your percentage of body fat and increasing your muscle strength provide the biggest bang for the buck when it comes to improving the pain and disability of arthritis, as well as reducing the initial risk. One of the best ways to do that is with strength training.

Concentrate on your quadriceps. These are the muscles in your upper thighs. The stronger they are, the more strain they take off your knees. Reducing the strain reduces the risk of injury to chondrocytes. Good exercises are squats, knee extensions, and step-ups (in which you use your stairs as exercise equipment).

Tilt your face toward the sun. Unless you live in a very northern climate, about 15 to 20 minutes a day should do it. Sunlight is your best source of vitamin D, which is required for healthy bones. Bone strength is important when it comes to arthritis because as cartilage tries to repair itself after injury, it triggers bone remodeling—loss or addition of bone cells. A Boston University study that evaluated vitamin D intake in 62 people with arthritic knees and 126 people with normal knees found that those with low D levels in their diet and blood were three times more likely to have arthritis than those with high levels. This finding is particularly important for older people, who are less able to absorb vitamin D from the sun as they age.

Habits Worth Breaking

Give up the high-heeled shoes. Harvard University researchers wondered if the fact that women are twice as likely to develop osteoarthritis might have something to do with the high-heeled shoes they wear. They studied 20 healthy women as they walked in their own high-heeled shoes and barefoot. Researchers found that walking in high heels increases pressure across a major joint in the knee called the patellofemoral joint and puts 23 percent more force on the inner part of the knee, both of which could lead to joint damage and osteoarthritis. You don't have to be wearing 4-inch spikes; even shoes with 1.5-inch heels lead to greater twisting of the knee.

Aim for 400 to 800 international units (IU) of vitamin D a day. In addition to sunlight, other good sources are fatty fish like salmon, mackerel, and sardines (about 345 IU in a 3.5-ounce serving), fortified cereals and cereal bars, beef liver (30 IU in a 3.5-ounce serving), and egg yolks (25 IU in a whole egg).

Boil some kale. Kale is high in vitamin K, which plays an important role in the normal development of cartilage and bone. When researchers evaluated the diets of 672 people with an average age of 65, they found that the higher the levels of dietary vitamin K, the lower the likelihood of hand or knee arthritis. About half the study population had low blood levels of the vitamin. That's not surprising given that studies conducted in the United States and United Kingdom found that people in both countries have low vitamin K levels. The best sources of vitamin K are leafy greens like spinach, turnip greens, collards, Swiss chard, and raw parsley. Just 1/2 cup of boiled fresh kale, for instance, provides 660 percent of the recommended daily value.

Best Ways to Reduce Arthritis Pain

Hit the pool. Swimming has long been recommended as a good exercise for people with arthritis; the weightlessness from the water reduces impact on your joints. But there's been very little research into the benefits of the therapy. Finally, a Taiwanese study confirms what anyone with arthritis has long suspected: Working out in water significantly improves knee and hip flexibility, strength, and aerobic fitness. Meanwhile, an Australian study found that such programs also resulted in less pain and better overall function. Contact your local YMCA or community pool and ask about water aerobic classes or other programs specifically designed for those with arthritis.

Walk barefoot. Going au naturel reduces the load on knee joints, minimizing pain and disability from osteoarthritis by 12 percent compared to walking with shoes. That's the finding from a study of 75 people with osteoarthritis conducted by researchers at Rush University Medical Center in Chicago. If barefoot isn't an option, find shoes that mimic the natural arch and heel contour, but don't lift up the heel, which puts more pressure on the joints. Orthotics might be another option.

Rub on some cream. If your stomach has rebelled against over-the-counter and prescription pain relievers, attack the pain at its source with capsaicin cream. The cream contains high levels of the same compound that gives hot peppers their bite, and works by depleting a chemical called substance P that contributes to pain perception. But be patient; you may need to apply it several times a day for a week to 10 days before you feel any relief.

Best Supplements for Arthritis

Whatever you think about herbs and supplements, the research results are clear: Several natural supplements do make a difference when it comes to arthritis relief. Here are four to seriously consider.

Glucosamine sulfate. You've undoubtedly heard about the benefits of glucosamine/chondroitin supplements for joint repair. The best evidence is for glucosamine, an amino sugar required to build the substances needed to maintain and grow healthy cartilage. Numerous studies find that it can reduce the symptoms of osteoarthritis. Although it isn't a cure, it may prevent further damage. Take 1,500 milligrams at one time or in three divided doses, and be patient. It may take four to six weeks before you notice any improvement. Glucosamine supplements come from seashells, so stay away if you're allergic to shellfish.

SAMe (S-Adenyl-L-Methionine). You're probably most familiar with this supplement for mild depression. But it also works well in osteoarthritis, likely because of its anti-inflammatory properties. An analysis of 11 studies involving 1,442 people found that it worked as well as nonsteroidal anti-inflammatory drugs like aspirin or ibuprofen in terms of reducing pain and improving function, with fewer adverse effects such as stomach problems. Take 600 to 800 milligrams, and take it along with a B-50-complex vitamin.

Devil's claw. Another anti-inflammatory herb, Devil's Claw significantly improves pain and other symptoms related to arthritis, with some studies showing that it works just as well as prescription drugs but with fewer side effects. Take

2.6 grams a day of an extract standardized to 3 percent iridoid glycosides in divided dosages.

Boswellia. This anti-inflammatory herb, *Boswellia serrata,* comes from the Boswellia tree, commonly found in India. In one study, 30 patients with osteoarthritis of the knee took the extract for eight weeks, then took a placebo for eight weeks (although neither they nor the researchers knew what the participants received). When taking the herb, participants had less knee pain, greater range of motion, and could walk farther than when taking the placebo.

The Exercise Cure for arthritis

Researchers from Tufts University in Boston randomly split 46 people with knee osteoarthritis into two groups. The first group was assigned a 16-week, home-based strength-training program; the second, a nutritional education program (they were the control group). The results are hardly surprising: Those doing the strength training reduced their pain by 43 percent and increased their physical function by 38 percent. The comparable improvements for the control group were 11 percent and 21 percent.

Without question, exercise—not sitting—is the right response to arthritis. But a simple walk, while an excellent start, isn't enough. In addition to regular aerobic exercise like walking or swimming (experts suggest doing 20 to 30 minutes a day, three to four days per week), you need both range-of-motion exercises and strength training. Flexibility exercises increase the length and elasticity of your muscles, helping reduce stiffness, increase joint mobility, and prevent contractures. Strength training reinforces the muscles that support the affected joints.

The fitness programs in this book incorporate both types of exercises: Try the Easy Does It routine (page 200) as a start. To get the most out your efforts, follow this advice.

Flexibility Exercises

● Perform stretching exercises before bed, when your pain and stiffness are likely to be at their lowest.
● Take a warm shower or apply moist heat to the painful joint before beginning your stretching exercises to warm and relax the muscle.
● Relax before you begin, perhaps with some deep breathing exercises or focused mental imagery (imagine your muscles warming, lengthening, and becoming more flexible before you even start the first exercise).
● If your joint is inflamed, go easier on the stretching but don't give it up altogether.

Strength Training

● Do not work your muscles to the point of fatigue. The exercises you perform should be challenging, but doable without feeling you've reached your limits.
● Start out with one set of 4 to 6 repetitions of each movement twice weekly, increasing about 1 repetition a week until you reach 12.
● Breathe through each muscle contraction. For instance, if you're doing squats, keep inhaling as you squat down and hold the position; this keeps oxygenated blood flowing throughout your body and prevents a spike in blood pressure.
● If your joints hurt an hour after a strength-training bout, you've done too much.

Osteoporosis

We've all seen her, and it breaks our hearts: The stooped old woman whose gaze is fixed on a spot just in front of her feet. The one who has to sit down and lean back to look you in the eye. They used to call the dome shape on the backs of women like this a dowager's hump. But it's certainly not relegated only to rich ladies—or even women—and it's not a hump, but the result of years of compression fractures that have left her spine inches shorter and her body twisted.

That woman has an extreme case of osteoporosis, the most common bone disease in most countries, and one that affects an estimated 50 percent of women and 20 percent of men over age 50. Once thought to be an inevitable consequence of aging, today we know that osteoporosis is a preventable disease, one that, even if it does occur, can be arrested in its development and even reversed.

The best way to understand what goes on with your bones as you age is to think about your retirement fund. You've likely been socking away money for years, watching it grow, counting the interest, anticipating the day when you'll finally start making withdrawals. The goal, of course, is to ensure you don't outlive your money. The same is true of bone.

Throughout your life, cells called osteoblasts busily build bone, using hormones, vitamins, and minerals in a complex metabolic process to create the densest bone possible. At the same time, however, other cells called osteoclasts break down bone to supply calcium for other parts of your body, particularly your brain, muscles, and nervous system. That's why calcium intake is so important throughout your life; not so much to build strong bone, as the dairy industry would have you believe, but to provide the valuable mineral for the *rest* of your body so osteoclasts don't have to dissolve bone to get it.

Throughout your first 50 years, the osteoblasts have it over the osteoclasts and you build more bone than you lose. But as you age, the osteoclasts begin gaining until you start losing more bone than you build. This isn't so much of a problem if you have dense bone to begin with, just as retirement-fund withdrawals are fine as long as the principal remains relatively intact.

But if you never laid down enough bone to begin with, or if you're following a lifestyle that makes it easier to break down bone and harder to build up bone, then at some point, you find yourself with a deficit. When this happens, your bones become lacelike, with holes and paper-thin spots, and you can fracture your wrist simply by pushing open a heavy door. That is osteoporosis.

Best Ways to Prevent Osteoporosis

If you were reading this 15 years ago, you'd have been lucky to be evaluated for osteoporosis, let alone diagnosed. That's because there was nothing doctors could do if you had the disease.

Today, however, a plethora of medications and a greater understanding of the impact of lifestyle and diet on bone health have made osteoporosis not only treatable but eminently preventable. Here's some advice to give you a great start at preventing or slowing the onset of this troublesome bone disease.

Stop smoking. Researchers helped 152 postmenopausal women who smoked at least 10 cigarettes a day to quit. After one smoke-free year, total hip bone mineral density increased by 1.52 percent, an amount more significant than it sounds. In addition, bone mineral density in the upper thigh bone increased 2.9 percent among quitters.

Hit the weight room. Strengthening exercises build up more than just muscle; they increase bone density, too. While walking and other aerobic exercises are important to maintain bone throughout your life, regular strength workouts, like those beginning on page 201, provide the most significant benefits.

Load up on calcium. Get it in your diet and, just for good measure, take a daily calcium citrate supplement. The seminal study on this involved 301 healthy postmenopausal women who took 500 milligrams per day of calcium citrate, calcium carbonate, or a placebo for two years. Those taking calcium citrate had small improvements in bone mineral density in their hip bones and less bone mineral density loss in their spines. Those taking calcium carbonate only maintained the bone mineral density in their hips and showed no change in the density of their spinal bone. As it turned out, calcium citrate is the form of the mineral best absorbed; take half in the morning and half at night.

Pop some D. Calcium is great, but it is just one part of the nutritional needs of bone. Without vitamin D, calcium can't get into your bones.

Taking Blood Thinners?

If you answered yes, and you believe you are at risk of developing osteoporosis, talk with your doctor. Older people taking the blood thinner warfarin (Coumadin) have a significantly increased risk of fractures from osteoporosis. The correlation is likely due to vitamin K, which affects bone strength. But warfarin interferes with your body's absorption of vitamin K, possibly affecting bone density. So ask your doctor about other options.

The results can be devastating. In one study of women with osteoporosis hospitalized for hip fractures, half had a vitamin D deficiency. Meanwhile, the Women's Health Initiative study, a 15-year-long investigation of the health of postmenopausal women, found that the more consistent women were in taking calcium and vitamin D supplements, the lower their risk of osteoporosis. It doesn't take long for the supplements to show a benefit, investigators found; just two to three years of consistent use reduced the risk of hip fracture by 29 percent. Although study participants took 1,000 milligrams of calcium carbonate and 400 international units (IUs) of vitamin D, the researchers suspect they would have seen an even larger benefit if the vitamin D supplement was upped to 600 IU. In addition to supplements, exposing your arms and legs, or hands, arms, and face to the sun two or three times a week for 5 to 10 minutes can also guarantee sufficient vitamin D intake.

Switch to decaf. A study of 96 women with an average age of 71 found that those getting more than 300 milligrams of caffeine a day (the amount in two to three cups of regular coffee) had much higher rates of bone loss than women getting less. The really interesting thing here is that the bone loss only occurred in women with

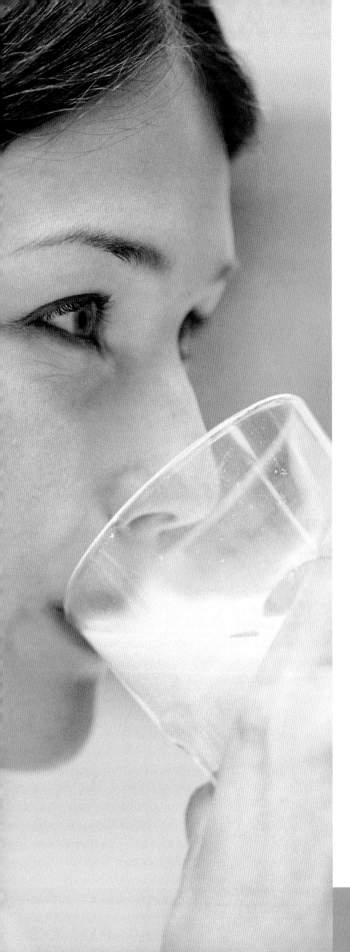

a certain gene that affects how the body uses vitamin D. If you have a family history of osteoporosis, you may have this genotype and could significantly benefit from cutting out caffeine.

Switch from soda to skim milk or water. When researchers measured the bone mineral density at the spine and hips of 1,413 women, they found that those who drank soda every day—whether regular, diet, or decaffeinated—had average hip bone mineral densities 3.7 percent lower and spine densities 5.4 percent lower than those drinking less than one soda a month.

Take an exercise class. Whether it's a resistance training, agility training, or general stretching class, it can reduce the risk of falling between 37 and 43 percent, according to Canadian researchers from British Columbia Women's Hospital and Health Center Osteoporosis Program. They found that the benefit persisted up to a year after the classes ended, even if the women didn't continue the exercise. This is critical because falling is the major cause of fractures in people with osteoporosis.

Shape up your cholesterol levels. High levels of "bad" LDL and low levels of "good" HDL increases the risk of fractures of the vertebrae in postmenopausal women. Plus, a study from researchers at Alberta University in Canada found that women with osteopenia (a forerunner of osteoporosis) or osteoporosis of the lower spine and hip were more likely to have high cholesterol levels. Meanwhile, other studies suggest that people taking statins, the most commonly prescribed medication for high cholesterol, have a 60 percent reduced risk of fracture.

Cholesterol levels are also important when it comes to prevention. When University of California, Los Angeles, researchers compared mice fed a high-fat diet designed to raise cholesterol levels with those fed a normal diet, they found a 43 percent decrease in mineral content and a 15 percent decrease in bone density in the leg bones of the high-fat-diet mice. One link between cholesterol and osteoporosis may be that free radicals resulting from oxidized cholesterol molecules prevent osteoblasts from functioning normally to build up bone.

Add a fruit or veggie to every meal. While calcium and vitamin D get all the glory when it comes to osteoporosis prevention, a Scottish study of 62 healthy women between ages 45 and 55 found that those who consumed the greatest amounts of foods containing zinc, magnesium, potassium, fiber, and vitamin C had the highest bone mineral density. Best sources of all these micronutrients? Fresh fruits and vegetables.

Munch on some dried plums. What used to be known as prunes may hold the key to restoring bone loss in postmenopausal women. A study from Florida State University found that supplementing your diet with about 9 or 10 dried plums a day improves markers of bone formation in postmenopausal women. Meanwhile, feeding dried plums to rats whose ovaries had been removed (putting them into menopause) significantly restored bone mass. Researchers don't know exactly why the dried fruit has such an effect but suspect that it's related to an increased rate of bone formation through some plant-based chemicals on osteoblasts.

Check your dental health. The only way to diagnose osteoporosis conclusively is with a bone mineral density test. One early clue that you're at risk, however, may be tooth loss and gum diseases. Conversely, if you *have* osteoporosis, you're at much higher risk of developing gum disease and tooth loss. If you're having dental problems, ask your doctor to test your bone mineral density.

Eat More Calcium

If the only time you buy milk is when you bake a cake or young children are visiting, don't despair! A glass of milk isn't the only way to get your calcium. In fact, it may actually be the *worst* form of calcium because it's so high in protein, which contributes to bone breakdown. Calcium goals are 1,200 milligrams a day. Here are some of the best nondairy dietary sources:

3/4 cup **whole-grain breakfast cereal**	1,104 mg
1 cup **cornmeal**	483 mg
1 cup **wheat** or **enriched white flour**	423 mg
1 cup of cooked **collards**	357 mg
1 cup cooked **rhubarb**	348 mg
3 ounces **sardines** with bone	325 mg
1 cup cooked **spinach**	291 mg

Vision Problems

What if you couldn't watch your grandchildren growing up, catch the latest movies at the theater, or even see well enough to drive your car? Once, low vision and even blindness were accepted as inevitable parts of growing older—with truly life-altering consequences.

The thieves of sight are still with us. There are four main ones:

- The first is the least troublesome: the loss of the ability to focus on close objects. Called presbyopia, it affects virtually all adults beginning in their forties; by the mid-fifties, the decrease usually ends, leaving many adults with reading glasses in their pockets, but no other significant damage done. Behind this problem is merely the loss of elasticity of the lens in your eye, along with the loss of power of the muscles that bend and straighten that lens.

- The second is cataracts, in which the normally clear lens in one or both of your eyes may grow so cloudy that your vision blurs. Half of all people over 80 develop cataracts.

- Third, you may develop age-related macular degeneration (AMD). A leading cause of blindness in developed countries, AMD slowly damages your retina, the thin lining on the back of the eye that collects visual images.

- Fourth, your optic nerve, which transmits images to your brain, may become damaged by too much fluid pressure inside your eyes—a condition called glaucoma. Once glaucoma's damage begins, you have a 50 percent risk of going blind in at least one eye within 20 years, unless you take action.

These are the same four concerns we've long known about—but thinking about them has changed significantly in recent years. Excuse the pun, but the future is brighter than ever when it comes to the health of your eyes!

New Thinking about Vision

Exciting new research proves that catching these problems early—sometimes before they've done even a tiny bit of damage—and treating them with newer, more-effective drugs and procedures could save the sight of millions of older women and men. Even more exciting: Pampering and protecting your eyes with smart eating, exercise, and even the kind of sunglasses you choose could slash your risk for ever having these conditions in the first place.

Rule #1: You must get eye exams regularly! Starting in your forties, you should be examined every two to four years until you're 64, then every one or two years after that—and it should be performed by an ophthalmologist or optician. The eye doctor should enlarge (dilate) your pupils by putting drops in your eyes. This is the only way to find some eye diseases that have no early signs or symptoms. The eye doctor should test your eyesight, your glasses, and your eye muscles.

And if your doctor does spot a problem, take action—pronto. There's no reversing the two leading causes of blindness in the world's developed countries: glaucoma and AMD. But the earlier they're caught, the more vision you can save. Prescription-only eyedrops can lower inner-eye pressure (doctors call it intraocular pressure) that destroys the optic nerve in glaucoma—in studies, these drops have significantly slowed or even halted the advance of this vision-robbing condition.

If your doctor says you have the more advanced "wet" form of AMD, a drug called Lucentis could give you a 90 percent chance of maintaining your vision. In one study, it significantly improved vision for 40 percent of study participants. In contrast, 60 percent of study volunteers who had a conventional treatment called photodynamic therapy still became blind after just one year.

Got cataracts? Consider surgery. Replacing the eye's clouded lens with a plastic, acrylic, or silicone version is one of the safest and most effective surgeries you can have. And while doctors once waited until cataracts were advanced, they now suggest having the surgery as soon as you have cataract-related vision problems, such as too much glare from oncoming traffic while driving at night. In fact, driving may be one of the best reasons to go ahead with this procedure. It could save your life or someone else's. In one study of older drivers, those who had cataract surgery were less likely to be involved in automobile crashes than those who didn't have the procedure.

Ways to Keep Your Vision Clear

You can lower your odds for ever having many common vision problems by following these smart lifestyle steps.

When to Get Help

Most of us see "floaters"—little spots that cross our field of vision, especially when outdoors in bright sunlight. This is entirely normal. But if they're accompanied by flashes of light, or suddenly become more numerous, call the doctor right away. It could be a sign of retinal detachment. That requires fast, vision-saving medical attention.

Order bouillabaisse or pasta with clam sauce the next time you dine out. Shellfish, such as clams, oysters, and mussels, are rich sources of zinc—a mineral known to protect against AMD. Other good zinc sources include lean meat, wheat germ, whole grains, and yogurt.

Start the day with Irish oatmeal. Packed with fiber, this breakfast cereal is especially adept at keeping your blood sugar on an even keel. Your eyes will thank you. In a study from Tufts University School of Medicine in Boston, 500 women, ages 53 to 73, who chose high-fiber foods such as oatmeal—and steered clear of white bread, sugary drinks, and high-sugar desserts—cut their risk for developing early signs of AMD in half, compared with women who ate high-sugar, refined-carbohydrate foods.

Cook up a dinner omelet. Fast and fresh, a two-egg omelet is a delicious evening meal. The bonus for your eyes: Egg yolks are the food world's richest, most easily absorbable and usable source of the eye-protecting antioxidants lutein and zeaxanthin. Lutein and zeaxanthin accumulate in the eye's lens and retina, creating a natural filter from the sun's ultraviolet rays. Sun damage is a leading cause of cataracts and AMD. People who get plenty of these healthy

Moisturize dry eyes

Your eyes naturally produce tears—a mix of water, oil, and mucus—to lubricate, clean, and nourish the outer surface of the eye. But wind and sun, aging and stress, even a variety of medications can reduce your eyes' natural production of tears. The result is a dry, scratchy, gritty feeling—and even pain, redness, eye damage, and a loss of vision.

The fix? Start with these items to protect and moisturize your eyes.

Sunglasses. They shield against wind, pollen, and airborne grit as well as sun—all factors that can dry out your eyes.

Fish oil and/or flaxseed oil capsules. A Harvard Medical School study of 32,470 women found that those who got the most good omega-3 fatty acids in their diets had the lowest risk of dry eyes. Many eye doctors recommend 1,000 milligrams of flaxseed oil a day, but fish-oil capsules are a more potent source of these good fats. Experts suggest getting 2 to 3 grams of omega-3s in fish-oil capsules daily. (Check the labels to see how many capsules you'll have to take; it varies by brand.)

Blinking. If you spend hours watching TV, surfing the Web, or working at a computer, you may not be blinking enough. Studies show that while people normally blink 12 times a minute, your "blink rate" may drop to 2 or 3 times in three minutes while you're watching a screen. Simply positioning your screen just below eye level could help minimize moisture loss, because you'll close your eyes a little bit to look down. But also schedule regular blink breaks.

A humidifier. Air-conditioning and heating systems can both dry out indoor air. If your eyes dry out at home, consider a humidifier to boost the moisture content of the air. Keep the filter and water tank clean to avoid mold and bacteria growth.

Artificial tears. Look for demulcent drops that moisturize your eyes—not types that remove redness (these can dry out eyes even more!).

A warm washcloth. If dry eyes is just an occasional concern, then soak a washcloth with water, wring it out, and warm it in a microwave oven for 20 seconds, or until soothingly warm. Then place over your eyelids for 5 to 10 minutes. This will provide instant relief and also will help get tears flowing again. You can repeat a few times a day if you wish.

antioxidants have a 20 percent lower risk for cataracts and a 40 percent lower risk for AMD.

Add a side of dark, leafy greens. Adding spinach, kale, Swiss chard, collards, or other greens to salads, soups, and sandwiches is a smart, eye-protecting move. They're also rich in the eye-protecting antioxidants lutein and zeaxanthin, as well as beta-carotene.

Wear sunglasses in the spring, summer, fall, and winter. Year-round protection from the sun's damaging UV rays can help lower your odds for major vision-robbing problems, as well as eye cancer, nerve damage, and even burns on your cornea. "Think of sunglasses as sunblock for your eyes." says Paul T. Finger, MD, director of Ocular Tumor Services at the New York Eye and Ear Infirmary.

Look for close-fitting shades (wraparound styles are best) that entirely block UVA and UVB rays. Good news: The price and the color of the lenses won't affect how well they deflect the sun's damage. If you already have sunglasses you like, get the UV protection level checked at an optical shop—most are equipped with a machine called a photometer that can gauge UV-blocking levels.

Add a broad-brimmed hat. You may be especially vulnerable to sun damage if your eyes are blue, if you spend lots of time outdoors—especially at the beach, on the water, or on snow, which all reflect and magnify sun exposure—or if you take sun-sensitizing drugs (ask your doctor about your prescriptions; many classes of drugs have this effect). If any of these apply to you, wear a broad-brimmed hat plus sunglasses for double protection.

Snack on an orange or red fruit or veggie at least once a day. A tangerine, a clementine, a handful of ripe strawberries, strips of red bell pepper … these high vitamin-C foods add

delicious sweetness and crunch to snack time and pack an eye-guarding bonus, say Tufts University researchers. In a study of 247 women, ages 56 to 71, those who got the most vitamin C over 10 years cut their risk for early signs of cataracts by 77 percent. Some researchers think that if more people ate high-antioxidant foods, including those rich in vitamin C, it would cut the need for cataract surgeries in half.

Have salmon burgers tonight for dinner. Yet another study has found that omega-3 fatty acids, and by extension, flaxseed, can reduce the risk of AMD. The results of a Harvard study, published in August 2001 in the *Archives of Ophthalmology*, showed that people with a high intake of omega-6 (vegetable oils) were more likely to develop macular degeneration, while those with a combination of lower omega-6 intake and higher omega-3 intake were less likely to have the disease

Ask about a vision-protecting supplement. If you have intermediate-stage AMD in one or both eyes, or advanced AMD in just one eye, ask your doctor about taking a well-studied supplement containing antioxidants, zinc, and copper. In a large study, this combo cut risk for AMD progression by 25 percent and reduced AMD-related vision loss by 19 percent. The winning combination contained 500 milligrams of vitamin C; 400 international units of vitamin E; 15 milligrams of beta-carotene; 80 milligrams of zinc as zinc oxide; and 2 milligrams of copper as cupric oxide (Copper is added to avoid copper deficiencies that can be the result of getting high levels of zinc.)

Don't take high-dose antioxidant supplements of C, E, and/or beta-carotene alone—studies show that without zinc, they don't seem to help. And if you smoke, skip this supplement completely. Studies show that smokers who take beta-carotene supplements may raise risk for lung cancer.

Ask about preventive eyedrops. If you have a family history of glaucoma or elevated eye pressure but no sign of nerve damage, using pressure-lowering eyedrops could drastically reduce your odds for developing glaucoma in the future, report researchers at the University of California, Davis, Medical Center. They found that people who used preventive drops for five years cut their odds for glaucoma-related optic-nerve damage in half.

Pamper your eyes. If you have diabetes, high blood sugar raises your risk for cataracts, glaucoma, and diabetic retinopathy—damaged blood vessels within the eye that lead to blindness. Controlling your blood sugar and getting a yearly eye exam in which the doctor dilates your pupils to look carefully at the inside of your eyes can greatly reduce your chances of future vision troubles.

Vision-Robbers to Avoid

Here are a few things you can control and that can hurt your vision as you age:

Sitting disease. When researchers tracked nearly 4,000 residents of a town in Wisconsin for 15 years, they found that those who climbed more than six flights of steps a day or walked more than 12 blocks were 70 percent less likely to develop advanced AMD than their more sedentary neighbors. Turns out a sedentary lifestyle—aptly called sitting disease—can even harm your eyes!

Smoking. Cigarette-smokers are up to four times more likely than nonsmokers to be blinded by AMD later in life.

Tight neckties. Seriously. Tight neckties raised the pressure of fluid within the eye—a risk factor for glaucoma—significantly in a study of 40 men conducted at the New York Eye and Ear Infirmary. And if you do have glaucoma, a snugly cinched tie could make it worse. If you wear neckties, you should be able to easily slip two fingers inside your collar. If you can't, loosen up your tie.

There is absolutely no reason why you can't have good eyesight at any age. Our knowledge of vision problems has grown deep—as has the menu of treatments.

Hearing Problems

Deep within your inner ear, tiny "hair cells" are dancing to the soundtrack of your life. Whether you're listening to the quiet strains of a solo violin or the roar of a chainsaw, these microscopic bristles quiver, quake, and shimmy—and convert sound waves into electrical signals for your brain. But when they die off—the result of too many rock 'n' roll concerts in your younger days, too many lawns mowed without ear protection, even too many nights with a snoring bed partner—they're gone. And so is some of your hearing.

A little hearing loss is inevitable as we grow older. By the time you're in your twenties, you may have already lost the ability to detect extremely high-pitched sounds—the reason high-school students are downloading ultra-high-frequency cell phone ring tones that most of their teachers can't even hear! In later years, as hair cells die a natural or unnatural death, you may have difficulty hearing lower tones as well. If you find yourself asking people to repeat themselves, frequently turn the volume up on the TV, or don't always notice that the telephone is ringing, you're in good company. Between 24 percent and 40 percent of adults over age 65 have difficulty hearing, as do up to half of people over age 75. By age 85, 30 percent are even deaf in one ear.

The truth is, some hearing loss can't be stopped. And once it's gone, you'll need hearing aids to get it back. The good news is that much hearing loss can be avoided—and it's never too late to preserve what you have.

If you're planning to use all the strategies at your disposal to live a long, happy, healthy life—from eating well to exercising frequently, from socializing often to keeping your mind active with cultural and educational activities—you'll need your ears. When University of Florida researchers checked the hearing and health of 152 people, ages 60 to 90, they found that those with more hearing problems were in poorer health. Other studies show that hearing loss contributes to feelings of depression, isolation, and anxiety, as well as no longer feeling in control or independent.

In contrast, a survey of 2,069 people with hearing problems and their families underscores how vitally important sharp hearing is for good health and a long life. Among those who made the decision to wear hearing aids, 71 percent said life was better, 35 percent felt more self-confident, 40 percent were involved in more social activities including sports and clubs, 53 percent had better relationships with grandkids and kids, 28 percent said their physical health improved, 35 percent were less dependent on others… and 13 percent said their sex lives improved.

14 Ways to Preserve Your Hearing

Most medical issues are complicated; hearing problems, by contrast, are pretty simple. In the majority of cases, they are caused by—you guessed it—prolonged exposure to loud sounds.

When to Get Help

Everyone over age 50 should have a hearing test performed by a licensed audiologist every few years. But don't wait if you have sudden or bothersome hearing loss.

- **Get emergency help if you suddenly lose most or all of your hearing in a short time**—such as three days or less. Doctors suspect that the cause of sudden hearing loss is a viral infection of the inner ear or of important nerves related to hearing.

- **Call the doctor if you seem to be having more difficulty hearing than in the past.** Make an appointment if you're having problems hearing people on the telephone, following conversations involving several people, understanding what's happening in a noisy room, having trouble hearing the speech of kids or women, if other people seem to be mumbling, or if family or friends tell you that you're turning the TV up too loud.

Sadly, modern living is decidedly noisy. Whereas most of man's history lacked engines, machines, and amplified music, today's life exposes us to a never-ending parade of loud sound. Some of that is lifestyle—living in an urban environment, a love of rock music, flying frequently. For many others, it's their jobs: merely a week as a firefighter, police officer, factory worker, farmer, construction worker, musician, or in the military or heavy industry can damage your hearing.

Your first move? Do all you can to protect the hearing you have right now. The first batch of tips are common sense—protect yourself from loud noises. But they may be the hardest to take action on: Many people worry that earplugs and hearing aids will make them look old or silly. False! With the rise of cell-phone usage and portable music devices, there's hardly any adult—or teenager—who doesn't have ear gear of some type. No one notices, and no one cares, if you have a hearing aid or sound-blocking tool in your ear! With that in mind....

Buy earplugs and keep them in your home, garage, car, and purse. Wear them when you'll be exposed to any sound over 85 decibels—such as lawn equipment, a loud concert, a wedding or social event with loud music, an afternoon hunting or target-shooting, even time in a loud health club. Don't rely on cotton balls or bits of paper stuffed in your ears; they'll only screen out about 7 decibels of sound, while foam earplugs can block up to 32 decibels. Need more protection? Look into custom-made earplugs from an audiologist, or special sound-deadening earmuffs.

Love your headphones? Ask a friend if they can hear the music, too. Your tunes are turned up TOO LOUD if others can hear the sounds from your earbuds or headphones. And only listen to music piped directly into your ears for about 1 1/2 hours a day at normal volume—just 5 minutes at top volume, suggest University of Colorado at Boulder researchers. Beyond that, you can cause hearing loss.

Change seats at a noisy event. If it's too loud where you are—at a concert, meeting, or social event—move. Do the same if you can't hear someone who's just two feet away, if you have to raise your own voice to be heard, or if the sounds around you begin to seem muffled. Again, there's nothing old-fashioned about removing yourself from overly loud situations. In fact, your conversation mates will be grateful.

Wear earplugs on holidays celebrated with a bang, too. Fireworks and loud, booming rockets are a staple of holiday events around the world. Enjoy them to the fullest—with your eyes. Meanwhile, keep earplugs firmly in place in your ears.

Keep earplugs on your bedside table. A small Canadian study found that bedmates of snorers suffered hearing loss in the ear closest to the person making all that night noise. Snoring can reach 80 decibels—as loud as someone yelling for help—or even 90 decibels—equivalent to truck traffic.

Get a med check. Many prescription and nonprescription medications can damage the ear and cause hearing loss. These include high doses of aspirin, anti-malaria drugs, and antibiotics, including erythromycin, vancomycin, tetracycline, gentamicin, and streptomycin.

Ask about earwax. Embarrassing but true: Sometimes, hearing loss is simply the result of a gradual accumulation of earwax. It can block the ear canal and prevent the transmission of sound waves. Ask your doctor to check your ears and remove any buildup.

Control your blood sugar. When University of Maryland researchers compared the blood sugar levels and hearing levels of 1,644 women and men, they found that those with diabetes were 30 percent more likely to have hearing loss than those without diabetes. High blood sugar damages tiny nerves and blood vessels in the ears—and throughout the body—giving people with diabetes one more reason to keep sugar levels healthy.

Snack on pumpkin seeds. In lab studies, magnesium deficiencies seem to stress cells in the ear. A two-month study of army recruits found that a little magnesium seemed to protect them from some permanent noise-related hearing loss. Pumpkin seeds are a rich source of magnesium, as is Swiss chard, halibut, flax seeds, brown rice, and navy beans.

Have a glass of orange juice at breakfast. In a Dutch study of 728 older women and men,

How Loud Is Too Loud?

Unprotected, your ears will be damaged by just one minute of exposure to a chainsaw—or any other sound at 110 decibels or higher. Your damage threshold is 15 minutes for sounds at 100 decibels and just a few hours at 90 decibels. A smarter plan: Always wear ear protection around these potential deafeners.

Gunshot (peak level)	140–170 decibels
Jet taking off	140 decibels
Rock concert, chainsaw, snowmobile, stereo headphones, diesel train	110–120 decibels
Motorcycle, lawnmower, shop tools, truck traffic	90 decibels
Snoring spouse	30–90 decibels

those who got 800 micrograms of folic acid a day had less hearing loss after three years than those who didn't. Split pea soup, whole-grain bread, spinach, and fortified breakfast cereals are also great sources of this important B vitamin.

Enjoy a glass of wine, in silence. Soothe—and protect—your ears at the same time. Some research suggests a little alcohol somehow slows age-related hearing losses.

Get moving! Exercise improves the flow of blood to every cell in your body—including the ever-so-delicate hair cells inside your ears. But don't listen to loud music on headphones while you walk or work out. A Swedish study found that even at a moderate volume, exercisers with headphones had hearing loss after just 10 minutes.

Stop the buzz of tinnitus. Ringing in the ears is a problem for 10 to 14 percent of older

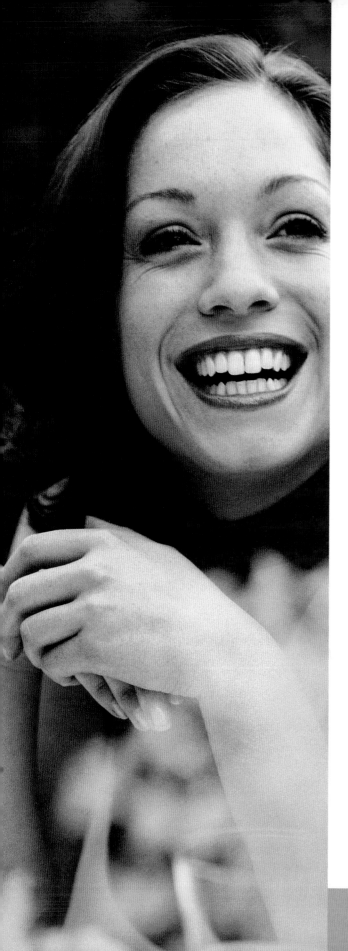

adults—and often, the head noise may sound like a squeal, a roar, or a whistle or a hiss. Controlling your blood pressure and lowering your cholesterol can help. So can avoiding alcohol, which increases blood flow to the inner ear. Quiet "white noise" like a fan or soft radio static can help mask the annoying buzz, too.

Have a bowl of vegetable soup and a fruit salad topped with nuts. In a lab study at the University of Michigan, extra vitamin A, C, and E seemed to protect against ear damage caused by exposure to loud noises. Skip the supplements, though. Get extra vitamin A from sweet potatoes, carrots, and turnip greens as well as mango, papaya, and apricots. Soak up extra E in almonds, pistachios, and wheat germ. For vitamin C, how about citrus, strawberries, and red bell peppers?

3 Hearing Thieves to Avoid

These three habits have been shown to have a particularly bad effect on your hearing.

Caffeine. Make your morning blend decaffeinated. Caffeine can worsen tinnitus, another ear problem associated with hearing loss.

Excess sodium. Choose low-sodium soups and frozen entrées, and rinse canned beans thoroughly. Take the saltshaker off the table, too. There's evidence that controlling your sodium levels can help reduce your odds for a vertigo problem called Ménière's disease, which is also linked with hearing loss. Too many high-salt foods can alter the pressure of fluids in your inner ear.

Cigarette smoke. Exposure to tobacco smoke—from your own cigarette or someone else's—raises your odds for more severe age-related hearing loss.

Diabetes

If you haven't heard the word "epidemic" linked to the word "diabetes," then you've clearly chosen to avoid TV news, the newspaper, or even the Internet. For few health stories have gotten so much coverage in recent years—and validly so—than the growing menace of type 2, or "adult-onset" diabetes.

As the World Health Organization—an international agency not known for its bold pronouncements—puts it: "Diabetes is a common condition and its frequency is dramatically rising all over the world." Today at least 171 million people worldwide have the disease, a figure likely to more than double by 2030 as populations age. And just who are these people? Primarily, those "above the age of retirement," according to the World Health Organization. In other words, older people. In fact, one out of five people age 75 and older have diabetes.

But let's be clear: Diabetes is not merely a side effect of aging. Yes, it's true that as we age, our bodies become less efficient at producing and using glucose and insulin—the two key factors in type 2 diabetes. But this natural decline isn't enough to cause the disease. Instead, look at the other major lifestyle issues of our time.

Not too long ago, many people—and doctors—blamed a diet high in sugar as the cause of type 2 diabetes. Today, we know that's not the real issue (though, yes, eating lots of refined sugar and refined carbohydrates does cause troublesome peaks and valleys in your blood sugar amounts that makes diabetes problems worse). More recently, doctors have shown that being overweight is a major risk factor for the disease.

But here's the breakthrough news, based on an increasing body of evidence: The amount you exercise—not just how much you eat—in large part determines your risk of developing diabetes or its precursor, insulin resistance. Put simply, sedentary living, coupled with excess body weight, are the real culprits. And you control both.

To prevent diabetes, then, you need to take action. And the first step is to become educated about the disease.

Understanding Insulin Resistance

To start, there are two types of diabetes. Type 1 starts in childhood and is usually related to a malfunctioning pancreas. It requires a lifetime of careful management, and often, daily insulin injections. Type 2 is far more common, and is the form of diabetes that is rising in epidemic proportions, due in large part to the growing unhealthiness of our daily lives.

Type 2 diabetes usually progresses along a predictable pattern. Before there is diabetes, there is insulin resistance. It works like this. Every time you eat, your body signals "beta" cells in your pancreas that it's time to pump out the hormone insulin. Insulin's job is to shepherd the energy extracted from your food—in the form of glucose, commonly called blood sugar—into each living cell of your body.

Insulin does this in a kind of lock-and-key process by fitting into molecules on the surface of cells called insulin receptors. Once "unlocked," the cell does its energy exchange, either pulling in glucose from the bloodstream to use or store, or sending out stored energy—in the form of either fat or glycogen (the stored form of glucose)—to be used by other parts of your body when they have depleted their own energy stores.

Once a cell is filled with fat or glycogen, or if the cell has been inactive for a long time, it moves the insulin receptors deep within, effectively making it impossible for insulin to reach them. But as the cell uses up its energy stores, it becomes thinner, and those insulin receptors move to the cell's surface again. And the cycle resumes, with the receptors ready to bond with insulin and usher in more glucose to the cell.

But if you're overweight and/or sedentary, more of those insulin receptors stay hidden within the cell. The result? Glucose and insulin build up in your bloodstream. Those high levels of glucose signal the beta cells in your pancreas to pump out more and more insulin, vainly trying to move that glucose into cells. Eventually, thanks to sheer numbers, some insulin links up with insulin receptors and some glucose gets in. But this process gets more difficult every year until, finally, your beta cells wear out like an overworked engine. Next thing you know, your body lacks the capacity to make enough insulin to carry energy to all your cells. And that is why many people with diabetes need insulin shots.

The relatively simple relationship between glucose and insulin becomes more complex as you age because of the presence of a second hormone called glucagon. While pancreatic beta cells react to high glucose levels by issuing insulin, their neighbors, alpha cells, react to low glucose levels by issuing glucagon. This hormone gloms onto receptors in the liver, telling it to release glucose into the bloodstream to provide energy for the rest of the body.

The thing is, alpha cells only learn about the state of blood glucose levels from signals they receive from beta cells. In older people with type 2 diabetes and insulin resistance, communication breaks down between alpha and beta cells in the pancreas. So even while beta cells are releasing insulin in response to high blood glucose levels, alpha cells are releasing glucagon, stimulating even more glucose to be released into the bloodstream. You can see where this would become a real mess. And this mess is called diabetes.

Once you have diabetes, you become subject to a range of complications as you age with it, including blindness, chronic nerve pain, nerve damage, incontinence, impotence, memory loss and, of course, the biggie: heart disease. If you have diabetes, you're more likely to have a heart attack than a lifelong smoker—even if you never took a puff yourself. Diabetes is also the strongest predictor of functional decline in older people, that is, handling the day-to-day tasks of life like walking, dressing, or housecleaning. You're more likely to be depressed or to develop dementia and Alzheimer's disease. And it means you're likely to be in the hospital and require other medical services at twice the rate of people your same age without diabetes.

6 Ways to Prevent Diabetes

The good news is that insulin resistance and, in some cases, type 2 diabetes can be reversed through generally healthy living, as prescribed throughout this book. Not only that but also the same kind of lifestyle can prevent the disease—

The Best diet

The issue of what and how to eat when you have diabetes is one that is constantly changing. At one time, people with the disease were forbidden any foods with sugar. At another, they were told to cut nearly all the fat from their diets. Today, the advice focuses more on an overall diet than on any specific food or food ingredient. The American Diabetes Association, a world leader in diabetes prevention and treatment guidelines, recommends the following:

If you're at risk of diabetes...

Focus on just one thing: Having a diet high in fiber (14 grams of fiber for every 1,000 calories). You should get at least half of all grains from whole grains like brown rice, whole-grain pasta, barley, and oat bran. Other top sources include green, leafy vegetables and beans.

If you have diabetes...

Your carbohydrates should come *only* from whole fruits and vegetables (*not* juices); whole grains; beans; and low-fat milk. This means no sugary desserts or breads made from refined flour. You should also eat fiber-rich foods like those listed above, keep saturated fats (butter, shortening, red meats) to less than 7 percent of your total calories; and get at least two servings of fish a week (not fried!). You should also stay away from trans fats and limit cholesterol intake from food to less than 200 milligrams per day, about the amount in one egg yolk.

If you wish to go to the limit...

Want a really powerful diet to control your blood sugar—and willing to drastically change the way you eat? Consider a vegan diet. A study published recently in the journal *Diabetes Care* found that a vegan diet, which eliminates all animal-based foods including dairy and eggs, dramatically improved blood sugar control, cholesterol, weight, and kidney function in people with type 2 diabetes. One advantage: No limits on calories, carbohydrates, or portions!

even if you already have insulin resistance. The following tips have been proven in studies to have particularly strong preventive powers.

Strengthen your muscles. Work out with hand weights, six days a week. It's the best thing you can do to prevent diabetes! See the fitness routines on page 200 to get a start. Every time you stress muscle cells with strength training, you increase their need for glucose, thus reducing insulin resistance. The more muscle you build, the more glucose they need. That means more insulin receptors on cells, and less glucose in your bloodstream.

Maintain your level of activity. If you're using aerobic activities like walking, playing tennis, and bicycling to maintain healthy glucose levels, don't let up. When you're young, the boost in insulin sensitivity you get from one bout of aerobic exercise can last up to four days. But once you pass age 40, that boost has a shorter and shorter time span. That makes it crucial that you get some type of activity most every day.

Drink tea. A compound in black, green, and oolong tea called epigallocatechin gallate substantially increases the ability of cells to take in insulin. Just skip the milk; adding just a teaspoon of 2 percent milk reduced the benefit by a third. Also stay away from nondairy creamers and soy milk, which also significantly reduced the benefits.

Get your grains. Whole grains—whether wheat, quinoa, rice, rye, or oats—should be considered diabetes prevention in a plant. Because these grains haven't been stripped of nutrient-containing components and fiber, they pack a powerful nutritional punch. How powerful? A study of nearly 43,000 male health professionals found those who had the greatest amount of whole grains in their diets were 42 percent less likely to develop type 2 diabetes than those who got the least amount of grains. Whole grains' benefits likely come from their ability to slow the release of glucose into the bloodstream, thus tempering that post-meal insulin spike. Thus, studies find, diets high in fiber naturally improve insulin sensitivity and reduce insulin secretion.

Load up on magnesium. Found in high amounts in whole grains (yet another reason for that morning bowl of oatmeal), magnesium influences the release and activity of insulin, and plays a role in your body's ability to use carbohydrates. When blood sugar levels are high, your body loses magnesium. Numerous studies, including two that followed more than 170,000 health professionals for up to 18 years, found that the risk of developing type 2 diabetes was much higher in men and women with low dietary levels of magnesium than in those with high levels. Other good sources include halibut, almonds, cashews, soybeans, and spinach. Just an ounce of almonds or cashews provides 20 percent of your recommended daily intake of magnesium.

Choose chicken. When researchers evaluated the diets of 69,554 women ages 38 to 63 over 10 years, they found that every 3-ounce serving of red meat increased the risk of diabetes by 26 percent, with an increased risk of 73 percent for every serving of processed meats (bacon, hot dogs, lunchmeat, and so forth). Lean chicken had no such affect.

5 Ways to Stabilize Blood Sugar

Already struggling with insulin resistance or diabetes? These five tips have been shown to have a wonderfully stabilizing effect on blood sugar levels.

Sprinkle cinnamon. On cereal, low-fat cottage cheese or yogurt, even over fruit. The fragrant herb contains numerous compounds called polyphenolic polymers that improve your cells' ability to use glucose, enabling them to pull more out of your bloodstream. It doesn't take much; in one study from the United States Department of Agriculture, less than a 1/2 teaspoon a day for 40 days significantly reduced blood sugar levels in 60 people with type 2 diabetes.

Switch to soba. Instead of pasta, ladle your tomato sauce and turkey meatballs over soba noodles, made with buckwheat. Canadian researchers found extracts of the grain reduced blood glucose levels by 12 to 19 percent in diabetic rats, and a similar affect appears to occur with people. You can find soba noodles in the Oriental food section of supermarkets.

Pop some cherries. These sweet-and-sour fruits are filled with powerful antioxidants called anthocyanins that can increase insulin production up to 50 percent, according to animal studies.

Get a good night's sleep. If you don't get enough sleep, or you toss and turn all night, don't be surprised to find your blood sugar levels higher than normal the next day. One study of 161 people with type 2 diabetes found 67 percent had poor sleep quality. Lack of sleep and poor sleep wreaks havoc with a multitude of hormones responsible for metabolizing glucose and regulating appetite, studies

Time to Supplement

Studies find that older people with diabetes tend to have low levels of magnesium and zinc. Taking supplements of these minerals has been proven to improve blood glucose control. Additionally, taking supplements of antioxidant vitamins such as vitamin C and E can help improve blood sugar control, likely by reducing inflammation and oxidation within your bloodstream. Talk to your doctor about the right amounts for you.

find, so much so that some researchers suggest our 24/7 society may, in part, be contributing to the current diabetes epidemic.

Try tai chi. Researchers from Taiwan had 32 people with type 2 diabetes participate in a 12-week tai chi program. The ancient Chinese martial art uses a combination of movement and breathing exercises to strengthen the body and mind. After 12 weeks, participants showed a significant decrease in their A1c levels, a marker of glucose levels, over time, and fewer pro-inflammatory chemicals.

Another study, this one from the University of Queensland in Australia, involved 12 people with type 2 diabetes who practiced Qigong and tai chi three times a week for 12 weeks. At the end of the study, participants' blood sugar levels had significantly improved, and they'd lost weight, were sleeping better, and had more energy.

Lung Disease

Chronic Obstructive Pulmonary Disease (COPD) is called the forgotten killer and is currently the fourth leading cause of death in the United States and the fifth leading cause of death in the world. In Canada, it kills more women than breast cancer. And throughout North America, it's the only common cause of death still increasing in prevalence. Yet when's the last time you heard of a fundraiser to fight for its eradication?

COPD is a collection of chronic lung diseases, including emphysema and chronic bronchitis, that blocks the airways and restricts oxygen flow throughout your body. The condition has long been linked with cigarette smoking, and smoking remains its top cause. But researchers now know that some cases of COPD are also the result of exposure to dust, fumes, and secondhand smoke; decades of living with asthma; poor diet; and even a wily bacteria that shifts just enough to continually outwit the antibiotics used to vanquish it.

Researchers also think COPD is more than just a disease of the lungs. In an editorial in the British medical journal *The Lancet*, doctors from the Netherlands and Italy suggested that in many people, COPD is part of a cluster of conditions, all related to chronic inflammation in the body. This systemic inflammation is likely responsible for the high blood pressure, diabetes, coronary artery disease, heart failure, and even cancer that tend to exist along with COPD. They recommend that people with at least three of the following be diagnosed with what they call Chronic Systemic Inflammation Syndrome, not just a single disease.

- Smoking for more than 10 pack-years (the equivalent of smoking 1 pack a day for 10 years; or 2 packs a day for 5 years)

- Symptoms and abnormal lung function of COPD
- Chronic heart failure
- Metabolic syndrome
- Increased levels of C-reactive protein, an inflammatory marker, in the bloodstream

Other evidence that COPD is often part of a broader syndrome comes from researchers in Great Britain, who found that people with the disease develop arterial stiffness, or atherosclerosis, far earlier than those without COPD. The researchers also found high levels of inflammatory chemicals in the arteries of people with COPD. All of which adds up to one thing: COPD, whether on its own or part of cluster of conditions, is scary stuff.

Best Ways to Prevent COPD

Who wants to lose their ability to breathe? As with so many other serious health conditions, the answer to that question is determined by how you choose to live each day. Lead a healthy, energized life, and the chances of COPD ever entering your life will be remote.

Stop smoking. Cigarettes are by far the number one cause of COPD. There are so many arguments for quitting, and this is yet another big one. If you continue to smoke, and want to stop, turn to page 58 for guidance.

Stick to smoke-free bars and restaurants. Even if you don't smoke, being around people who do significantly increases your risk of COPD. Chinese researchers estimated that the equivalent of 40 hours a week of such "passive smoking" for five years made people who never smoked nearly 50 percent more likely to develop COPD than those who weren't around the smoke.

Follow a Mediterranean diet. This approach to eating, with its emphasis on fruits, vegetables, healthy oils, fish, and whole grains, can reduce your risk of COPD by 25 percent. In contrast, following a typical American diet high in refined grains, cured and red meats, desserts, and French fries increases the risk by 31 percent. Meanwhile, other studies find that diets high in starches and sodium also significantly increase the risk of developing COPD. The Mediterranean diet's anti-inflammatory effects may be one reason for its impact on COPD risk.

Live fit. Exercise, particularly aerobic exercises like walking, biking, or swimming, help your lungs become more efficient at providing your body with the oxygen it needs. Not only do your heart and lungs benefit by the more robust breathing but so do all the muscles and connective tissues in and around your lungs. If you get winded easily, it's time to take daily walks and build up your aerobic fitness.

Become a healthy breather. Too many people take lots of small breaths as they go about their business. Rapid breathing also becomes the norm in stressful times. But for better lung health—and overall health, for that matter—learn to breath more deeply and less frequently.

The Wrinkle Factor

If you smoke and are still on the fence about quitting, look at yourself in the mirror. Is your face heavily lined with wrinkles? If yes, then you really need to quit. A study from researchers at the Royal Devon & Exeter National Health Service Foundation Trust in England found that middle-age smokers with heavily lined faces were five times more likely to have COPD than smokers with fewer wrinkles. They were also three times as likely to have more severe emphysema than those with less-lined faces.

If you still insist on smoking, make sure that you're getting as much exercise as possible. A study from researchers in Barcelona, Spain, evaluated the chances that 928 smokers would develop COPD over 11 years; those who got moderate to high levels of physical activity were 21 percent less likely to develop the lung disease than the couch-potato smokers.

Inhale through your nose slowly and fully; your chest and abdomen should move together. If only your chest moves, your breathing is too shallow. Exhaling should take twice as long as inhaling. The more you clear your lungs out with strong exhalations, the healthier and fuller your inhalations will be! While there's no agreed upon standard, try to reduce the number of breaths you take in a minute to just six. Deep breathing not only improves lung function but can also lower blood pressure and provide relaxation, even in stressful times.

Natural Remedies for COPD

If you have COPD, chances are good that your doctor has prescribed various medications and programs to help you cope. But there are simple lifestyle improvements you can also make to battle back against the disease.

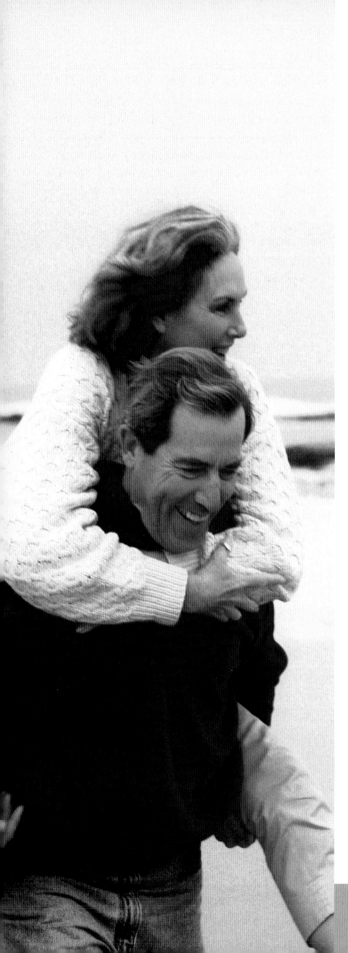

Ventilate your indoor spaces. High levels of indoor air pollution caused by smoking, indoor fires, and indoor toxins can significantly exacerbate COPD symptoms, say researchers from Aberdeen, Scotland. The scientists measured concentrations of indoor air pollutants in the homes of 148 people with COPD. They found that indoor air pollution levels were up to four times the levels that experts say is acceptable. The higher the levels of indoor air pollution, the worse the individual's COPD. As expected, the highest pollution levels were found in homes in which someone smoked.

Get at least 20 minutes a day of moderately intense exercise. It could be riding a stationary bicycle, briskly walking, or swimming. Not only will this improve your breathing capabilities but, chances are, you'll feel sharper mentally afterward. That's what researchers from Ohio State University found when they evaluated the effects of just one session of exercise on 58 adults, half with COPD and half healthy. The COPD group was able to process and retain information better than before they exercised, while the healthy subjects didn't show any improvement. The improvement in the COPD group was probably due to the fact that the exercise increased their lung capacity—sending more oxygen to their brains. The healthy group already had good lung capacity; a 20-minute exercise session wasn't going to affect them that much. A follow-up study in which participants were tracked for a year found that those who continued exercising maintained their cognitive gains, while those who didn't lost physical, cognitive, and psychological functioning.

Pop some fish oil. Two grams a day should do it. Take half in the morning and half in the evening. When Japanese researchers had 64 people with COPD supplement their diets with about 400 calories a day of an omega-3-

rich supplement or one without omega-3 fatty acids for two years, they found numerous indicators of improved lung function in the omega-3 group, with no change in the placebo group. They also found much lower levels of inflammatory chemicals called cytokines in the omega-3 group. Omega-3 fatty acids are potent anti-inflammatories; their ability to quell the inflammation of COPD likely prevented further lung damage during the study.

Maintain a healthy weight. Being overweight puts more pressure on your heart and lungs, increasing breathlessness. It also makes it harder to exercise. But being underweight—a common problem as COPD progresses and eating a full meal becomes more difficult—is linked to an increased risk of death. You should aim for a body mass index (BMI) of 25 or 26. If you're having trouble maintaining your weight:

- Ask for a referral to a nutritionist
- Add calorie supplements like Ensure to your diet
- Eat several small meals throughout the day rather than three large ones
- Increase the calories in each meal. For instance, if you eat yogurt, eat full-fat yogurt.

Mind over Breath

Shortness of breath, or **dyspnea**, is one of the most debilitating and frightening symptoms of **COPD**. People describe it as a sensation of chest tightness, suffocation, not getting enough air, and smothering. The fear of dyspnea leads many with COPD to cut their activities and do as little as possible, one of the worst things they can do. If you feel that horrible sensation of not being able to breathe, don't panic. That only makes the feeling worse. Instead, slowly close your eyes and focus on your breathing. Then envision a calming, peaceful place that makes you happy. Don't just see it in your mind, however; try to engage all your senses. For instance, if you picture the ocean, let yourself hear the waves, taste the salt, feel the grittiness of the sand. This is guided imagery relaxation, and numerous studies find it can help people with COPD reduce the number of episodes of breathlessness and the severity. One way in which it does this is by stimulating your body to release natural brain chemicals called endorphins. They activate part of your nervous system to relax your body and reduce your blood pressure, respiration, and heart rate.

Most people don't breathe healthfully. Take longer, deeper breaths, and exhale slowly. Shallow, rapid breathing does not serve your health nearly as well.

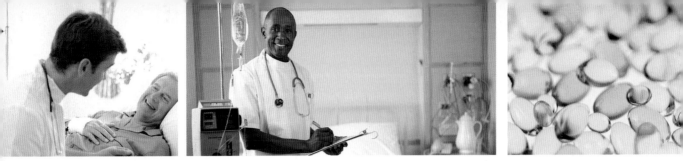

Get the Most from Your Health Care

A compassionate doctor. An early, insightful diagnosis. Effective drugs and treatments that work, with minimal side effects. You deserve all this—and more—from your health-care system.

But the reality can be far different: Your doctor's appointment may be shorter than a television commercial break; your physician may interrupt you brusquely and have no interest in listening to you; in the hospital, the doctors and nurses who care for you may forget to wash their hands—raising your risk for a hospital-acquired infection; and you may receive prescriptions that cause unwanted side effects or that interact with other medications and remedies you're taking. Like any other service industry, there are many terrific doctors and hospitals, but plenty of mediocre ones, too, and, on any given day, someone is going to a make a mistake.

But there's the other side of the health-care equation. As patients, we don't always hold up our end of the bargain. Studies show that half of us don't take prescription drugs as directed, and many of us skip them entirely. One in three of us are reluctant to ask questions. And many of us withhold important information from the doctor, either intentionally or without giving it a second thought. "We're ultimately responsible for our health," notes University of Alabama at Birmingham communications expert Jonathan Amsbary, PhD. "It's the patient who speaks up who lives longer and gets their treatment needs met."

Your first step in making sure you receive top-quality health care? Believe that you deserve it. "Don't dismiss health problems you're having as simply signs of aging," says Buffalo geriatrician Robert Stall, MD. "You can be healthy and active as you get older—provided you take care of problems that come up as readily as you would have at a younger age, or even sooner."

Your second step? Follow these strategies to get the care you need—and deserve.

Doctor Visits That Work

By now, it's a world-famous statistic: Experts have found that doctors tend to interrupt patients just 20 to 30 seconds after they begin speaking during an office visit. But the truth is, bossy doctors are just one reason you may feel shortchanged when you leave your physician's office. Your visit itself may feel way too short: In a study published in the *British Medical Journal*, Belgian researchers found that the typical office visit in Germany and Spain lasted less than 8 minutes; in the United Kingdom and the Netherlands, around 10 minutes; in Belgium and Switzerland, about 15 minutes. Other researchers have found that American office visits last a relatively lengthy 20 minutes ... but that's still barely enough time to discuss something as important as your health.

Meanwhile, we don't always use our time with the doctor to our best advantage. A Dutch study found that half of all visitors to the family doctor hadn't decided in advance what they wanted to talk about; 77 percent did absolutely nothing to prepare for their visit; and 80 percent didn't bring a list of questions with them.

Given the brevity of most doctors' appointments, being ready to give—and get—information should be your top priority. "Having a good relationship with your doctor is important. You should be comfortable discussing your lifestyle and health history so your doctor can best address your health concerns and keep you healthy," says Caroline Rudnick, MD, PhD, a Saint Louis University physician. "Information is a powerful weapon, and if I'm armed, I can do a better job helping a patient fight to stay healthy."

Here's how you can prepare for your visit, and feel confident about asking questions during your appointment.

Study up before your visit. Research your medical conditions and concerns by reading reputable Web sites. Generally, government health Web sites and those maintained by medical associations, large nonprofit groups dedicated to a single medical condition, and university medical centers have the most trustworthy, up-to-date medical information. Make notes and create questions. However, don't hand your doctor a huge sheaf of printouts and expect her to respond to them during your visit. Nor should you try to diagnose your symptoms or self-prescribe your remedies. It's still up to your doctor to do that.

Make a list of questions, then prioritize them. You'll feel more confident when talking

Beyond the Doctor

Your doctor is the point person on your health-care team: She makes the diagnosis, decides on medications and treatments, and oversees your progress. But she's not the whole team. You'll get better sooner when you're ill, live better with chronic conditions, and avoid medical problems if your team includes some (or all!) of these health-care all-stars.

A nurse practitioner or physician's assistant. Often, these highly trained medical folks can devote more time to your appointment and may seem more approachable.

A nutritionist. If you have diabetes or heart disease, meeting with a registered dietitian is an important way to find out what you should be eating on a daily basis—and how to come up with strategies to make it happen. A nutritionist should also be on your team if you're overweight or underweight, have trouble eating due to an illness, or if you're having trouble sticking with a healthy eating plan.

Physical therapist or exercise physiologist. If you have back pain, joint pain, or chronic muscle pain, a physical therapist or exercise physiologist can help you work your muscles in ways that ease the ache and build strength so that you'll stay pain-free.

Pharmacist. This unsung member of the team can check for potential drug interactions when you get a new prescription filled—but only if you give all your prescription-drug business to one pharmacy (a highly recommended move). Pharmacists are willing to discuss side effects to watch out for and can help suggest alternatives if a medication is too expensive (he can put in a call to your doctor, but can't prescribe an alternative himself.)

with your doctor—and you'll get the answers and info you need. The bonus: In one review of 33 office-visit studies, researchers found that people who brought checklists even got more time with their doctors.

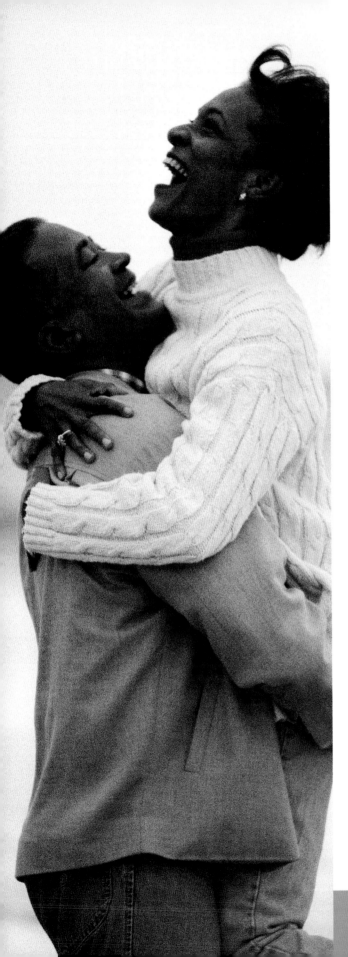

Once you're in the exam room, don't be afraid to give your doctor the list. "I always ask to see it, so that I can be sure that important questions aren't left for the last minute of our visit," Dr. Stall says. "It's okay to give your list to your doctor—and okay to ask him or her to give it back so that you can refer to it."

Rehearse. In one study, older people who practiced their questions just before a doctor's appointment were nearly twice as likely to speak up during the visit than people who didn't rehearse. Ask your spouse, another relative, or a close friend to play doctor while you voice your health concerns, and ask every question on your list, out loud. The best time to do it is in the hours just before your appointment.

Bring a family member or friend along. Another person who knows about your health and your concerns can help you listen carefully, take notes, ask the right questions, and even help you make important decisions during a doctor's appointment.

Carry a tape recorder. Replaying an audiotape of your visit could assist you in better understanding instructions and information that you may have missed or not fully understood at the time. Just let the doctor know you are recording for that purpose.

Bring in your meds. Get a canvas tote bag and designate it as your "medicine tote." Several times a year, toss in all your prescription drugs as well as herbal supplements, vitamins, and over-the-counter remedies and bring it to your doctor's appointment. This will help your doctor understand if you're experiencing any problems with drug interactions or if you're taking any drugs you really don't need.

At your annual visit, put these health issues on the must-discuss list. Yes, you should schedule an annual checkup even if you're in tip-top shape. Be sure to talk with your doctor about these important health risks every year.

- Your blood sugar levels. A high reading could suggest insulin resistance or metabolic syndrome, which are risk factors for diabetes, heart disease, stroke, and even some forms of cancer.

- Screenings for chronic diseases. This includes diabetes, cancers (such as breast cancer, skin cancer, prostate cancer, and more), and heart disease.

- Your mental health. It's important to open up to your doctor about issues like anxiety, depression, and sources of stress in your life.

- The quality of your sleep. The amount of sleep you are getting can affect other health issues, and don't forget to mention snoring or other signs of sleep apnea to your doctor.

Be sure that your doctor knows these three important things about you. If you haven't done so already, give your doctor your past health history, your family's health history, and your own lifestyle history at your next annual checkup. When discussing your own past, include major illnesses, allergies, and drug reactions. Family history? Summarize major illnesses your first-degree relatives (parents, aunts and uncles, grandparents) have had, and pay special attention to medical conditions such as diabetes that seem to run in the family. Clue your doctor into your own lifestyle—tell her how much you exercise, how you eat, whether you have a pet you enjoy, how stressed you are, whether you smoke tobacco or drink alcohol, any over-the-counter or prescription drugs (from another doctor) that you take regularly. Do you bungee-jump, skydive, or ski down the expert slopes? Include any risky sports you enjoy, too.

Evaluate your doctor. Is she too bossy? Is he too deferential? Does your doctor interrupt or not take your views as seriously as you'd like? Try discussing your concerns first, and make a good-faith effort to build a relationship of trust and respect with your physician. But if it's not working out, don't feel obligated to stay. Patients who don't trust their doctors simply don't get well as quickly, studies show, probably because they're less motivated to follow their advice and treatments. Ask to see another doctor in the same practice, or ask friends and family for recommendations for a new doctor.

Get the Right Dose

It was an eye-opening study: When University of California, Los Angeles, researchers listened in on recorded conversations between 44 doctors and 185 patients, they uncovered a dangerous silence about prescription drugs. Though physicians prescribed medications, they neglected to mention drug side effects 65 percent of the time, didn't tell patients how long to take a new drug 66 percent of the time, skipped instructions on how often to take it 42 percent of the time, and didn't explain the drug's purpose 23 percent of the time. They even left out the name of the drug 26 percent of the time!

"Patients who receive less counseling about their medication may be less likely to adhere to their prescribed regimen, in part because they may not understand how to take their medications," notes lead study author Derjung M. Tarn, MD, PhD, an assistant professor of medicine at UCLA.

This communication gap helps explain why half the time, people don't follow directions when taking medications. The danger? One in

Maintaining

your own health-care records will make it easy for you to provide your doctor with important information—and could even save your life. You can store your medical info in this simple, color-coded file folder system, or opt for a high-tech software to keep records on your computer or even online. The best system: The one that's easiest for you to complete and maintain. Here's what to include.

Red **Folder**

MUST-HAVE INFORMATION

Keep this folder of basic and emergency information at the front of your medical records.

Contact information for your health-care team: Get a business card from each doctor and specialist you see. Staple or tape them to a separate sheet of paper and keep it in your files.
Your health insurance information: Photocopy the front and back of your insurance cards. Add additional data as you acquire it, such as customer service phone numbers, names of helpful staff members, and online addresses for the company.
Emergency health information: Keep a list of life-threatening allergies or other health conditions that medical personnel should know about immediately in case of an emergency. Put this info into the folder, label it "EMERGENCY INFO", and make sure it's the first file in your folder of medical records.
Emergency contact information: List the names, phone numbers, and addresses of relatives and friends who should be contacted in case you or your spouse has a medical emergency.
Copies of advanced-care directives: If you have appointed someone else to make medical or health-care decisions for you if you cannot make them for yourself, or if you have written out a living will, signed a do-not-resuscitate order, or want to be an organ donor, include copies of this important paperwork in your folder.

Blue **Folder**

DOCTOR'S RECORDS

This is where you'll keep information about doctor visits, hospital stays, procedures, and test results. From now on, ask for copies of reports on tests, procedures, and important doctor visits as they happen. That way, your own file will be up-to-date.

Current records: Ask each of your current doctors for copies of your health records. If you've seen one doctor for many years, ask if the office can create a summary for you. Include your dentist, eye doctor, and any specialists you see on a regular basis.
Reports from specialists: Often, doctors cannot release information provided by other physicians. Go back to specialists you've seen for tests or consultations and ask for copies of their reports.
Immunization records: Include current immunizations and, if possible, immunizations from your past.
Eyeglass prescription: This is the place for a copy of your vision prescription.
Test results: Keep copies of x-rays, blood tests, and other results in a separate file.
Doctor's reports on medical procedures: If you've had outpatient or inpatient hospital treatments, surgeries, or other procedures, ask the institution for copies of records.

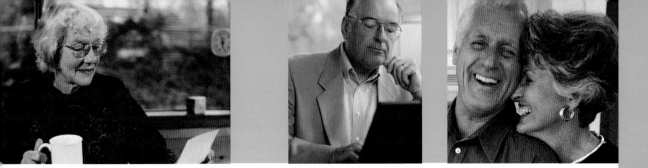

Green **Folder**

MEDICATIONS, REMEDIES, AND SUPPLEMENTS

Copies of prescription-drug label info. For each drug you take, file a copy of the pharmacy receipt that looks like the drug label—it should contain the drug's name, when the prescription was filled, dosage, directions for taking it, and contact info for the pharmacy.

Over-the-counter remedies: Keep a list of any that you use on a regular basis, such as low-dose aspirin. If you see your doctor for a specific health complaint, be sure to bring along any nonprescription remedies you've been taking along with your prescription drugs.

Vitamins and other supplements: Keep a list of supplements—such as multivitamins, calcium, vitamin D, fish oil, or herbal supplements—that you take on a regular basis. Note the brand name and the amount you take each day.

Side effects list: On a separate sheet of paper, note anything you've taken that's caused side effects. Include the name of the drug, remedy, or supplement; when and how much you took; details about the side effects; other drugs and remedies you were using at the same time.

A list of drugs you've been told *not* to take. If you've ever been told you have an allergy or serious reaction to a drug, make a note of it. Include any test results or other info here, too.

Yellow **Folder**

YOUR OWN HEALTH NOTES

Here's the place to track vital stats, like your weight, as well as the results of ongoing home testing—such as blood sugar tests for diabetes, home cholesterol checks, home blood pressure checks, and so on. Your yellow folder should include:

Your height and weight, tracked over time. Log in both four times a year. Watch for diminishing height—a warning sign of osteoporosis of the spine. Take weight changes seriously, too. Unintended weight gain or weight loss could be a sign of an underlying health problem and warrants a call to your doctor.

Your waist measurement. Experts now know that your waist circumference can help determine whether you're at risk for metabolic syndrome—a collection of symptoms and conditions that raise your risk for heart attack, stroke, diabetes, and more. You're in the danger zone if your waist measures more than 35 inches (for women) and more than 37 inches for men. A waist more than 40 inches is a serious threat.

Your BMI. Short for body mass index, this is a number that assesses whether your weight is healthy for your height. A BMI of 18.5 to 24.9 is healthy; 25 to 29.9 is overweight; 30 and above is obese. The best way to figure out your BMI is with an online calculator (the math's a little bit complex). Most major health Web sites have one.

Results of ongoing home testing. Keep track of your blood sugar levels, blood pressure, cholesterol levels, and other common health measurements, whether taken at home, at work, at the doctor's office, or elsewhere. This will help you notice trends and provide info you can show your doctor in case the numbers move in an unexpected direction.

ten hospital visits are the result of medication problems, says the *Merck Manual of Medical Information*

Meanwhile, older people may face a second peril when the doctor scrawls a prescription: Drugs with dangerous side effects for the elderly. A study from the Centers for Disease Control and Prevention in Atlanta has found that this happened 1 out of every 12 times that a person over age 65 visits the doctor—and even more often for women and for anyone taking multiple drugs. Top drugs to watch were the pain reliever propoxyphene, the antihistamine hydroxyzine, the anti-anxiety agent diazepam, the antidepressant amitriptyline, and the urinary tract relaxant oxybutynin.

So get the full story when your doctor prescribes a new drug by asking these crucial questions.

1. What is the name of the drug? Is it a name-brand drug or a generic?
2. Why is it being prescribed?
3. How, when, and for how long should I take it?
4. Will I need a refill? How can I get one?
5. What are the side effects, and what should I do if I have any adverse effects?
6. How soon should it start working? How will I know?
7. Will I need a smaller dose because of my age or because I'm a woman?
8. Do I need to take it all, or can I stop when I feel better?
9. Should I avoid any foods, beverages (including alcohol), medications, or supplements while taking it?
10. What if I miss a dose?
11. How should I store it?
12. What is the cost? Will my health insurance pay for it?

The next step in smart medicine management: Get all your prescriptions filled at one pharmacy. Your pharmacist can serve as a central point to maintain a list of all your medicines and can screen for drug interactions to avoid harmful situations.

Survive Your Hospital Stay

Each year, a surprisingly large number of people die in hospitals—not as a result of a medical condition but due to medical mistakes such as a wrong diagnosis, inappropriate treatments, or hospital-acquired infections. Hospital errors are the eighth leading cause of death in the United States alone, ahead of car accidents, breast cancer, even AIDS. These steps can help you prevent something from going awry the next time you require overnight medical care.

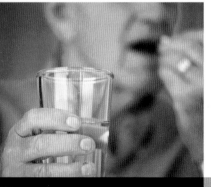

Medicine is serious business. Ask your doctor every conceivable question, and make sure your pharmacist filled your prescription correctly!

Choose the best hospital in your area.

Before there's an emergency (or a scheduled procedure), check out local hospitals covered by your insurance. Among the questions to ask:

- Does the hospital employ "intensivists"—physicians who specialize in intensive care—and "hospitalists"—doctors who manage your total care during your stay, then brief your family doctor before you leave? Many believe these dual-doctor arrangements provide better care.

- How safe is it? Good signs include: A hospital that includes a pharmacist on daily rounds (this lowers drug errors), uses a computerized physician order entry system for in-hospital prescriptions, and one that has a lower nurse-to-patient ratio (there's no magic number, but lower is better).

Look for a "high-volume" surgeon.

New studies show that doctors who have more experience performing specific procedures really do get the best results. In research published in the *Journal of the National Cancer Institute*, prostate cancer patients treated by highly experienced surgeons were much more likely to be cancer-free five years after surgery than patients treated by surgeons with less experience. Ask your doctor how many times he performs the procedure in a year, and how many in his career.

And a study of more than 11,000 older women treated for breast cancer found that those who went to high-volume hospitals were less likely to die than those whose surgeries were performed at lower-volume hospitals.

Before a procedure, confer with your physician.

Find out what kinds of tests, drugs, and processes to expect—and whether there are any drugs you should avoid. Write down what you find out. During your stay, you or a trusted family member or friend should consult the list each time you're given a drug, a doctor's review, or a treatment. If its not on the list, find out more about what it is and why you need it. Not satisfied? Ask for a delay while hospital staff consult your doctor.

Find out who will be taking care of you.

Once you're in your room, find out from your nurse which doctors and other nurses will be taking care of you. Later, if a nurse or intern is doing something that you're not sure is right for you, you can find out who ordered it. If the doc's name isn't on your list, the procedure may be meant for someone else.

Ask questions.

Always ask about any procedure or treatment that seems unusual.

Read your chart.

Yes, you *do* have the right to see it. Check to see if treatments on the chart match what your doctor told you to expect. If they don't, find out why—and if need be, ask the hospital staff to call your doctor.

Make them scrub up.

Less than half of all hospital nurses and physicians clean their hands between patients—one reason millions of people contract hospital-based infections each year. Studies show that its more likely that health-care professionals will wash up, and even use more soap, if someone asks them to. In Canada, government agencies recently launched a "wash your hands" campaign in the nation's hospitals, aimed at cutting infection rates by 10 to 30 percent. Don't wait—start your own campaign next time you're in the hospital.

Don't leave without instructions.

Before you're discharged, ask the doctor caring for you for written instructions on how you should care for yourself. Look over the instructions and ask questions, or have a friend or family member do it for you.

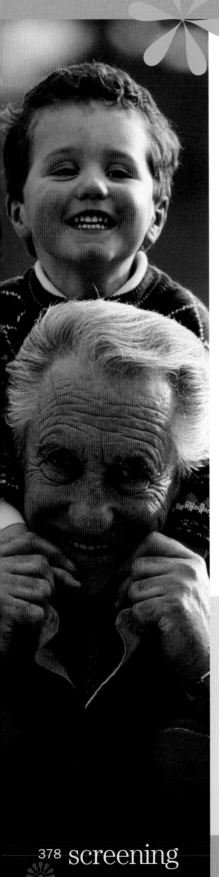

SCREENING SMARTS

Diseases don't just happen, like the switching on of a light. They develop gradually and imperceptibly. By the time you finally feel or observe a symptom, they likely have been progressing for a long time. It's a scary thought.

But we live in an amazing time. Doctors have the know-how to tell if a disease is developing in us long before a major symptom has occurred. Today, we can catch cancer early and even destroy or remove abnormal cells before they have time to become cancer. This is a time when a simple blood test can tell more about what's happening within your body than open-heart surgery, and when sophisticated imaging machines and procedures can identify microscopic abnormalities long before they cause any damage.

Even better—you don't always need a doctor to provide the kind of top-to-bottom checks that can assure your health over the next 40 years. You can conduct many screening tests yourself, in the privacy of your own home. Yet 9 out of 10 adults age 65 and older fail to get or perform recommended health screenings.

To help you remember, refer to these handy charts. If you're technologically savvy, enter the reminders into your cell phone, PDA, or computer calendar now; if you're more the paper type, make a copy and stick it on the front of your refrigerator next to your grandkids' pictures. Just seeing their sweet faces every morning will keep you motivated to stick around as long as possible—by getting regular screenings.

Do I Need an
annual checkup?

The short answer is no—if you're under 65. Every two to five years is generally enough for a full physical if you're healthy and are getting the screenings recommended here. Once you reach age 65, however, experts recommend that you see your doctor for a full physical every year or two. Whenever you go for a checkup, make sure you bring all the prescription and over-the-counter medications, vitamins, and herbal and nutritional supplements you're taking so your doctor can see if you still need to be on them, check for potential interactions, and adjust your dosages.

Daily Checks

Check your …	Why?
Weight	Weighing yourself daily keeps you attuned to the small 1- to 2-pound weight gain that could signal a problem with your diet or physical activity levels. A sudden weight gain could also be a sign of a more serious problem, like fluid retention due to congestive heart failure.
Feet	This is particularly important if you already have diabetes, but even if your blood sugar is perfectly fine, give your tootsies a once over for any unexpected sores, ingrown toenails, or blisters that could develop into a problem if left untreated.
Fingernails	Your fingernails are a window into your health. For instance, heart valve infections can cause red streaks in the nail bed, kidney and liver diseases can damage nails, and low thyroid levels can cause brittle nails.
Tongue	You should scrape it daily to reduce bad breath, but you should also take a good look at it. A shaking tongue could be a sign of an overactive thyroid or certain neurological disorders; while a very red tongue (redder than normal) could be a sign of nutritional deficiencies.
Urine	It should be clear and light yellow, nearly straw-colored. If it's dark, you're either not getting enough fluids or you may have some blood in your urine.
Stool	It should be a medium brown. If it's black and tarry, or there are signs of blood, let your doctor know.

Every Month

Check your …	Why?
Breasts (women only)	While most breast cancers are found on a mammogram or during a breast exam from your doctor, enough are found by women themselves to make this monthly check worthwhile. Also make sure you know how your breasts normally feel and let your health-care provider know about any changes. A good idea is to check your breasts in the shower on the same day of the month, usually a week after your period begins.
Testicles (men only)	To check for testicular cancer. Feel for any unusual bumps or lumps.
Moles	Examine any moles for changes in size, shape, or color, which could signify cancer.

Every Year

Have a ...	Why?
Dental exam and cleaning	Gum disease and tooth decay not only hurt your smile and your breath but also can lead to the type of low-level inflammation that increases your risk of a host of health conditions, including heart disease. Twice a year checks are even better!
Stool guaiac test beginning at age 50	This test, also called fecal occult blood test, checks for blood in your stool, providing an early indication of colon cancer.
Screening mammogram, beginning at age 40 (women only)	The majority of breast cancers are diagnosed on screening mammograms, which studies find have significantly reduced the death rate from the disease. Once you reach age 75, it's up to you and your doctor if you want to continue having mammograms.
Clinical breast exam (women only)	Your doctor is experienced in identifying any breast abnormalities or changes that might indicate an increased risk of breast cancer or even a potential cancer.
Prostate-specific antigen (PSA) test, beginning at age 50 (men only)	Not everyone agrees on the need for annual PSA testing, so talk to your doctor. If you have a high risk of prostate cancer (African-American men and men with one or more first-degree relatives [father, brothers] diagnosed before age 65), talk to your doctor about beginning testing at age 45.
Pap test and pelvic exam (women only)	To screen for abnormalities that could indicate pre-cervical cancer. If you are over 30 and have a normal Pap *and* a normal HPV test (which tests for the virus that causes most cervical cancers), you do not need to be tested again for 3 years; or if you've had three normal Pap tests in a row, you can skip the next 2 or 3 years. Check with your doctor is you are over 70.

7 Symptoms *never* to ignore

1. Sudden worst-I've-ever-had-in-my-life headache. Could signify an aneurysm, or bleeding in the brain. Get to an emergency room immediately.

2. Black, tarry stools or blood with a bowel movement. Could indicate internal bleeding. Call your doctor.

3. Slurred speech, weakness or paralysis (particularly on one side of your body), numbness, confusion. Could be a stroke. Get to an emergency room.

4. Vaginal bleeding after menopause. Could be a sign of uterine cancer. Call for a doctor's appointment.

5. Sudden weight gain or loss with no change in eating habits. Could indicate liver disease, overactive thyroid, diabetes, or cancer. Call your doctor.

6. Sudden flashes of light. Could indicate that your retina is becoming detached. Have someone drive you to the emergency room immediately.

7. Never-before-experienced pain in your chest, throat, jaw, shoulder, arm, or abdomen. It could be a heart attack. Get to the emergency room immediately.

Other Tests and Screenings to Schedule

Get this	Every ...	Because ....
Blood pressure screening	2 years in your doctor's office	There are no signs or symptoms of high blood pressure. The only way to know you have it is with a formal test.
Cholesterol screening	Every 5 years after 35; age 20 if you have a family history of heart disease, or smoke.	High cholesterol levels are one of the top markers for heart disease in the present or future.
Bone density screening	At least once beginning at age 65; earlier depending on your risk for osteoporosis.	Osteoporosis is a silent disease in which bones become thin and filled with holes.
Fasting plasma glucose test	3 years beginning at age 45; more often or earlier if you're overweight or at risk for diabetes.	To provide an early warning sign of high blood sugar levels, which could represent an increased risk for diabetes.
Rectal exam/ colonoscopy	5 to 10 years for rectal exam; 10 years for colonoscopy	It can find polyps that could turn into colon cancer. Doctors can remove the polyps during the test.
Abdominal aortic aneurysm test (Men age 65 to 75 who have ever smoked)	One time only between age 65 and 75 if you have ever smoked	It provides an early warning sign of a very dangerous condition in which the aortic artery becomes abnormally large or balloons outward.
Thyroid test (women only)	5 years beginning at age 35	The signs of an underactive thyroid (hypothyroidism) mimic those of middle age: fatigue, weight gain, heavy periods, depression. A blood test is the only way to know if your levels are normal.
Skin exams	3 years beginning at age 20; annually beginning at age 40	Years you spent working on a good tan can come back in the form of skin cancer.
Hearing test	Once every 10 years until age 50; then once every 3 years.	You're often the last to notice you're losing your hearing. Regular testing will provide an early heads up.
Eye exam	At least once from ages 20-29; at least two exams from ages 30–39; then every 2 to 4 years until age 65; annually thereafter.	The exam should test your vision and screen for glaucoma and macular degeneration.

index

environmental toxins, 44, 56, 101, 135, 265

epigallocatechin gallate, 364

epinephrine, 256, 278

Epsom salts, 287

erectile dysfunction, 180

erythromycin, 359

esomeprazole (Nexium), 278

esophageal cancer, 51, 58, 64, 276, 330, 331, 332

esophagus, heartburn and damage to, 276

estrogen, 332
  for incontinence, 306

evening primrose, 297

exercise, 15, 24–25, 38–39, 45, 56, 61, 62, 67, 71, 87, 89, 90, 91, 105, 106, 111, 158, 172–235, 236, 280, 299, 309, 312, 313, 314, 327, 339, 373
  Antidote-to-Aging program for, 198, 199, 212–23
  as antidote to pain, 334
  for back pain, 289
  balance and, 182, 191–92, 195, 262–63
  cancer and, 328, 332
  cold prevention and, 266
  constipation and, 278
  in daily living, 182, 194, 195
  dementia and, 340
  diabetes and, 361, 364
  Easy Does It routine for, 198, 199, 200–211
  endurance in, 175, 179, 182–84, 185, 189, 193, 195
  falling and lack of, 265
  fatigue and, 280–81
  fitness pyramid for, 195
  flexibility in, 182, 189–91, 193, 195
  goals for, 197
  hearing loss and, 359
  inner motivation and, 196
  lack of, 41, 42, 43, 44
  low-impact, 285
  lung disease and, 367, 368
  moderation in, 53
  natural ways to, 183
  recovery time and, 188
  repair and, 38–39, 40
  repetitions in, 187
  sets in, 187
  short- and long-term goals for, 186
  Spread Stopper program for, 198, 199, 224–35

strength training in, *see* strength training
  television and, 62
  ten reasons for, 176–81
  understanding, 182
  weight-bearing, 197
  when not to, 193

exercise balls, 179, 263
  inflatable, 190

exercise bands, 184, 195

exercise classes, 178–79, 196, 350

exercise gear, 190

exercise physiologists, 371

exercise tests, graded, 186

exfoliation, 296

extracorporeal magnetic innervation chair, 308

eye cancer, 355

eye doctors, 79

eyedrops, 353, 354
  preventive, 356

eye pressure, elevated, 356

eyes, 118, 124, 322
  dry, 354
  exams of, 352, 381
  lens of, 39

F

falling, 24, 74, 102, 175, 178, 191, 262, 265, 350
  balance training and, 197
  reasons for, 265
  reducing risk of, 264–65

family, 28–29, 183, 251

famotidine (Pepcid), 279

farsightedness, 15

fast food, 43, 45, 76–77, 91, 134, 165

fasting blood sugar check, 327

fasting plasma glucose test, 381

fat cells, 180–81

fatigue, 113, 150, 193, 280–83, 287, 301
  lack of fuel as cause of, 282

fats, 38, 69, 75, 76, 78, 86, 91, 108, 131, 150, 151, 292, 336
  added, 119
  animal, 146
  bad, 134, 162–64, 316
  density of, 185–87
  good, 41, 110, 111, 114, 128, 134–38, 150, 162, 316, 318, 335
  monunsaturated, 114, 135, 138, 147, 162, 252, 318
  processed, 317

saturated, 19, 63, 121, 131, 138, 146, 160–62, 170, 292, 316, 317–18, 363
  "see it, lose it" rule for, 149
  trans, *see* trans fats
  unsaturated, 316

fatty foods, 45, 312

fava beans, 120

fecal occult blood test, 380

feet, 379
  in PAD, 291
  tingling, 113

fertility, 15

fertilizers, 97

fever, 193, 269

fiber, 75, 78, 102, 110, 114, 128–29, 131, 132, 150, 151, 152, 158, 162, 164, 317, 319, 325–26, 336, 339, 351, 353, 363
  constipation prevented by, 276–77
  insoluble, 129, 130
  recommended servings of, 128
  soluble, 129, 320

fibrinogen, 244

fibromyalgia, 336

fifties:
  hearing tests in, 358
  signs of aging in, 15
  sleep patterns in, 299

figs, dried, 145

filberts, 145

fillings, 271

financial advisors, 29

fingernails, 379

fish, 78, 108, 111, 134, 136, 146, 163, 165, 316, 318, 355, 363, 367
  canned, 136
  fatty, 114, 135, 335, 341–42, 345
  frozen, 136, 171

fishing, 195

fish-oil capsules, 115, 165, 169, 285, 297, 318, 320, 342, 354, 368–69

fitness instructors, 197

fitness pyramid, 195

fitness test, real life, 177

Flamingo (exercise), 219

flatbreads, 131

flavonoids, 118, 123

flavonols, 163, 341

flaxseed, 137, 250–51, 323, 336, 355

flaxseed oil, 138, 354

flexibility, 24, 99, 175, 178, 179, 189–91, 195

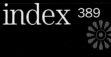

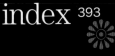

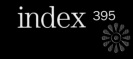

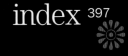

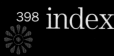